Pa[...] [...] Ph. D.
Prof[...]
University of Texas [...] Science
Center at Houston
P. O. Box 20186
Houston, Texas 77025

Pa[...]
Pro[...]
University of Texas [...] Science

United States Environmental Protection Agency	Health Effects Research Laboratory Research Triangle Park NC 27711	EPA/600/1-83/015e September 1987
Research and Development		Pesticides and Toxic Substances

U.S. Cancer Mortality Rates and Trends, 1950-1979

Volume IV: Maps

by

Wilson B. Riggan, Ph.D.*
John P. Creason, Ph.D.*
William C. Nelson, Ph.D.*
Kenneth G. Manton, Ph.D.**
Max A. Woodbury, Ph.D.**
Eric Stallard**
Alvin C. Pellom, Ph.D.***
Jefferson Beaubier, Ph.D.****

*Environmental Epidemiology and Biometry Division
Health Effects Research Laboratory
U.S. Environmental Protection Agency
Research Triangle Park, North Carolina 27711

**Center for Demographic Studies
Duke University
Durham, North Carolina 27706

***Northrop Services, Inc.
Research Triangle Park, North Carolina 27709

****Exposure Evaluation Division
Office of Toxic Substances
U.S. Environmental Protection Agency
Washington, DC 20460

For Sale by the Superintendent of Documents, U.S. Government
Printing Office, Washington, DC 20402

Disclaimer

This document has been reviewed in accordance with U.S. Environmental Protection Agency policy and approved for publication. Mention of trade names or commercial products does not constitute endorsement or recommendation for use.

Foreword

The many benefits of our modern, developing, industrial society are accompanied by certain hazards. Careful assessment of the relative risk of existing and new man-made environmental hazards is necessary for the establishment of sound regulatory policy. These regulations serve to enhance the quality of our environment in order to promote the public health and welfare and the productive capacity of our Nation's population.

The complexities of environmental problems originate in the deep interdependent relationships between the various physical and biological segments of man's natural and social world. Solutions to these environmental problems require an integrated program of research and development using input from a number of disciplines. The Health Effects Research Laboratory, Research Triangle Park, NC and Cincinnati, OH conducts a coordinated environmental health research program in toxicology, epidemiology, and clinical studies using human volunteer subjects. Wide ranges of pollutants known or suspected to cause health problems are studied. The research focuses on air pollutants, water pollutants, toxic substances, hazardous wastes, pesticides and non-ionizing radiation. The laboratory participates in the development and revision of air and water quality criteria and health assessment documents on pollutants for which regulatory actions are being considered. Direct support to the regulatory function of the Agency is provided in the form of expert testimony and preparation of affidavits as well as expert advice to the Administrator to assure the adequacy of environmental regulatory decisions involving the protection of the health and welfare of all U.S. inhabitants.

This atlas, volume 4 in our series, which supplements the county tabulations presented in the first three volumes, an important Laboratory product, provides EPA and other governmental agencies, state and local health departments, universities, and environmental control agencies with an historic data base and ready reference containing maps which show spatial and temporal patterns of cancer mortality.

This report contains maps of the conterminous United States which show the geographic variation in cancer mortality rates for each of the three decades between 1950 and 1979 as well as the variation in the trends (i.e. the changes in these rates between the first and third decade). It supplements the three volume tabulation of cancer mortality rates and trends previously published in cooperation with the National Cancer Institute. With each map are graphs of the data distribution and corresponding national rates. The maps use five class intervals for the cancer rates, represented by grey tones ranging from black for the highest class to white for the lowest.

These maps and the information they provide about the geographic and temporal patterns in cancer mortality may be used in a number of ways in epidemiological investigation, such as aiding in the formulation of hypotheses about the environmental determinants of human cancer or standing as a ready reference for researchers and other concerned groups.

F. Gordon Hueter, Ph.D.
Director
Health Effects Research Laboratory

iii

Abstract

The reduction in deaths from contagious disease during the past century, and the reduction in deaths from cardiovascular disease during the past decade and a half, increase the relative importance of cancer mortality. With over 450,000 deaths in 1984 cancer mortality ranks second only to deaths from heart disease [1].

This atlas supplements the county tabulations in the first three volumes. The maps show patterns of cancer mortality rates for each of the four race-sex groups, for the three decades 1950-59, 1960-69, and 1970-79, as well as change maps reflecting the changes in rank between the first and third decades. More common cancers among the white population are mapped at the county level while the less common cancers and non-white cancers are mapped at the state economic area (SEA) level.

Spatial variation of site-specific cancer mortality at the county or state economic area level can provide insights into possible etiologic or environmental factors and/ or the bases for more detailed epidemiological studies. One complication with such studies, especially for rare cancer types, is that unstable local area rate estimates, resulting from small population sizes, can obscure the underlying spatial pattern of disease risk. These cancer maps use more stable rate estimates by statistically weighting the local area estimates toward the national level. Details of this procedure have been presented in a recent journal article by Manton et al. [2].

Cancer mortality data as arranged in these maps have many uses. For example, the geographic and temporal differences are useful in developing and examining hypotheses about the influence of various environmental factors. The consistency of such differences across race, sex and age groups can provide insight into other possible causes. For local communities concerned about a specific cancer situation, these maps provide both a spatial and temporal historic context in which to evaluate the local conditions.

The continuing improvement and steadily declining cost of all aspects of microcomputer operation, especially processing power, storage capacity, and graphic output quality, have recently provided the means to produce inexpensive, high quality maps at the county or state economic area level. Maps such as these should become even more important in the future as a valuable tool in assessing spatial and temporal variation in cancer mortality.

Contents

*WM = White male
 WF = White female
 NM = Non-white male
 NF = Non-white female

Acknowledgment

We wish to acknowledge and thank Dr. Thomas Mason, National Cancer Institute, for his helpful suggestions, consultation, and long-term support for and interest in our work.

We wish to acknowledge support and help of other USEPA scientists, especially Drs. Jack Griffith and Carl Hayes, EEB, EEBD, Dr. Thomas Curran, Warren Freas, III, William F. Hunt, Jr., OAQPS, and Dr. R. Clifton Bailey, AED, OWRS.

We wish to acknowledge support and help of Dr. Gene Lowrimore, formerly with USEPA, and now with Duke University and an independent consultant. Also, we thank Gregory and Sue Woodbury of Duke for their help especially with our mapping program and the generation of the maps.

We wish to acknowledge other scientists for their technical review and helpful suggestions, especially Dr. Kenneth Bridbord, International Studies Branch, Fogarty International Center, NIH, Dr. John F. Finklea, Department of Public Health, University of Alabama in Birmingham, Dr. Jean French, CDC, NIOSH, Atlanta, Dr. Roy Ing, Center for Environmental Health, Atlanta, Dr. Michael D. Lebowitz, University of Arizona College of Medicine, Dr. Clifford H. Patrick, U.S. Veterans Administration Medical Center, in Durham, Dr. James H. Stebbings, Jr., Center for Human Radiobiology, Argonne National Laboratory, and Dr. Marvin A. Schniederman retired from the National Cancer Institute and currently a private consultant.

We thank the many scientists who commented and provided valuable suggestions during and following presentation of the statistical stabilization of mortality rates and the mapping procedure used in this atlas. We made these presentations at local, national, and international seminars and professional meetings.

Dedicated to the Late John Van Bruggen

who directed the data management activity and who painstakingly collected, verified, and validated each data entry over a 20 year period. He looked forward to the publication of these maps.

Section 1

Introduction and Summary

Introduction

The reduction in deaths from contagious disease during the past century and from cardiovascular disease during the past decade and a half, increase the relative importance of cancer mortality. With over 450,000 deaths in 1984, cancer mortality ranks second only to deaths from heart disease [1,3,4]. The increase in the relative importance of cancer mortality during the past three decades has been accompanied by an unparalleled growth in urbanization, industrial expansion, increased use of private automobiles and other modes of transportation, and growth in chemical production. There have also been major changes in life style and occupation, and many advances in the knowledge, detection, and treatment of cancer [3,5,6,7]. However, the lag time between the inception of the disease and the clinical diagnosis suggests that the relevant exposure leading to current cancer deaths may vary from a very short period of time for some leukemias up to 20 or more years for lung cancer.

The geographic distribution of cancer has been used for various epidemiologic purposes. U.S. CANCER MORTALITY BY COUNTY: 1950 -1969 by Mason and McKay provided twenty year average cancer mortality rates by county [8]. In this and two companion atlases by Mason et al., the importance of analyses of county mortality data is discussed [9,10].

In U.S. CANCER MORTALITY RATES AND TRENDS, 1950-1979: Volume 1-3 containing tables, not maps, we used a strategy similar to that used by Mason and McKay for screening county mortality data, but in place of twenty year averages, we presented rates by county for each of the three decades 1950-59, 1960-69 and 1970-79, as well as the trends, defined as the percent change from 1950-59 to 1970-79 [11]. The above publications have been most useful in identifying high risk areas, facilitating correlational analyses to suggest potential risk areas and selecting areas for further study [12].

Recently NCI published ATLAS OF U.S. CANCER MORTALITY AMONG WHITES: 1950-1980, by NCI Epidemiology and Biostatistics Program scientists Linda W. Pickle, Ph.D., Thomas J. Mason, Ph.D., Robert Hoover, M.D., and Joseph F. Fraumeni, Jr., M.D., and by Neil Howard, ORI, Inc., under contract to NCI. [13]. This atlas is an update of an earlier NCI atlas by Mason et al. [9]. This publication should be even more useful than NCI's previous atlases by Mason et al. in generating etiologic clues and identifying geographic areas where cancer investigators and public health officials might direct special attention. NCI's latest atlas not only updates their previous publications, adding a third decade to the time period, but also provides an advancement in the graphic presentation of quantitative mortality data over time and space. By presenting the mortality data separately by decade the format is similar to that used by us in [11].

The current atlas is very similar to and complements NCI's with differences reflecting the difference in the mission of the two agencies. NCI is interested in developing clues to the etiology of cancer and developing strategies to prevent and/or cure cancer, while EPA is interested in providing information with which to protect the population from the harmful effect of environmental pollutants. As with the NCI atlas, we hope this atlas will continue to stimulate research and serve as a tool to better understand the true cause of cancer.

This atlas, volume 4 in our series, which supplements the county tabulations presented in the first three volumes, illustrates the geographic patterns of cancer mortality with maps, for males and females, whites and non-whites, for the three decades just described. Changes occurring in county or SEA ranking between 1950-59 and 1970-79 are also mapped. More common cancers among the white population are mapped at the county level, while less common cancers and all non-white cancers are mapped at the state economic area (SEA) level.

Cancer mortality data as arranged in these maps have many uses. For example, the geographic and temporal differences are useful in developing and examining hypotheses about the influence of various environmental factors. The consistency of such differences across race, sex and age groups can provide insight into other possible causes. For local communities concerned about a specific cancer situation these maps provide both a spatial and temporal historic context in which to evaluate local conditions.

Spatial variation of site-specific cancer mortality at the county or state economic area level can provide insights into possible environmental factors and/or provide the bases for more detailed epidemiological studies, or environmental monitoring. One complication with such studies, especially for rare cancer types, is that unstable local area rate estimates, resulting from small population sizes, can obscure the underlying spatial pattern of disease risk. These cancer maps use more stable rate estimates by statistically weighting the local area estimates toward the national level. Manton et al. presented the procedure in a recent journal article [2].

We used a two-step process to generate the maps. First, we statistically adjusted the data to stabilize the rates using an empirical Bayes procedure developed by EPA and the Duke University Center for Demographic Studies [2,14]. We provide a more detailed explanation in Section 2.B. We then downloaded the data to a microcomputer-based mapping system that imaged the maps, text, and two supplemental graphs on a desktop laser printer. The first graph presents the frequency distribution of areas by rate for the rate maps. The second graph presents the national age specific rates. For the trend maps, the second graph presents the national rates for each of the three decades.

The continuing improvement and steadily declining cost of all aspects of microcomputer operation, especially processing power, storage capacity, and graphic output quality, have recently provided the means to produce inexpensive, high quality maps at the county or state economic area level. Maps such as these should become even more important in the future as a valuable tool in assessing spatial and temporal variation in cancer mortality.

Uses of These Maps

Mapping and the analysis of geographic patterns is not new in epidemiological investigation. John Snow, in his classic study of 1854, mapped individual cases of a cholera epidemic in London, revealing a strong circular pattern centered on the Broad Street water pump. Even though the epidemic peaked prior to the removal of the pump's handle, this is an important historic example of an epidemiologist analyzing geographic patterns of morbidity or mortality in the epidemiological investigation of an epidemic—be the epidemic from environmental exposure or from contagious disease. Many books on planning epidemiological studies include a discussion of Snow's studies [15].

The maps of mortality rates in this volume may be used for various epidemiologic studies and purposes. These maps may be used to identify counties or groups of counties with high cancer mortality rates, large shifts in rank of areas over time, or both. Investigation into possible causes can then proceed. Or, approaching the problem from the other end, the maps may be used to locate counties with unusual demographic, environmental, industrial characteristics, or employment patterns and determine whether they exhibit elevated rates or unusual trends that might be attributed to these characteristics. Since these maps are sex specific, it is possible to compare the mortality among males and females. High rates in both sexes suggest a possible relation to environmental exposure or other factors unrelated to sex, while high rates among men only suggest occupational or other sex-related factors. This report may be used along with other secondary information such as data on ambient environmental pollution levels, emission data, employment patterns, and demographic characteristics as part of a systematic cancer research approach as described by Blot, et al. [12,16].

Researchers may use this report to identify counties and groups of counties for developing and implementing a detailed monitoring program of ambient environmental pollutants, or for performing field work such as case-control studies. Whether the study is an environmental monitoring or an epidemiological field study, this report provides a method of screening cancer mortality data to select areas most suitable for study. Another important use of these maps will be as a graphic reference for the EPA and other governmental agencies, state and local health departments, universities, and citizens' groups. For local communities concerned about a specific cancer situation, this report provides both a spatial and temporal historical context in which to evaluate the local condition.

An EPA publication, THE CANCER MORTALITY ATLAS DATA MANAGEMENT SYSTEM by Pellom et al., contains the computer programs used to generate the stabilized rate for the mapping system, their complete documentation and instructions for running the programs. A professional computer programmer should be able to prepare the data to be used in generating the maps. These programs will be available from the National Technical Information Service (NTIS) [17].

Another EPA publication, THE CANCER MORTALITY ATLAS MAPPING SYSTEM, by Pellom et al., contains the computer programs, documentation, and instructions to run the programs. This publication includes the specification of the desktop laser printer to generate the maps [18].

These programs, their documentations, and their instructions will provide interested researchers in epidemiology, biostatistics, geography, demography, and related departments a rapid and inexpensive means of generating maps. We hope these maps will stimulate additional research into the underlying causes and the prevention of cancer.

Data Characteristics

Several characteristics of the cancer mortality data mapped here can affect interpretation and should be kept in mind. These are the accuracy and completeness of the death certificate information, the effect of changes in classification over time, coding and population characteristics, the effects of migration, and the long latency period for many kinds of cancer.

Several studies have compared the diagnostic classification information on the death certificate to diagnostic information from other sources such as hospital records and autopsy results [19,20,21,22]. These studies have generally shown the overall agreement between diagnosis and underlying cause of death to be very high for the most frequent causes of mortality. Studies of completeness and consistency of the demographic information on the death certificate have also shown high agreement [20,22]. Although these results are very encouraging, the user should be aware of potential limits in interpretation.

Studies of temporal trends in cancer mortality require recognition of possible effects of the decennial revisions of the International Classification of Diseases (ICD) during the thirty year span of our study [23]. We discuss our treatment of the comparability issue in Section 3.C. Check the Cancer Site Comparability Table's footnote on code 156 ICD 6 and 7, and code 193 ICD 6. We generated equivalent codes for the sixth, seventh, eighth and ninth editions of the ICD. In Section 3.A, we discuss our method of establishing fixed equivalent county boundaries over the thirty years.

The rapid development of diagnostic procedures over the term of this study has increased the precision with which site-specific cancers are identified, but at the level of aggregation used in this report, diagnostic practice should have little effect on the results for most sites.

Population distribution by age, sex, and race affect cancer mortality. In Section 3.B, we present the U.S. standard million population for 1970 which we used for direct age standardization of mortality. Populations differ for these characteristics not only across county boundaries but also over time within counties due to migration, births, deaths and possible changes in competing causes of death [22,24]. The effect of these changes is complicated for most types of cancer by the long time between exposure to a suspected carcinogen and the appearance of the disease. Cause and effect cannot be determined from these maps without additional data and investigation.

A final reminder is that these cancer mortality maps are presented in terms of geographic risk. Our major purpose is to examine the spatial and temporal differences in order to generate hypotheses about possible environmental factors. In this respect, this report differs from studies concerned with the temporal trends such as Pollack and Horm [4]. The maps presented in this volume are a prime source in documenting geographic patterns of cancer rates and trends over the 30 year period. Despite the constraints on interpretation imposed by the data characteristics mentioned above and discussed more fully elsewhere [19-22], we believe these maps can contribute significantly to many aspects of cancer research.

Section 2

Materials and Methods

A. Source and Description of Data

These maps use data from the National Center for Health Statistics (NCHS) and the Bureau of the Census.

1. Death Records: General Characteristics

   ● Years available: We have virtually all cancer death records for 1950-1979.

   ● International Classification of Diseases: We used ICD codes from the ninth revision for 1979 mortality for our maps and the table of contents. NCHS used the ICD adapted for use in the U.S., the ICDA, instead of the unmodified ICD codes from the eighth revision to classify and code the underlying cause of death for 1968-1978 [25]. The comparability tables follow NCHS practice in the use of the ICD for editions 6, 7, and 9, and the ICDA for edition 8 [25]. We have used ICD in place of ICDA when referring to editions in general discussion.

   ● Each death record contains the county of residence, year and month of death, age in years, race (white or non-white), sex, and ICD rubric. For more detail on death records, see the Technical Appendix from Vital Statistics of the United States 1979 and other years [26].

2. Death Records: Special Characteristics

   ● Mortality data coded for 1952 combined the five boroughs of New York City. We used the average ratio for 1950, 1951, 1953, and 1954 to estimate 1952 deaths in each borough [27].

   ● New Jersey did not code race in 1962 or 1963 [28]. F. W. McKay of the National Cancer Institute gave us the estimates he used in their publications [8,9,10].

   ● We included all cancer deaths during 1972 even though Vital Statistics of the United States 1972 used only a fifty percent sample in their publication [29].

   ● Over the 30 years covered in this report, the International Classification of Disease [ICD] has undergone four revisions: sixth, seventh, eighth, and ninth [23]. We have included a table of comparative ICD codes from each revision. Also in the table codes from the sixth and

seventh revision are grouped together because for our purposes they are essentially identical. For comparability over the thirty years, we did not include Polycythemia Vera or Myelofibrosis [ICDA 208,209] since only the eighth edition classified these as cancer.

3. Population Records

   ● Census years: 1950, 1960, 1970, and 1980.

   ● Detail: By county, race, and sex, 5 year age groups through 84 and 85+.

   ● Population 1950 census: The 1950 Bureau of Census populations for each county, race, and sex were for 5 year age groups through 74, 75-84 and 85+. In order to make the 1950 county counts consistent with 1960, 1970, 1980 data, we used the U.S. race and sex specific counts for age 75-79, and 80-84 from the U.S. Bureau of Census 20% enumeration sample to estimate the percent of age 75-84 who were in the 75-79 age group. Using this percentage we estimated the county counts in the 75-79 age group and assigned the remainder to the 80-84 age group.

   ● Interpolation between census years: We used simple linear interpolation between census years to generate mid-year population estimates.

4. Geographic Detail

   ● "County" as used in these maps refers to a county, a parish in Louisiana, an independent city, or to a combination of counties as shown in the Technical Notes.

   ● Through the years political boundaries have changed. Therefore to keep a consistent geographic framework, we adopted a standard definition for counties and adjusted the data to it. The Technical Notes give details on these inconsistencies and their resolution [30].

B. Statistical Methodology

1. Local Area Mortality Rates and Their Variation

   ● We used area in referring to county or SEA in the statistical discussion on the generation of stabilized rates.

- One concern in creating these maps was the variability of county cancer death rates accumulated over a decade. For example, in [14] we ranked counties for white male bladder cancers by deciles for each decade. We found that between 1950-59 and 1960-69, 40 counties out of 306 shifted from the lowest to the highest decile and 38 shifted from the highest to the lowest decile. Contrast this with the case for lung cancer for which the corresponding numbers are 11 and 9.

- Variability in the mortality rates for many cancer sites is largely due to the small number of deaths involved. The chance occurrence or non-occurrence of a single death can have a disproportionate effect on the rate for a rare disease or for an area with a small population. Such statistical instability makes the identification of "extreme" rates difficult and tends to conceal patterns by breaking up clusters of counties or SEAs with similar rates. We increase the stability of these rate estimates by combining the event rate in the local area population with information from the event rate in the total population [31]. For these reasons, our stabilized rates are generally better risk indicators than the observed rates.

- We used a two-stage empirical Bayes (EB) procedure to create the stabilized (composite) rate estimates used for the maps [2,14]. In the first stage empirical Bayes estimates are obtained from the observed standarized mortality ratios (SMRs) by assuming that the number of deaths for each area i is distributed as a Poisson distribution, conditional on the unobserved true standardized mortality ratio k_i. The true standardized motality ratio k_i is assumed to be gamma distributed with mean 1 and variance b. This leads to the familiar negative binomial marginal distribution for the number of deaths in an area. Because the Poisson and the gamma distribution are conjugates the empirical Bayes estimates of k_i are given by:

$$k_i = B_i(SMR_i) + (1-B_i)(1)$$

a linear combination of the observed standardized mortality ratio and the mean of the standardized mortality ratio prior distribution. The weight estimates, B_i, depend on the variance parameter b which is obtained by maximum likelihood from the marginal negative binomial distribution. The second stage empirical Bayes estimates of age and county specific death rates are obtained by assuming a model in which the true death rates for individuals are independently gamma distributed with (1) mean values which are dependent on both area i and age group a [i.e., $k_i(m_{+a})$] and (2) variances that are proportional to mean values.

- The empirical Bayes age adjusted death rate ($EBDR_i$) for each area is a composite of three age adjusted mortality rates: (1) the direct method age adjusted death rate ($DMDR_i$); (2) the indirect method age adjusted death rate ($IMDR_i$); (3) the national age adjusted death rate (NDR).

- The weighting function eq. (1) is:

$$EBDR_i = W(DMDR_i) + (1-W)$$
$$[B_i (IMDR_i) + (1-B_i)NDR]$$

Where i indexes area, for county i = 1,...,3061, or for SEA i = 1,...,507. B_i is the first stage empirical Bayes weight which varies by area reflecting the different stability in rates for areas of different sizes. The second stage empirical Bayes weight W is constant over areas because it reflects the residual variation in age specific death rates after the first stage statistical adjustment. This weight depends on the proportionality constant in the residual variance expression which is obtained by maximum likelihood from the second stage conditional negative binomial distribution.

- We have as part of the stabilizing procedure a statistical test of the negative binomial coefficients to determine whether we have sufficient information in the data for meaningful maps. This provides a very high probability that none of the maps will be based on random data.

- We define:

  y_{ia} = the number of deaths in area i, age group a (within any selected category of race, sex, decade, and site),

  n_{ia} = the number of person-years of exposure associated with y_{ia},

  $m_{ia} = y_{ia}/n_{ia}$
  = the observed age specific death rate in area i, age group a,

  N_a = the number of persons in the standard (million) population age group a (see Section 3.B),

- In conventional summation notation, we replace the index i or a with + to denote summation over the range of the index. Hence,

  $y_{+a} = \Sigma\ y_{ia}$
  = the observed number of deaths in the national population in age group a,

  $n_{+a} = \Sigma\ n_{ia}$
  = the number of person-years of exposure associated with y_{+a},

$y_{i+} = \Sigma\, y_{ia}$

= the observed number of deaths in area i,

$n_{i+} = \Sigma\, n_{ia}$

= the number of person-years of exposure associated with y_{i+},

$N_+ = \Sigma\, N_a$,

= the number of persons in the standard (million) population.

- We use an asterisk to replace the index i or a in designating the marginal death rates. Hence,

$m_{*a} = y_{+a}\, /\, n_{+a}$

= the observed national death rate in age group a,

$m_{i*} = y_{i+}\, /\, n_{i+}$

= the observed death rate in area i.

- Using the above notations, the component adjusted mortality indexes are defined as,

$DMDR_i = \Sigma\, m_{ia}(N_a)\, /\, N_+$,

$NDR = \Sigma\, m_{*a}(N_a)\, /\, N_+$,

$IMDR_i = SMR_i(NDR)$,

where the observed standardized mortality ratio is defined as,

$SMR_i = y_{i+}\, /\, \Sigma\, m_{*a}(n_{ia})$.

- The EB-estimate of the "true" death rate in area i, age group a, is obtained as,

$u_{ia} = W(m_{ia}) + (1 - W)k_i(m_{*a})$

$\quad = W(m_{ia}) + (1 - W)(m_{*a})[B_i(SMR_i) + \quad (1 - B_i)(1)]$

where B_i and W are obtained by maximum likelihood described above.

- The final empirical Bayes estimate is obtained by direct method age adjustment of the set of EB-estimates u_{ia}, using N_a from the standard (million) population,

$EBDR_i = \Sigma\, u_{ia}(N_a)\, /\, N_+$,

which yields (1).

- For full mathematical details see [2,14] and their references. Also, the raw data, the programs used to stabilize the rates and to prepare the data for the mapping system, and a test data set will be available from National Technical Information Service (NTIS) [17,18].

C. The Maps

1. General Description

- The maps present statistically stabilized directly age adjusted mortality data for 31 site specific cancers for males and females, whites and non-whites for the three decades 1950-59, 1960-69, and 1970-79.

- The maps are grouped into sites, sex, and race. The four maps comprising each set consist of three rate maps, one for each decade, and a trend map displaying the changes in area rank between 1950-59 and 1970-79.

- The rates can be read as the number of deaths per hundred thousand. The trends are expressed as changes in color code between 1950-59 and 1970-79.

- The more common sites among the white population are mapped at the county level while the less common sites among the white population and all sites among the non-white population are mapped at the state economic area (SEA) level.

- The county base map is on page 362 and SEA base map is on page 363.

2. How to read the maps

- Except for obvious differences between the rate and trend maps, the maps presented in this atlas are identically organized. We have therefore decided to remove what would otherwise be redundant labelling and document common features of the maps in this section.

- The maps are grouped into sets by site, sex, and race. The maps comprising each set are organized so that the rate maps for 1950-59 and 1960-69 are on facing pages and the rate map for 1970-79 and the trend map are on the following pair of facing pages.

3. Mortality Rate Maps

- Percentiles were computed separately for the areas in each rate map as:

$pctl_i = 100\,[\, r_i\, /\, (n + 1)\,]$

where

$pctl_i$ = percentile for area i in the specified decade in ascending order,

r_i = rank for area i, when sorted by rate,

n = number of ranked areas (3061 counties or 507 SEAs)

- For the rate maps, the data are divided into five classes based on percentiles and represented by a unique gray tone. The class intervals in percentiles, and the color assigned to each class are

Class	Percentile	Color
1.	0 - 74	white
2.	75 - 89	light gray
3.	90 - 94	medium gray
4.	95 - 97	dark gray
5.	98 - 99	black

- A graph of the density distribution occupies the lower left of the map window. The length of the two color bars are proportional to the value range. The partitioning of the lower bar and the scale beneath it define the classes in terms of percentiles. The partitioning of the upper bar and the labels beneath it define the actual value range of each class. The small black pointers denote the national rate; one in terms of its numeric value, the other in terms of percentiles.

- For the rate maps, the lower right of the window contains a graph of the national age-specific rates. For the trend maps, this position contains a table of the national adjusted rates by decade.

- Below both graphs are two labels. One identifies the disease(s) affecting the site by their ICD (9th revision) code(s). The other identifies the map as by county or by state economic area.

4. Mortality Trend Maps.

- The trend maps are based on changes in rank of areas between 1950-59 and 1970-79.

- We define the coding variables as follows:

C_{50} = color class for each area 1950-59;
C_{70} = color class for each area 1970-79;
TC = trend class for each area of the trend map;
TC = C_{70} - C_{50}

- The five class intervals for the trend maps and the color assigned to each class are:

Class	TC Class	Color
1.	-4	white
2.	-3,-2	light gray
3.	-1,0,1	medium gray
4.	2,3	dark gray
5.	4	black

- For trend maps the lower left window contains a table which shows the relationship of the trend map color codes to the C50 and C70 color classes. The medium gray on the trend maps indicates little or no change in area rate between 1950-59 and 1970-79. The color black indicates the maximum increase in rate between 1950-59 and 1970-79. Color white indicates the maximum decrease in rate between 1950-59 and 1970-79. Hence, darker colors on the trend maps indicate relative deterioration over time and lighter colors indicate relative improvement.

Section 3

Technical Notes

A. Area Recodes and Combinations of Counties

Changes in boundaries during the 30 year period made it necessary to combine counties and cities to have a defined area which would not change over the period. When changes in boundaries involve negligible percentage of the population in the areas, we did not combine the areas. Virginia with independent cities located outside and frequently between counties, required the most adjustment. We combined the following areas.

1. Colorado

    a. Denver includes Arapahoe County.

2. Georgia

    a. Muscogee County includes Chattahoochee County.

3. Montana

    a. Park County includes the Montana portion of Yellowstone National Park.

4. South Dakota

    a. Dewey County includes the former Armstrong County.

    b. Jackson County includes the former Washabaugh County.

5. Virginia-Counties

    a. Albemarle County includes Charlottesville.

    b. Alleghany County includes Clifton Forge and Covington.

    c. Arlington County includes the city of Falls Church.

    d. Augusta County includes the cities of Staunton and Waynesboro.

    e. Bedford County includes Campbell County and the cities of Lynchburg and Bedford.

    f. Carroll County includes Galax City and Grayson County.

    g. Chesterfield County includes the cities of Richmond and Colonial Heights.

    h. Dinwiddie County includes Prince George County and the cities of Petersburg and Hopewell.

    i. Fairfax County includes the cities of Alexandria and Fairfax.

    j. Frederick County includes Winchester City.

    k. Greensville County includes the city of Emporia.

    l. Halifax County includes the city of South Boston.

    m. Henry County includes Martinsville City.

    n. James City County includes York and New Kent Counties, and the cities of Williamsburg and Poquoson.

    o. Montgomery County includes Radford City.

    p. Pittsylvania County includes Danville City.

    q. Prince William County includes Manassas and Manassas Park.

    r. Roanoke County includes Roanoke and Salem cities.

    s. Rockbridge County includes the cities of Buena Vista and Lexington.

    t. Rockingham County includes Harrisonburg City.

    u. Southhampton County includes Franklin City.

    v. Spottsylvania County includes Fredericksburg City.

    w. Washington County includes Bristol City.

    x. Wise County includes Norton City.

6. Virginia-Cities

    a. Chesapeake includes the counties of Norfolk and Princess Anne, and the cities of Norfolk, Portsmouth, South Norfolk, and Virginia Beach.

    b. Hampton City includes Elizabeth City County.

    c. Newport News City includes Warwick.

    d. Suffolk City includes Nansemond County.

7. Wisconsin

    a. Menominee County includes Oconto and Schwano Counties.

8. Wyoming

    a. Park County includes Teton County and the Wyoming portion of Yellowstone National Park.

B. Standard Million Population

Population used is the 1970 U.S. population as shown below.

United States
Standard Million Population by Age for 1970

Age	Population
All ages	1,000,000
< 5	84,416
5-9	98,204
10-14	102,304
15-19	93,845
20-24	80,561
25-29	66,320
30-34	56,249
35-39	54,656
40-44	58,958
45-49	59,622
50-54	54,643
55-59	49,077
60-64	42,403
65-69	34,406
70-74	26,789
75-79	18,871
80-84	11,241
85+	7,435

Source: U.S. Bureau of the Census of Population: 1970, General Population Characteristics, Final Report PC(1)-B

C. Constructing Equivalent Cause of Death Categories Across Years

The maps in this volume cover 30 years spanning four editions of the ICD, raising the problem of comparing periods when different rules of classification of underlying cause of death were in effect. We did not want to create artificially increased rates by attributing deaths to a site specific cancer solely because of a change in classification rules. To avoid this potential artifact, we developed comparability codes for translation between the 6th, 7th, 8th, and 9th edition (revision) of the International Classification of Diseases (see table below).

Several authors have attempted to create equivalencies between editions of the ICD [32,33]. The National Center for Health Statistics conducted the most intensive studies to test comparability by generating comparability ratios. However, for some cancer sites no absolute equivalence can ever be achieved. At the level of aggregation we are using, this should present few problems since whatever effects remain should apply equally to all counties. However, users of these maps should keep in mind the potential problems relating to coding in equivalencies.

Cancer Site Comparability Table

Cancer Site	ICD 9	ICDA 8	ICD 6 & 7
Oral cavity incl. tongue	141,143-146, 148,149	141,143-146, 148,149	141,143-146, 147,148
Nasopharynx	147	147	147
Esophagus	150	150	150
Stomach	151	151	151
Large intestine	153,159.0	153	153
Rectum	154 except 154.3	154	154
Liver & gall bladder including bile ducts	155,156	155,156, 197.8	155*
Pancreas	157	157	157
Larynx	161	161	161
Trachea, bronchus & lung, incl. pleura & other resp. sites	162,163,165	162,163.0, 163.9	162,163
Bone including jaw	170	170	196
Connective and soft tissue	164.1,171	171,192.4, 192.5	197,193.3 193.4**
Malignant melanoma of skin	172	172	190
Non-melanoma skin cancer	173,154.3	173 except 173.5	191
Breast	174,175	174	170
Cervix uteri	180	180	171

Cancer Site Comparability Table

Cancer Site	ICD 9	ICDA 8	ICD 6* & 7
Chorion, uterus & uterus not otherwise specified	179,181,182	181,182	172,173,174
Ovary, fallopian tube & broad ligament	183	183	175
Prostate	185	185	177
Bladder & other urinary organs	188,189.3	188,189.9	181
Kidney & ureter	189 except 189.3	189.0,189.1, 189.2	180
Brain & other parts of the nervous system	191,192	191,192 except 192.4, 192.5	193 except 193.3,193.4**
Thyroid gland	193	193	194
Lymphosarcoma & reticulum cell sarcoma including other lymphoma	159.1,200, 202.0,.1,.8,.9	200,202	200,202,205
Hodgkin's disease	201	201	201
Multiple myeloma	203 except 203.1	203	203
Leukemias	204-208, 202.4,203.1	204-207	204
Secondary, site unspecified & not previously listed cancers	152,158, 159.2-.9, 164.2-.9,184, 187,195-199, 202.2,.3,.5,.6	152,158,159, 163.1,173.5, 184,187,195, 196,197.0-.7, 197.9,198,199	152,156,158, 159,164,165, 176,179,198, 199
All cancers	140-208	140-207	140-205

*Code 156, ICD 6 and 7 secondary and unspecified cancers cannot be separated. For this reason, death rates for 1950-59 and 1970-79 are not comparable and the comparison should not be made.
**Code 193, ICD 6 cannot be subdivided. For this reason, deaths from malignant neoplasm of the brain and other parts of the nervous system for the years 1950-1957 contain deaths from malignant neoplasm of peripheral nerves and sympathetic nervous system.

References

1. National Center for Health Statistics: Advance report of final mortality statistics, 1984. Monthly Vital Statistics Report, Vol. 35, No. 6, Supp.(2). DHHS Pub. No. (PHS) 86-1120. Public Health Service. Hyattsville, MD Sept. 26, 1986.

2. Manton, K. G., E. Stallard, M. A. Woodbury, J. P. Creason, W. B. Riggan, and A. C. Pellom. Empirical Bayes Procedures for Smoothing Trend Maps of U.S. Cancer Mortality Rates. J. Amer. Statist. Assoc.,(In Review).

3. Toxic Substances Strategy Committee, Toxic Chemicals and Public Protection—A Report to the President. Council on Environmental Quality. U.S. Govt. Print. Off., Washington D.C., May 1980.

4. Pollack, E. S. and J. W. Horm. Trends in Cancer Incidence and Mortality in the United States, 1969-1976. J. Natl. Cancer Inst., 64, 5:1091-1103, 1980.

5. Schottenfeld, D. and J. F. Haas. Carcinogens in the Work Place. Amer. Cancer Soc., 1978.

6. Shabad, L. M. Circulation of Carcinogenic Poly-cyclic Aromatic Hydrocarbons in the Human Environment and Cancer Prevention. J. Natl. Cancer Inst., 64, 3:405-410, 1980.

7. Cederlof, R., R. Doll, B. Fowler, L. Friberg, N. Nelson, and V. Vouk, editors. Air Pollution and Cancer: Risk Assessment Methodology and Epidemiological Evidence. Report of a Task Group. Environ. Health Perspect., 22:1-2, 1978.

8. Mason, T. J. and F. W. McKay. U.S. CANCER MORTALITY BY COUNTY: 1950 - 1969. DHEW publication (NIH) 74-615, U.S. Govt. Print. Off., Washington DC, 1973.

9. Mason, T. J., F. W. McKay, R. Hoover, W. T. Blot, and J. F. Fraumeni, Jr. ATLAS OF CANCER MORTALITY FOR U.S. COUNTIES: 1950 -1969. DHEW publication (NIH) 75-780, U.S. Govt. Print. Off., Washington, DC, 1975.

10. Mason, T. J., F. W. McKay, R. Hoover, W. T. Blot, and J. F. Fraumeni, Jr. ATLAS OF CANCER MORTALITY AMONG NON-WHITES: 1950 - 1969. DHEW publication (NIH) 76-1204, U.S. Govt. Print. Off., Washington, DC, 1976.

11. Riggan, W. B., J. Van Bruggen, J. F. Acquavella, J. Beaubier, and T. J. Mason. U.S. Cancer Mortality Rates and Trends, 1950-1979, Vol. 1-3, Pub. No. EPA-600/1-83-015a. U.S.Govt. Print. Off., Washington, DC.

12. Blot, W. J., J. F. Fraumeni, Jr., T. J. Mason, and R. N. Hoover. Developing Clues to Environmental Cancer: A Stepwise Approach with the Use of Mortality Data. Environ. Health Perspect., 32:53-58, 1979.

13. Pickle, L. J., T. J. Mason, N. Howard, R. Hoover, and, J. F. Fraumeni, Jr. Atlas of U.S. Cancer Mortality Among Whites: 1950-1980. Washington, DC: U.S. Govt. Printing Office. (DHHS Publication No. (NIH) 87-2900), 1987.

14. Manton, K. G., E. Stallard, M. A. Woodbury, W. B. Riggan, J. P. Creason, and T. J. Mason. Statistically Adjusted Estimates of Geographic Profiles. J. Natl. Cancer Inst., 78, 5:805-815,1987.

15. MacMahon, B., T. F. Pugh, and J. Ipsen. Epidemiologic methods, Little Brown and Company, Boston, MA, and other similar text books on methods.

16. Blot, W. J., B. J. Stone, J. F. Fraumeni, Jr., and L. E. Morris. Cancer Mortality in U.S. Counties with Shipyard Industries During World War II. Environ. Res. 18:281-290,1979.

17. Pellom, A. C. and E. Stallard. The Cancer Mortality Atlas Data Management System. EPA publication available from the National Technical Information Service (in preparation).

18. Pellom, A. C., G. F. Woodbury, and S. Woodbury. The Cancer Mortality Atlas Mapping System. EPA publication available from the National Technical Information Service (in preparation).

19. Percy, C., E. Stanek, and L. Gloeckler. Accuracy of Cancer Death Certificates and Its Effect on Cancer Mortality Statistics. Amer. J. Public Health, 71, 3:242-250, 1981.

20. Marcus, S. C. Some Limitations in the Use of Cancer Mortality Data in Epidemiological Studies. PROCEEDINGS OF THE 71st ANNUAL MEETING OF THE AIR POLLUTION CONTROL ASSOCIATION, paper 78-6.2:1-12, 1978.

21. Glasser, J. H. The Quality and Utility of Death Certificate Data. Amer. J. Public Health (editorial), 71, 3:231-233, 1981.

22. Myers, G. C., and K. G. Manton. Accuracy of Death Certification. SOCIAL STATISTICS PROCEEDINGS OF THE AMERICAN STATISTICAL ASSOCIATION, 321-325, 1983.

23. World Health Organization. International Classification of Diseases, fifth, sixth, seventh, eighth, and ninth revision. Geneva, 1940, 1953, 1957, 1967, 1978.

24. Polissar, L. The Effect of Migration on the Comparison of Disease Rates in Geographic Studies in the United States. Amer. J. Epidemiol., 111:175-182, 1980.

25. U.S. Department of Health, Education, and Welfare. International Classification of Diseases adapted for use in the United States, eighth revision, PHS publication 1693, 1967.

26. U.S. Department of Health and Human Services. VITAL STATISTICS OF THE UNITED STATES, 1979, Volume II - Mortality, Part A. DHHS Publication (PHS) 84-1101, U.S. Govt. Print. Off., Washington, DC., 1984.

27. U.S. Department of Health, Education, and Welfare. VITAL STATISTICS OF THE UNITED STATES, 1952, Volume II - Mortality Data, U.S. Govt. Print. Off., Washington, DC., 1955. (See page 418 table 54 footnote 1.)

28. U.S. Department of Health, Education, and Welfare. VITAL STATISTICS OF THE UNITED STATES, 1962, Volume II -Mortality Part A, U.S. Govt. Print. Off., Washington, DC., 1964. (See Section 6 page 6-9.)

29. U.S. Department of Health and Human Services. VITAL STATISTICS OF THE UNITED STATES, 1972, Volume II - Mortality, Part A. DHHS Publication (HRA) 76-1101, U.S. Govt. Print. Off., Washington, DC., 1976 (see Technical Appendix.)

30. U.S. Bureau of Census, Census of population: 1960, Final Report PC(1)-A, and reports for 1970 and 1980 on the number of inhabitants, (Footnote in table - Population and Land Area of Counties).

31. Manton, K. G. and E. Stallard. Methods for the analysis of mortality risk across heterogeneous small populations: Examination of space-time gradients in cancer mortality in NC counties. Demography, 18:217-230, 1981.

32. Klebba, A. J. and J. H. Scott. Estimates of Selected Comparability Ratios Based on Dual Coding of the 1976 Death Certificates by the Eighth and Ninth Revisions of the International Classification of Diseases. National Center of Health Statistics MONTHLY VITAL STATISTICS REPORT, 28, 11, February 29, 1980 (supplement).

33. Nectoux, J. Comparison of the 7th and 8th Revisions of the ICD and Tables of Equivalence in chapter IV of CANCER INCIDENCE IN FIVE CONTINENTS, Volume III. J. Waterhouse, P. Correa, C. Muir, and J. Powell, editors. Agency for Research on Cancer, Lyon, 25-38, 1976.

U.S. CANCER MORTALITY RATES AND TRENDS 1950-1979

Volume IV: Maps

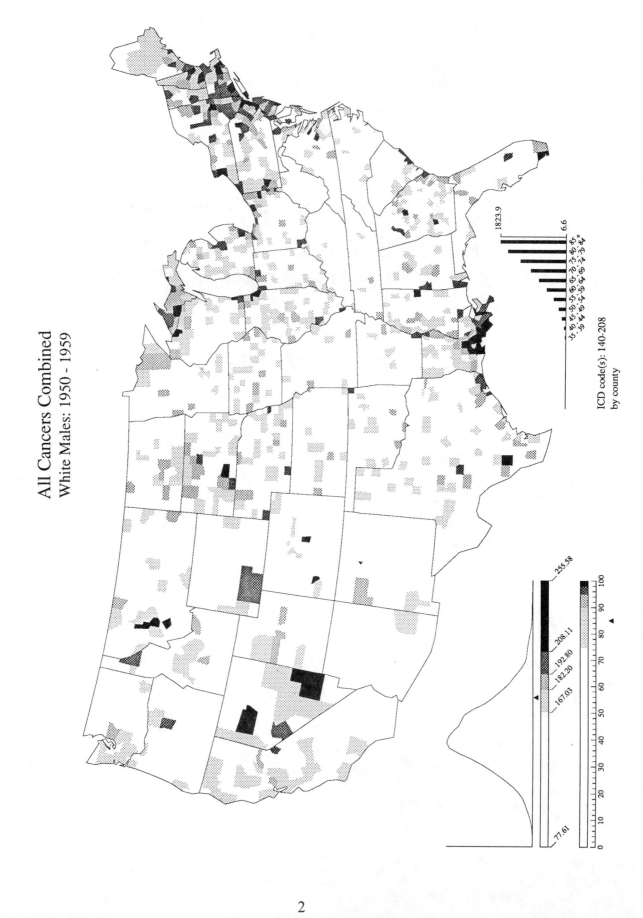

All Cancers Combined
White Males: 1950 - 1959

ICD code(s): 140-208
by county

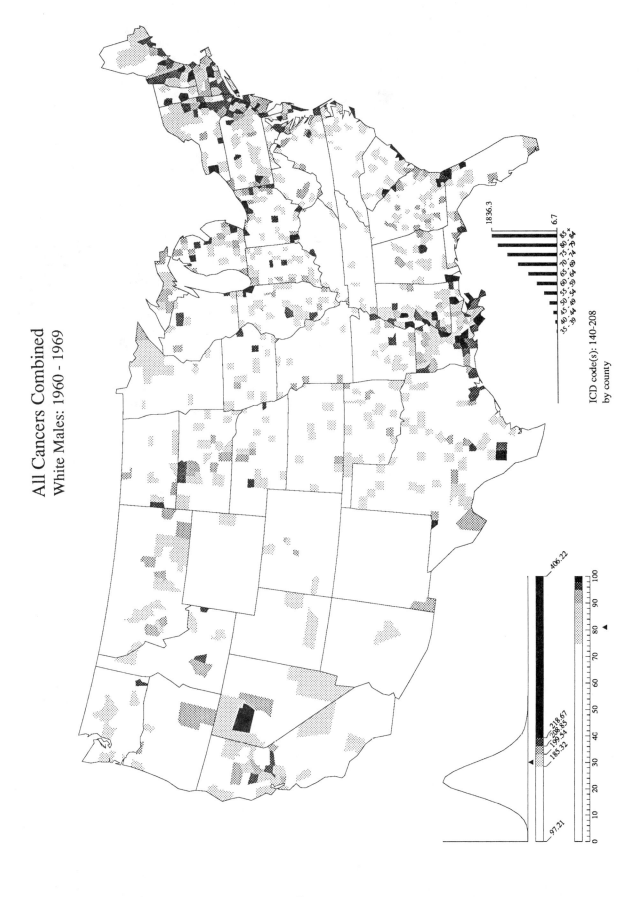

All Cancers Combined
White Males: 1960 - 1969

ICD code(s): 140-208
by county

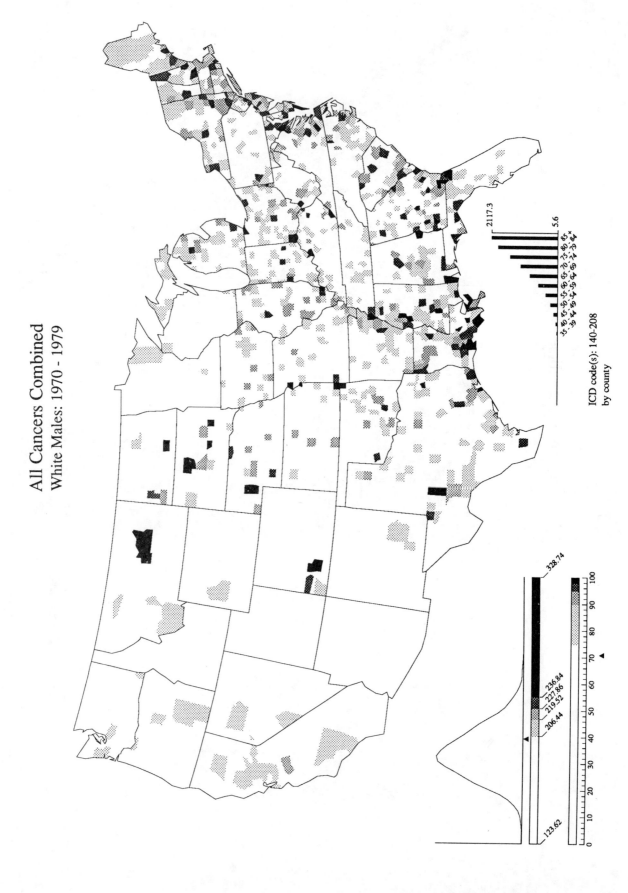

All Cancers Combined
White Males: 1970 - 1979

2117.3

85
80-84
75-79
70-74
65-69
60-64
55-59
50-54
45-49
40-44
35-39
5.6

ICD code(s): 140-208
by county

328.74

236.84
227.86
219.52
206.44

123.62

100
90
80
70
60
50
40
30
20
10
0

All Cancers Combined
White Males: Relative Change

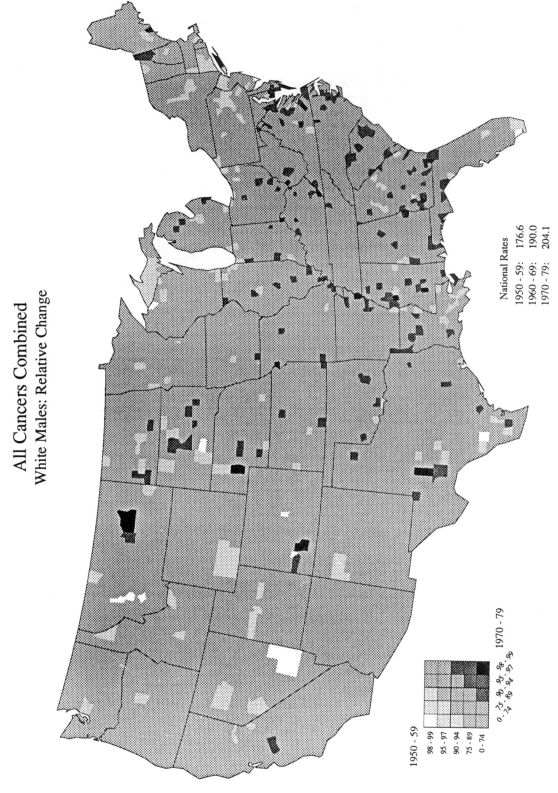

National Rates

1950 - 59:	176.6
1960 - 69:	190.0
1970 - 79:	204.1

ICD code(s): 140-208
by county

1950 - 59

98 - 99
95 - 97
90 - 94
75 - 89
0 - 74

1970 - 79

98 - 99
95 - 97
90 - 94
75 - 89
0 - 74

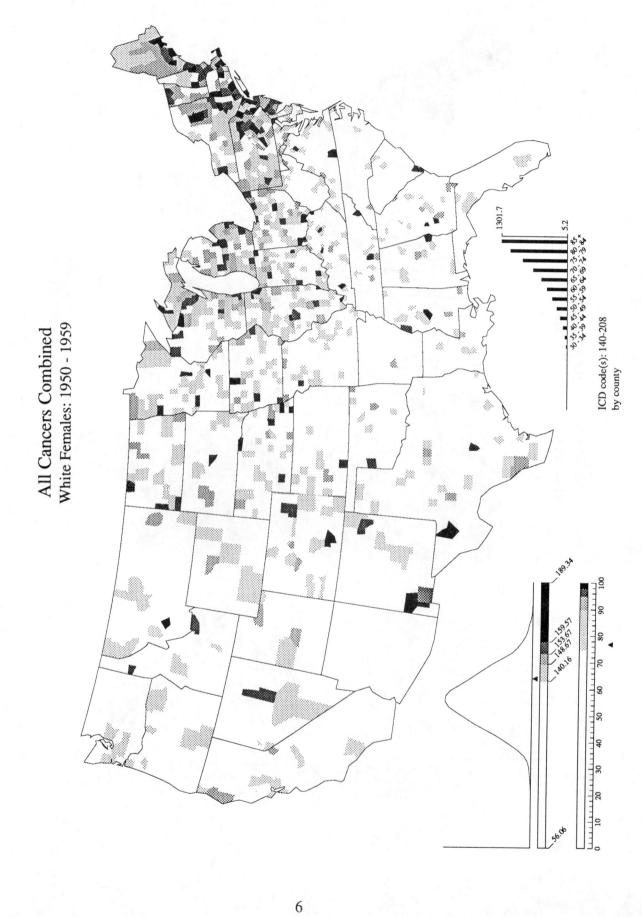

All Cancers Combined
White Females: 1950 - 1959

ICD code(s): 140-208
by county

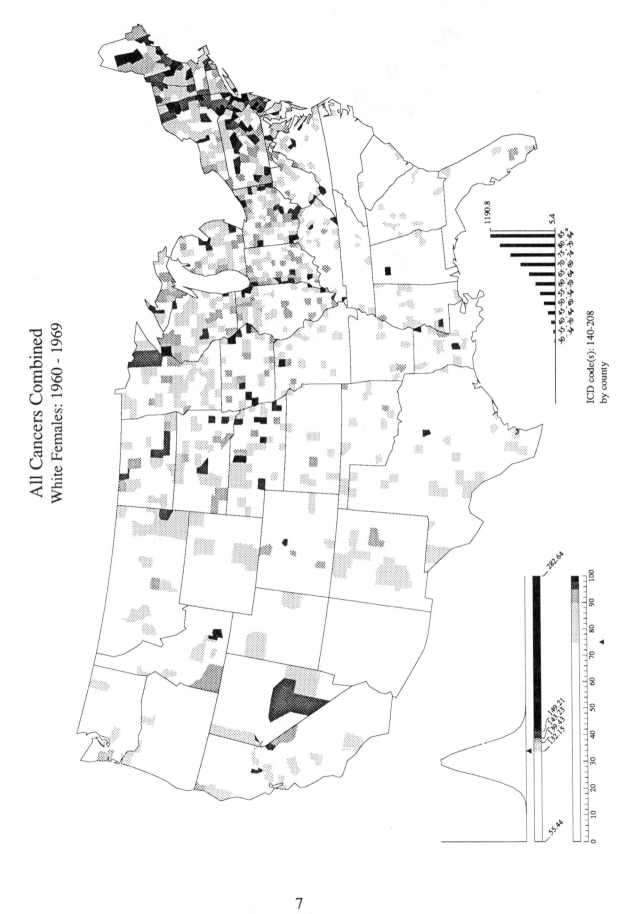

All Cancers Combined
White Females: 1960 - 1969

ICD code(s): 140-208
by county

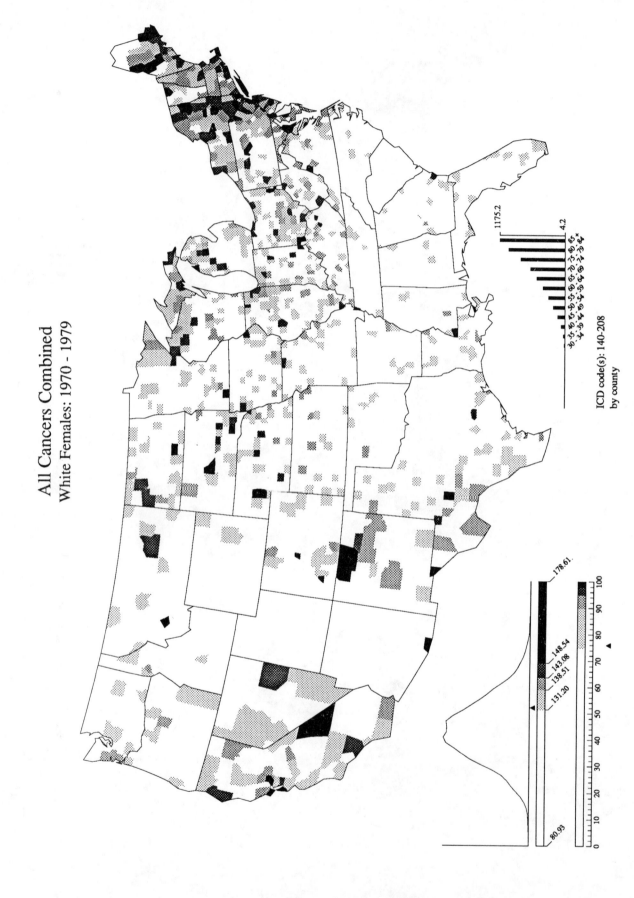

All Cancers Combined
White Females: 1970 - 1979

ICD code(s): 140-208
by county

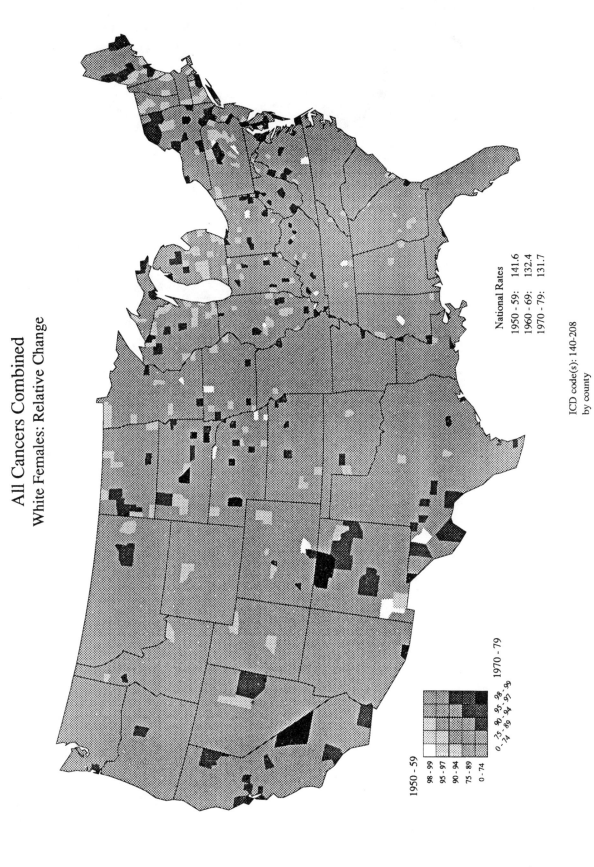

All Cancers Combined
White Females: Relative Change

National Rates

1950 - 59:	141.6
1960 - 69:	132.4
1970 - 79:	131.7

ICD code(s): 140-208
by county

1950 - 59

98 - 99
95 - 97
90 - 94
75 - 89
0 - 74

1970 - 79

98 - 99
95 - 97
90 - 94
75 - 89
0 - 74

9

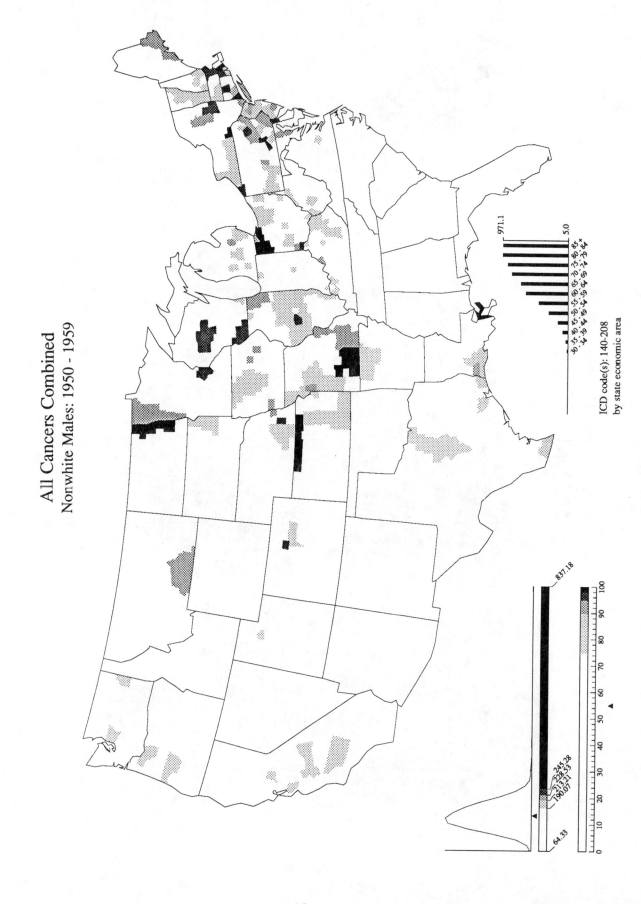

All Cancers Combined
Nonwhite Males: 1950 - 1959

ICD code(s): 140-208
by state economic area

All Cancers Combined
Nonwhite Males: 1960 - 1969

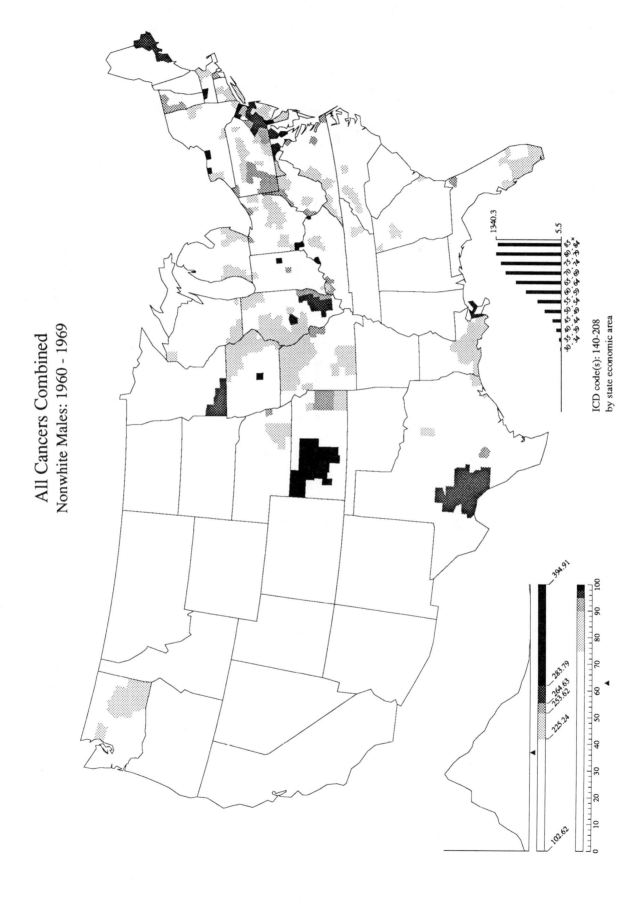

ICD code(s): 140-208
by state economic area

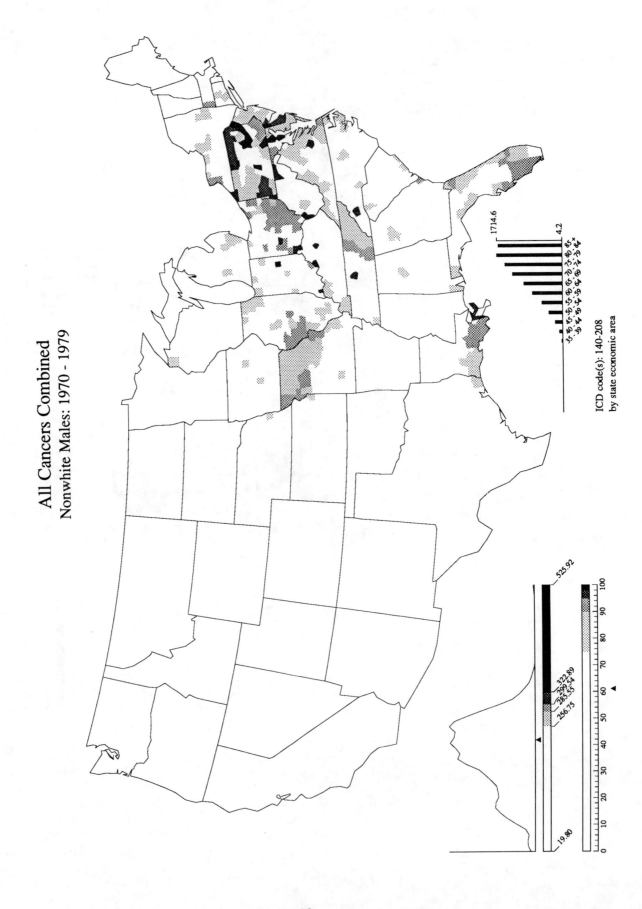

All Cancers Combined
Nonwhite Males: 1970 - 1979

ICD code(s): 140-208
by state economic area

All Cancers Combined
Nonwhite Males: Relative Change

National Rates

1950 - 59:	166.3
1960 - 69:	209.5
1970 - 79:	231.6

ICD code(s): 140-208
by state economic area

1950 - 59

98 - 99
95 - 97
90 - 94
75 - 89
0 - 74

1970 - 79

98 · 99
95 · 97
90 · 94
75 · 89
0 · 74

13

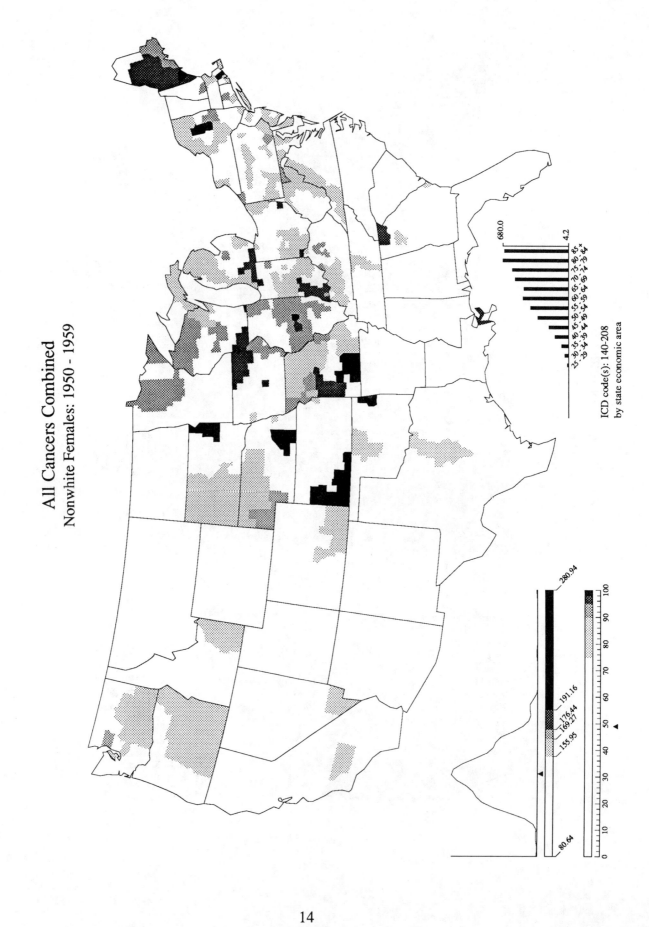

All Cancers Combined
Nonwhite Females: 1950 - 1959

ICD code(s): 140-208
by state economic area

All Cancers Combined
Nonwhite Females: 1960 - 1969

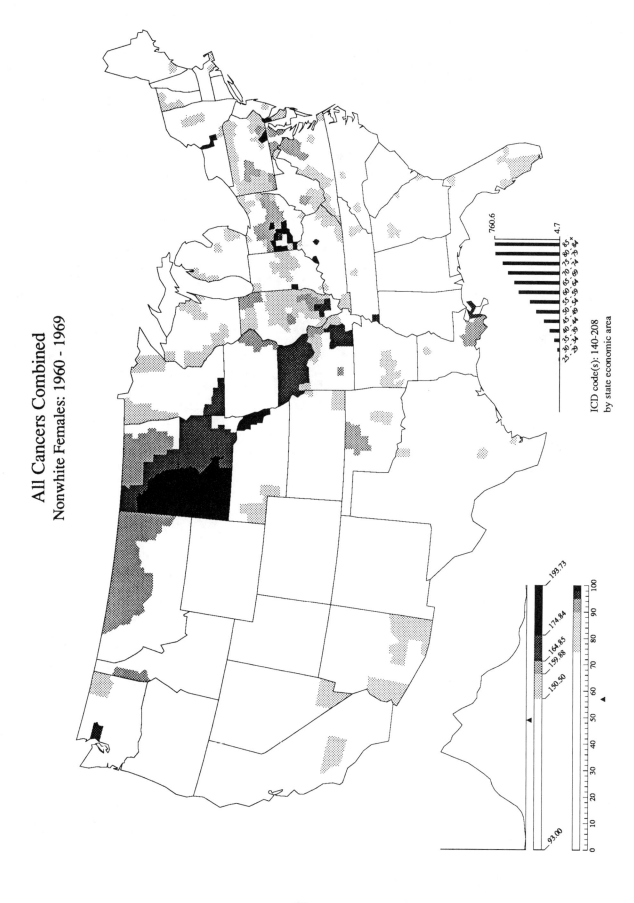

ICD code(s): 140-208
by state economic area

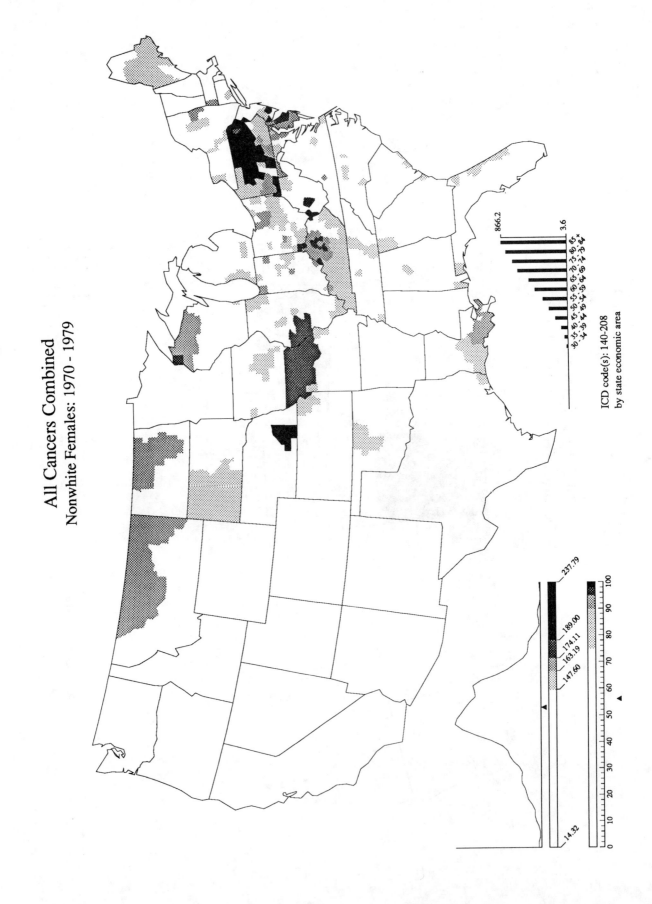

All Cancers Combined
Nonwhite Females: 1970 - 1979

ICD code(s): 140-208
by state economic area

All Cancers Combined
Nonwhite Females: Relative Change

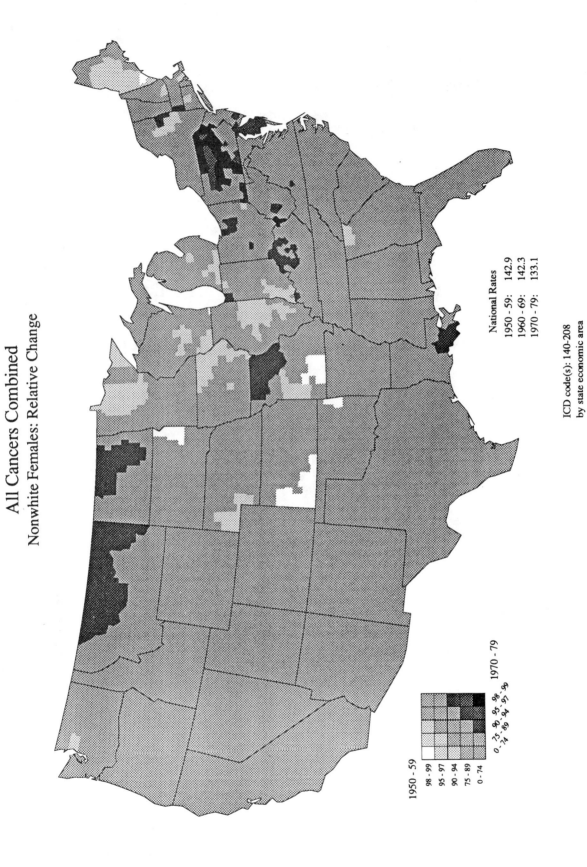

National Rates

1950 - 59: 142.9
1960 - 69: 142.3
1970 - 79: 133.1

ICD code(s): 140-208
by state economic area

1950 - 59

98 - 99
95 - 97
90 - 94
75 - 89
0 - 74

1970 - 79

0 - 74 75 - 89 90 - 94 95 - 97 98 - 99

17

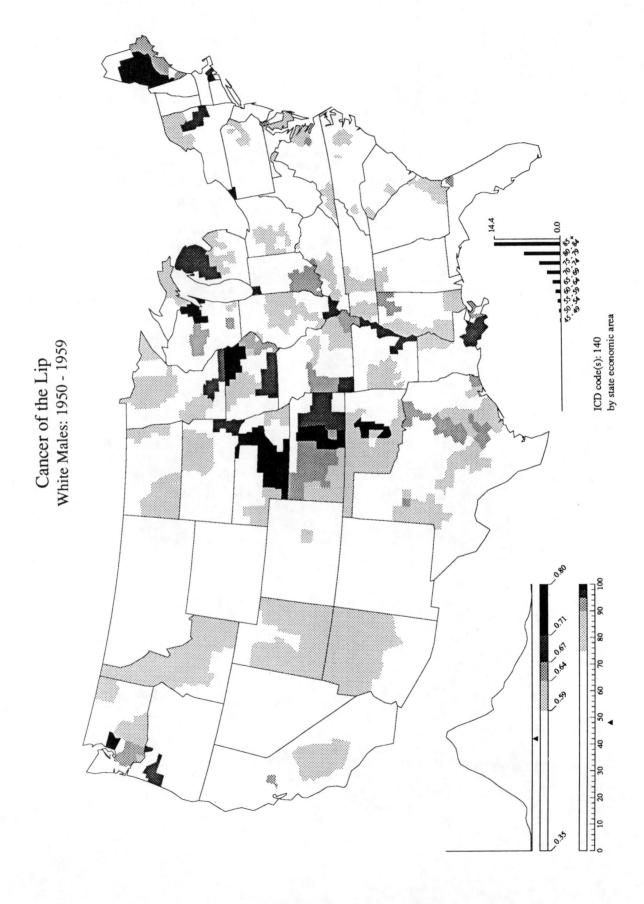

Cancer of the Lip
White Males: 1950 - 1959

ICD code(s): 140
by state economic area

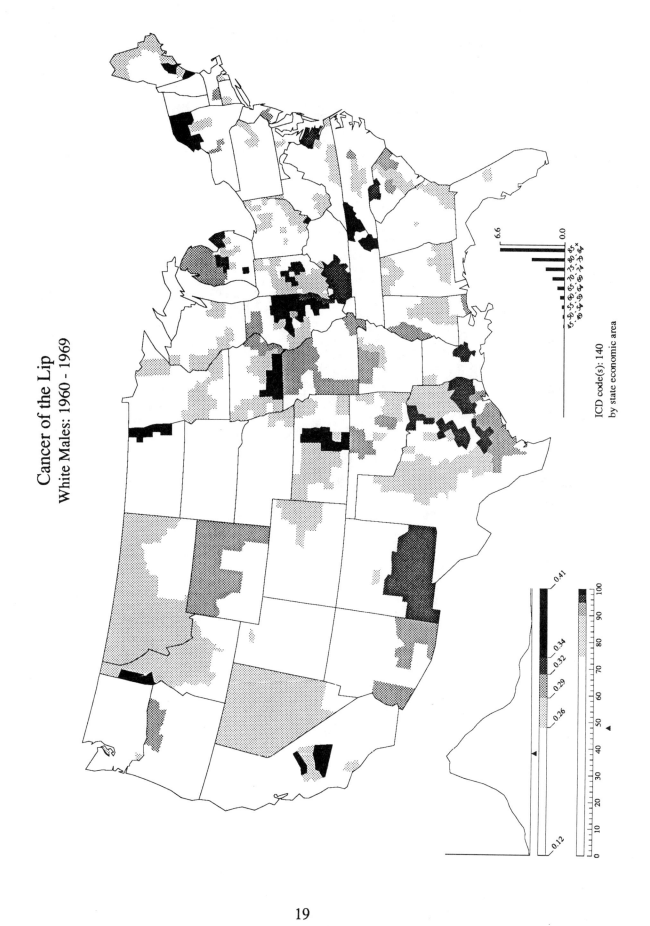

Cancer of the Lip
White Males: 1960 - 1969

ICD code(s): 140
by state economic area

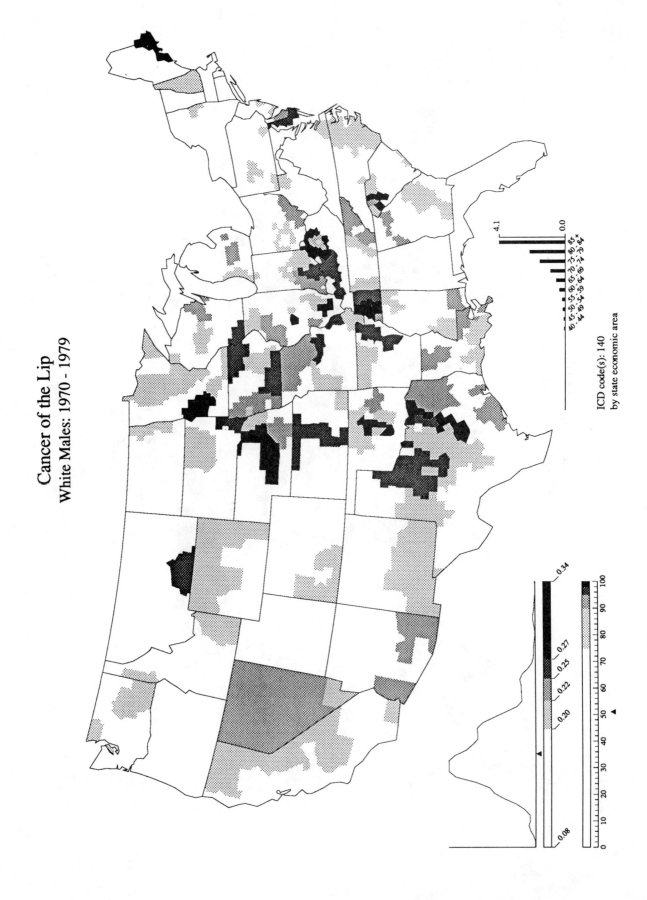

Cancer of the Lip
White Males: 1970 - 1979

ICD code(s): 140
by state economic area

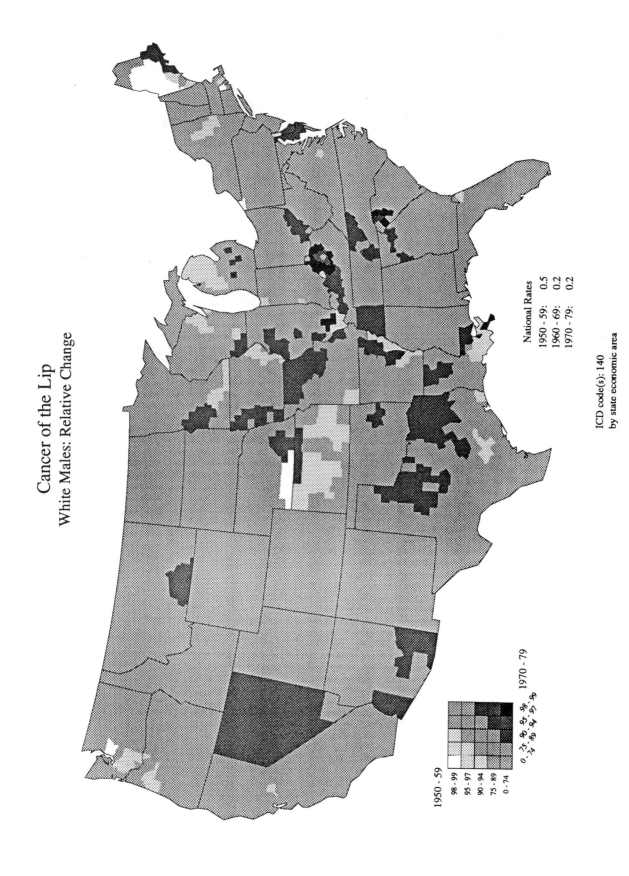

Cancer of the Lip
White Males: Relative Change

National Rates

1950 - 59: 0.5
1960 - 69: 0.2
1970 - 79: 0.2

ICD code(s): 140
by state economic area

1950 - 59

98 - 99
95 - 97
90 - 94
75 - 89
0 - 74

1970 - 79

0 - 75 - 90 - 95 - 98 - 99
74   89   94   97   99

Cancer of the Oral Cavity including Tongue
White Males: 1950 - 1959

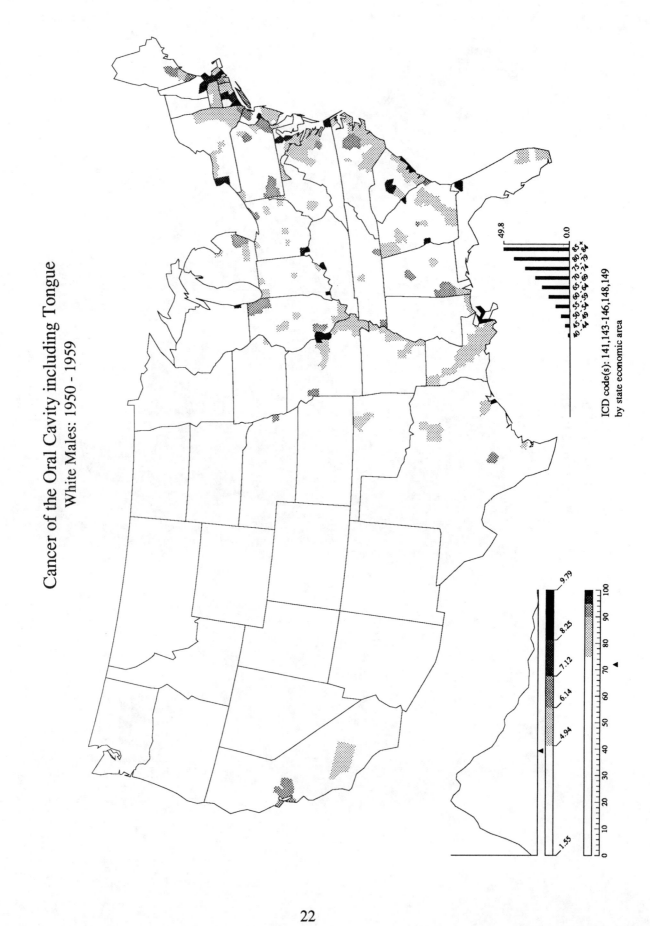

ICD code(s): 141,143-146,148,149
by state economic area

Cancer of the Oral Cavity including Tongue
White Males: 1960 - 1969

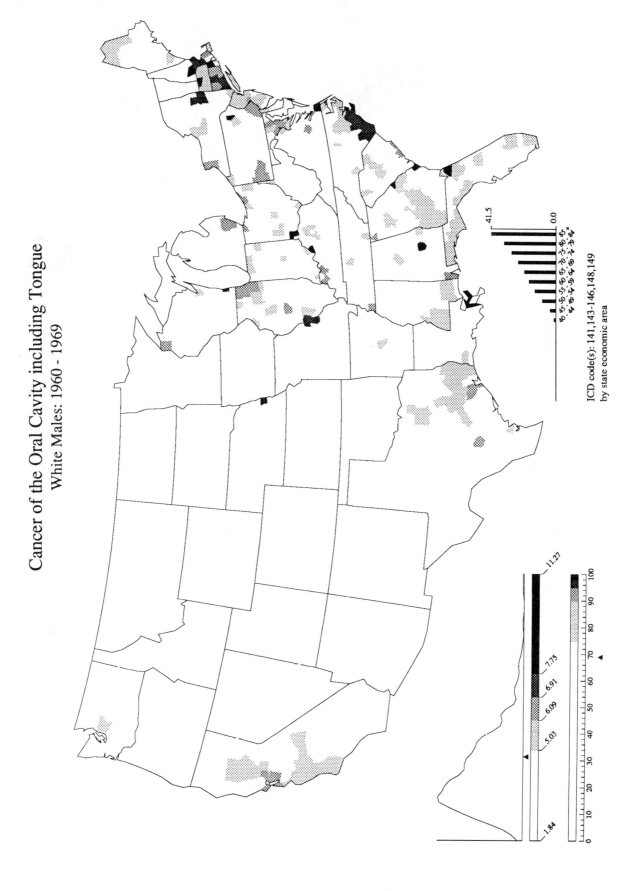

ICD code(s): 141,143-146,148,149
by state economic area

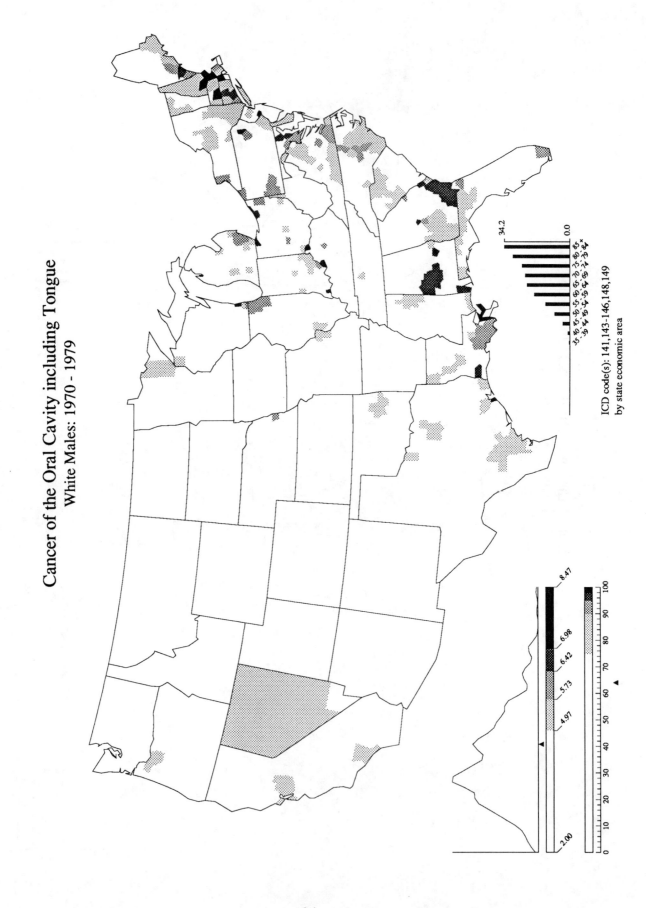

Cancer of the Oral Cavity including Tongue
White Males: 1970 - 1979

ICD code(s): 141,143-146,148,149
by state economic area

24

Cancer of the Oral Cavity including Tongue
White Males: Relative Change

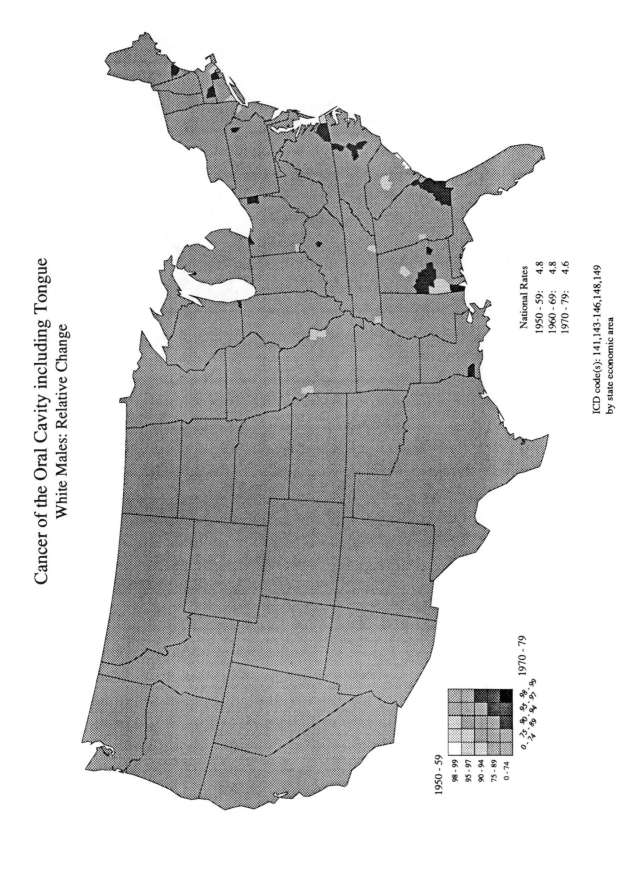

National Rates

1950 - 59: 4.8
1960 - 69: 4.8
1970 - 79: 4.6

ICD code(s): 141,143-146,148,149
by state economic area

1950 - 59

98 - 99
95 - 97
90 - 94
75 - 89
0 - 74

1970 - 79

0 - 74
75 - 89
90 - 94
95 - 97
98 - 99

Cancer of the Oral Cavity including Tongue
White Females: 1950 - 1959

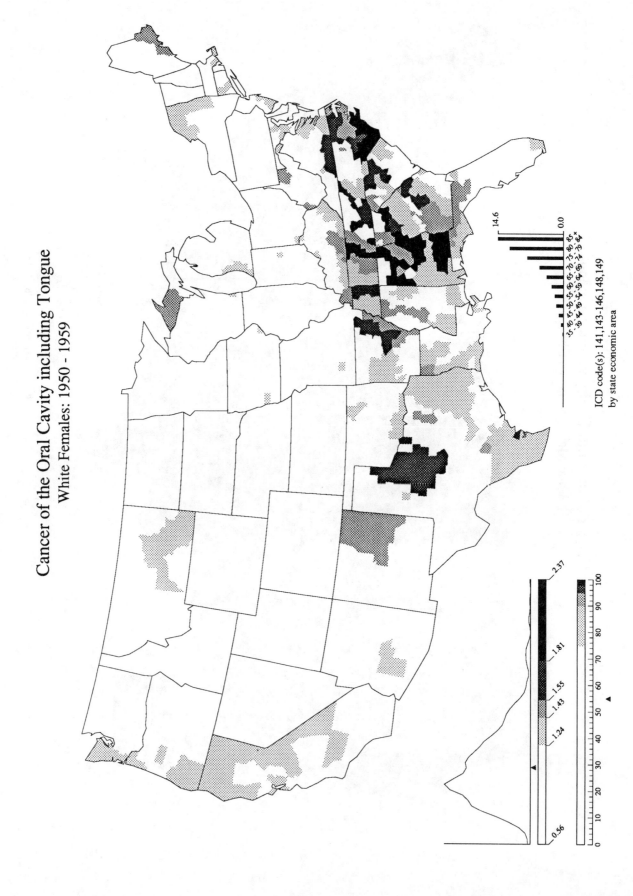

ICD code(s): 141,143-146,148,149
by state economic area

26

Cancer of the Oral Cavity including Tongue
White Females: 1960 - 1969

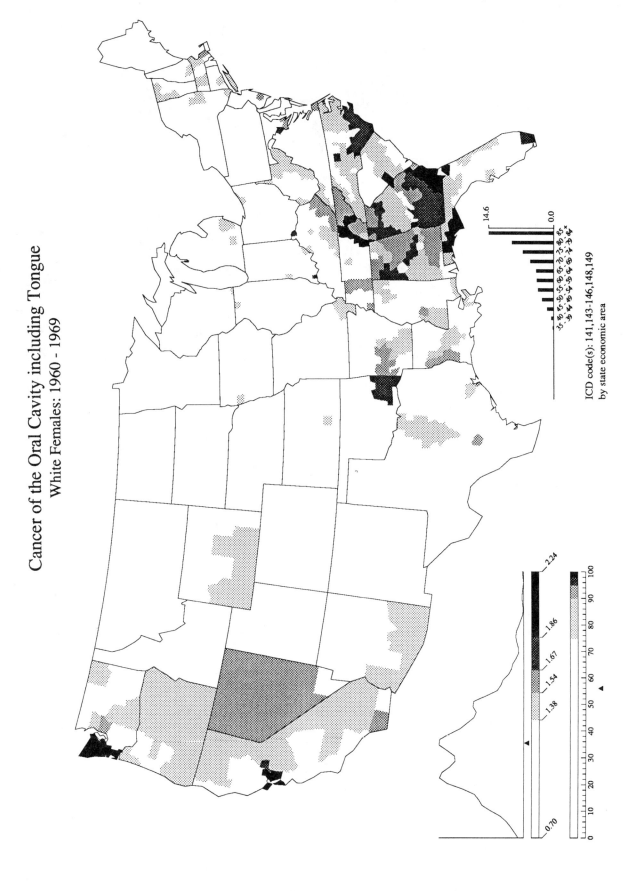

ICD code(s): 141,143-146,148,149
by state economic area

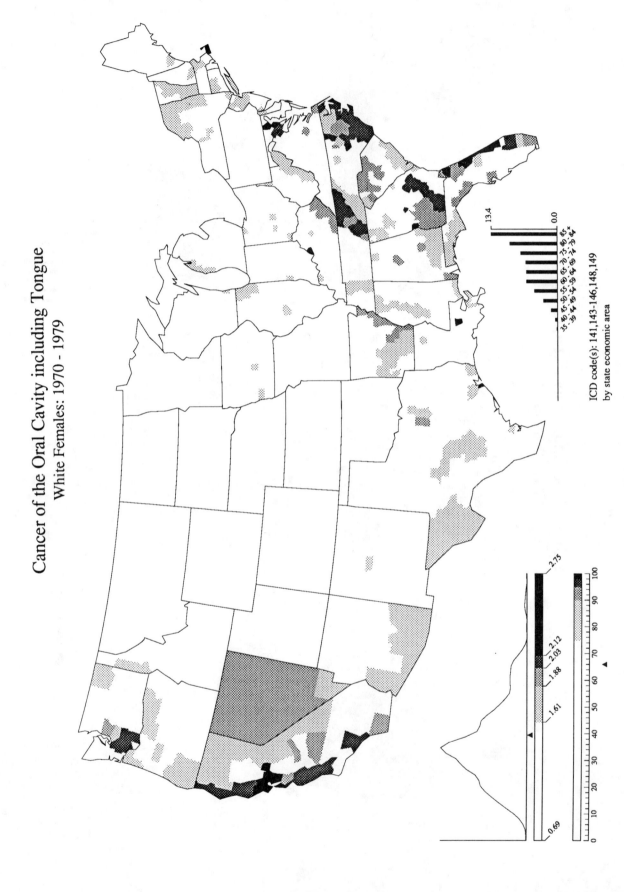

Cancer of the Oral Cavity including Tongue
White Females: 1970 - 1979

ICD code(s): 141,143-146,148,149
by state economic area

Cancer of the Oral Cavity including Tongue
White Females: Relative Change

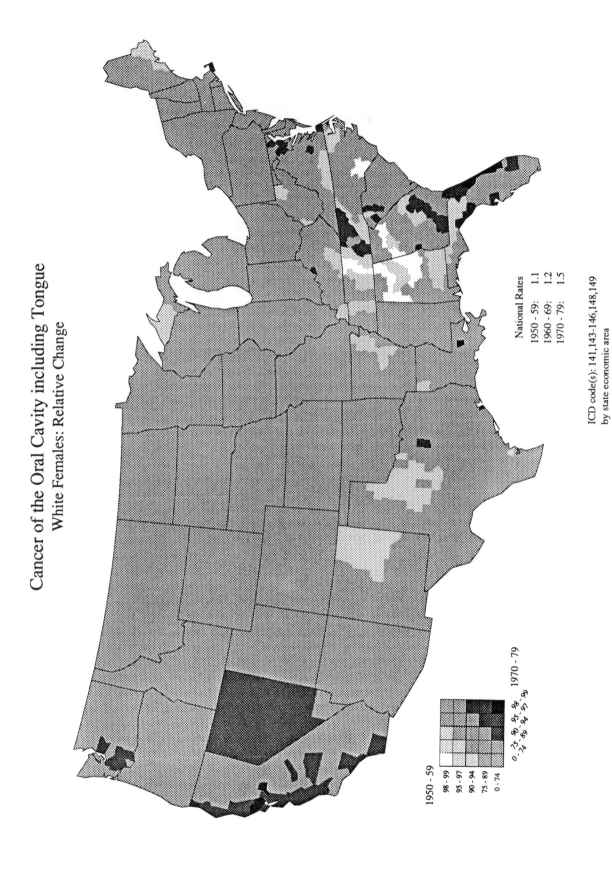

National Rates

1950 - 59: 1.1
1960 - 69: 1.2
1970 - 79: 1.5

ICD code(s): 141,143-146,148,149
by state economic area

1950 - 59

98 - 99
95 - 97
90 - 94
75 - 89
0 - 74

1970 - 79

98 - 99
95 - 97
90 - 94
75 - 89
0 - 74

Cancer of the Oral Cavity including Tongue
Nonwhite Males: 1950 - 1959

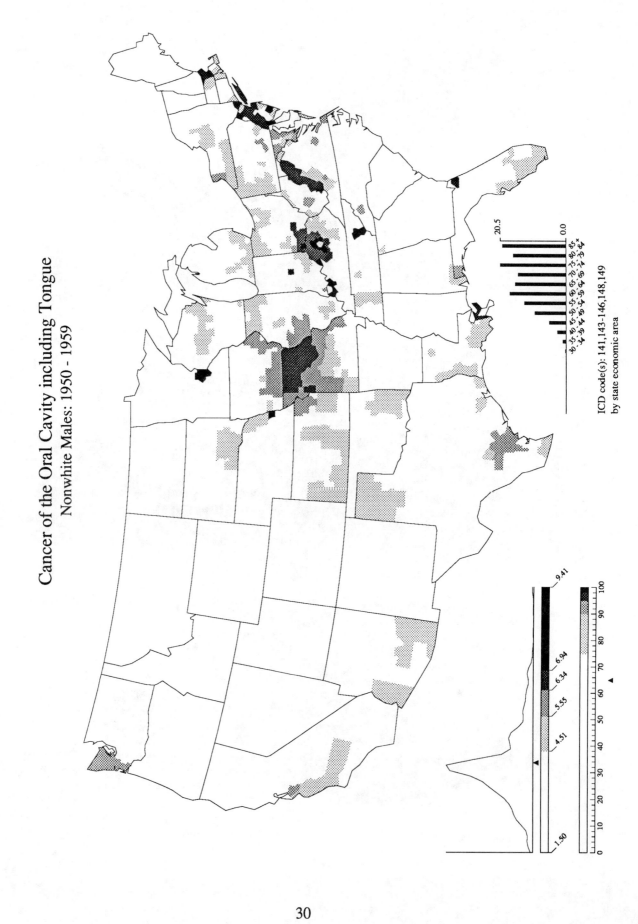

ICD code(s): 141,143-146,148,149
by state economic area

Cancer of the Oral Cavity including Tongue
Nonwhite Males: 1960 - 1969

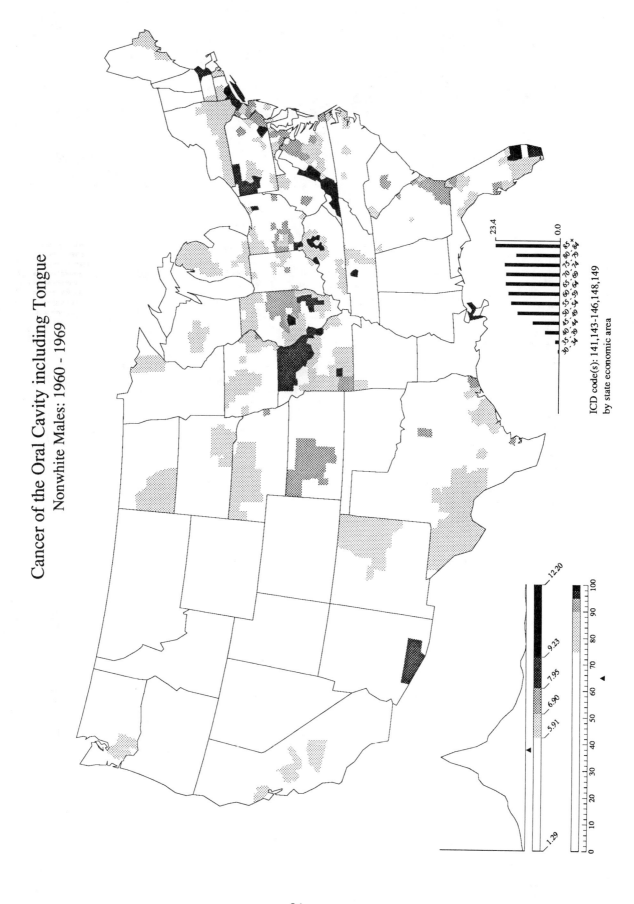

ICD code(s): 141,143-146,148,149
by state economic area

Cancer of the Oral Cavity including Tongue
Nonwhite Males: 1970 - 1979

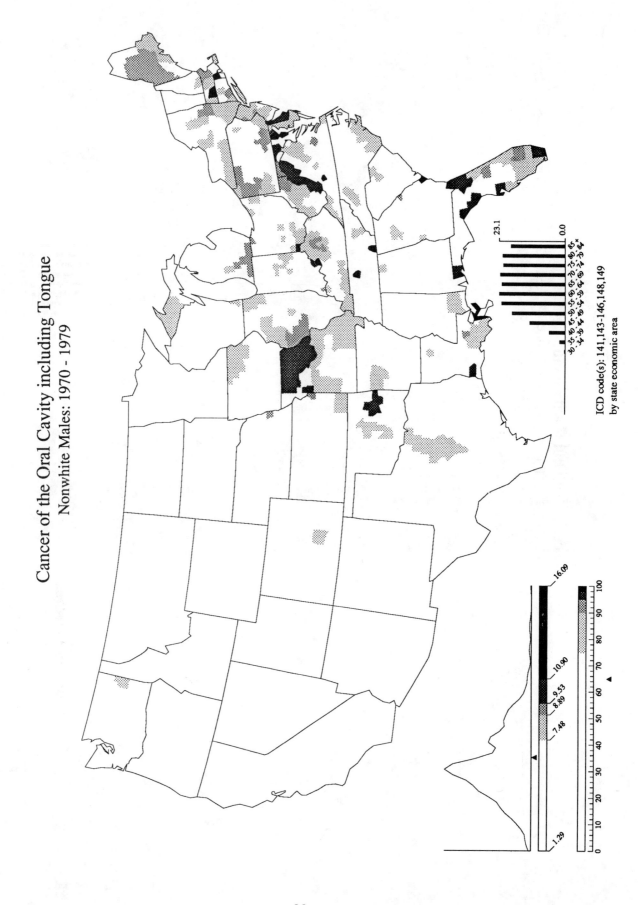

ICD code(s): 141,143-146,148,149
by state economic area

Cancer of the Oral Cavity including Tongue
Nonwhite Males: Relative Change

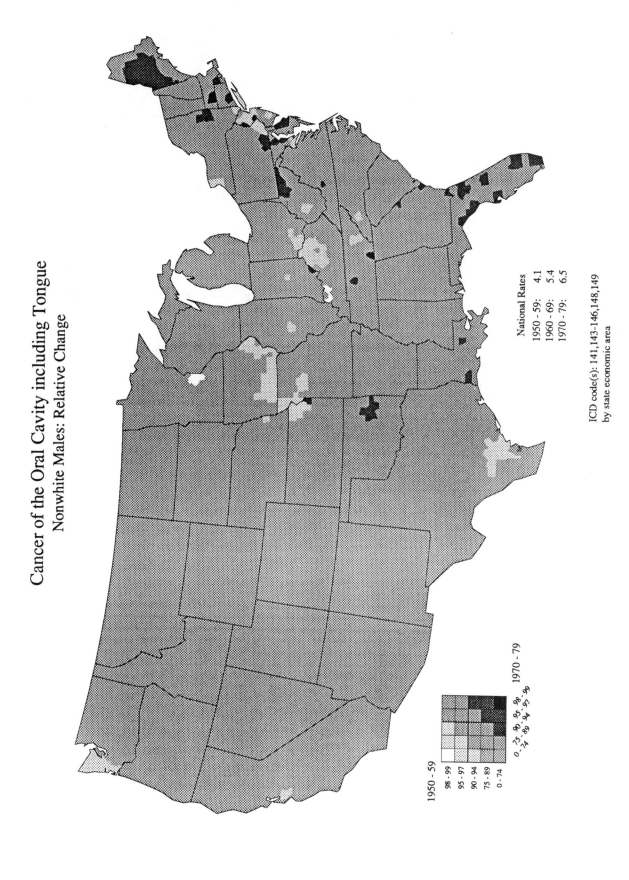

National Rates

1950 - 59:	4.1
1960 - 69:	5.4
1970 - 79:	6.5

ICD code(s): 141,143-146,148,149
by state economic area

1950 - 59

98 - 99
95 - 97
90 - 94
75 - 89
0 - 74

0 - 74   75 - 89   90 - 94   95 - 97   98 - 99   1970 - 79

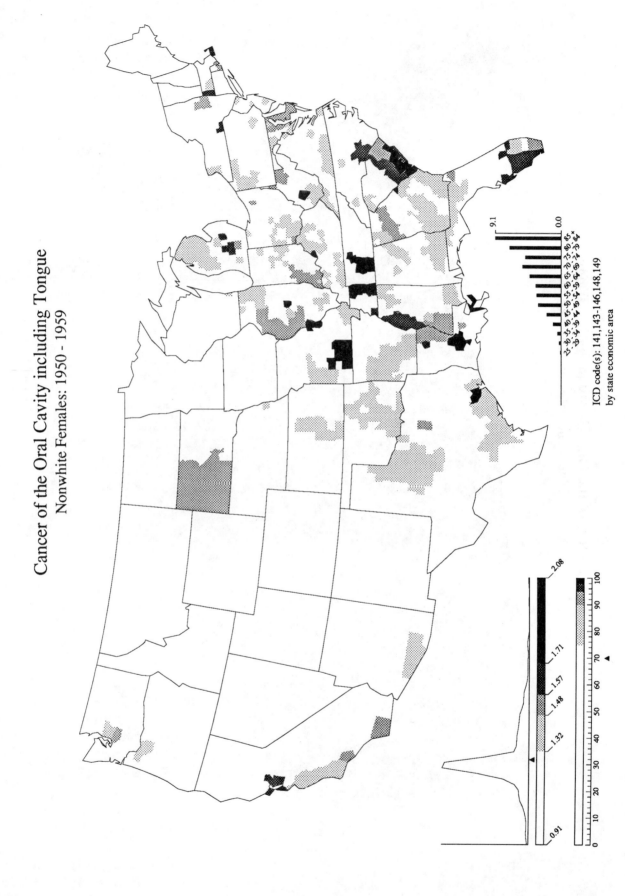

Cancer of the Oral Cavity including Tongue
Nonwhite Females: 1950 - 1959

ICD code(s): 141,143-146,148,149
by state economic area

Cancer of the Oral Cavity including Tongue
Nonwhite Females: 1960 - 1969

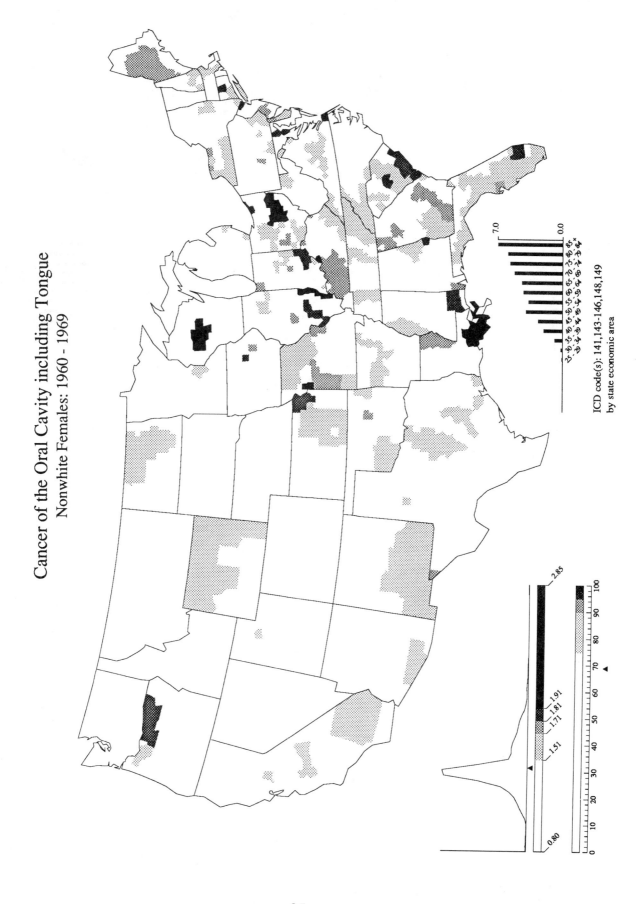

ICD code(s): 141,143-146,148,149
by state economic area

7.0

0.0

2.85

1.91
1.81
1.71
1.51

0.80

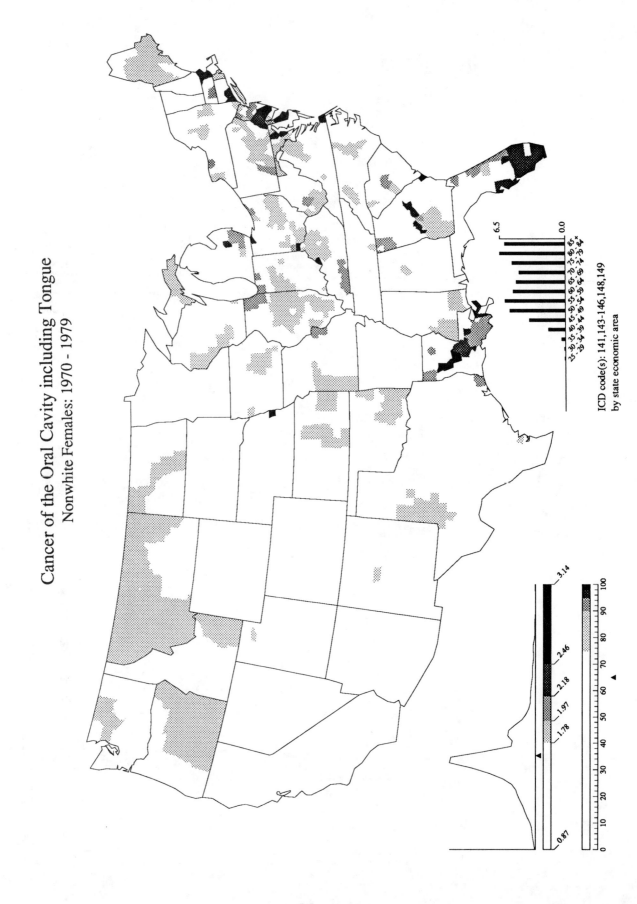

Cancer of the Oral Cavity including Tongue
Nonwhite Females: 1970 - 1979

ICD code(s): 141,143-146,148,149
by state economic area

36

Cancer of the Oral Cavity including Tongue
Nonwhite Females: Relative Change

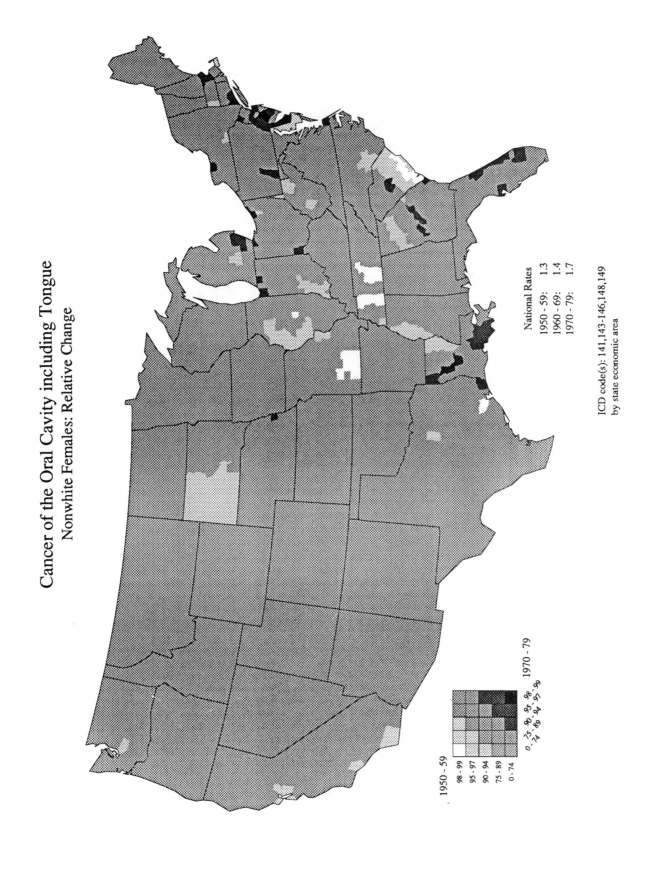

National Rates

1950 - 59:	1.3
1960 - 69:	1.4
1970 - 79:	1.7

ICD code(s): 141,143-146,148,149
by state economic area

1950 - 59

98 - 99
95 - 97
90 - 94
75 - 89
0 - 74

0 - 74 89 94 97 99
75 - 90 - 95 - 98 -

1970 - 79

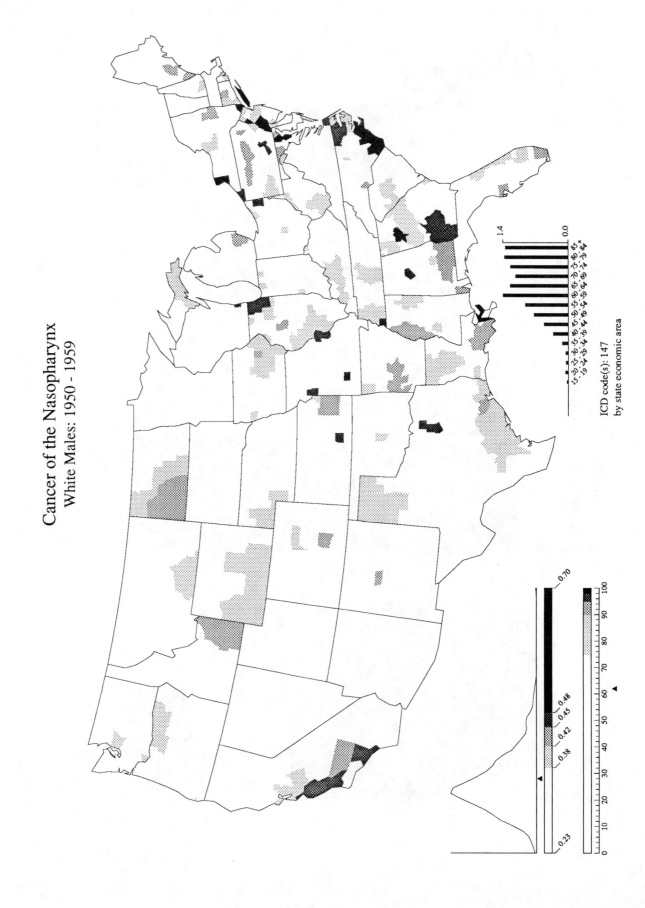

Cancer of the Nasopharynx
White Males: 1950 - 1959

ICD code(s): 147
by state economic area

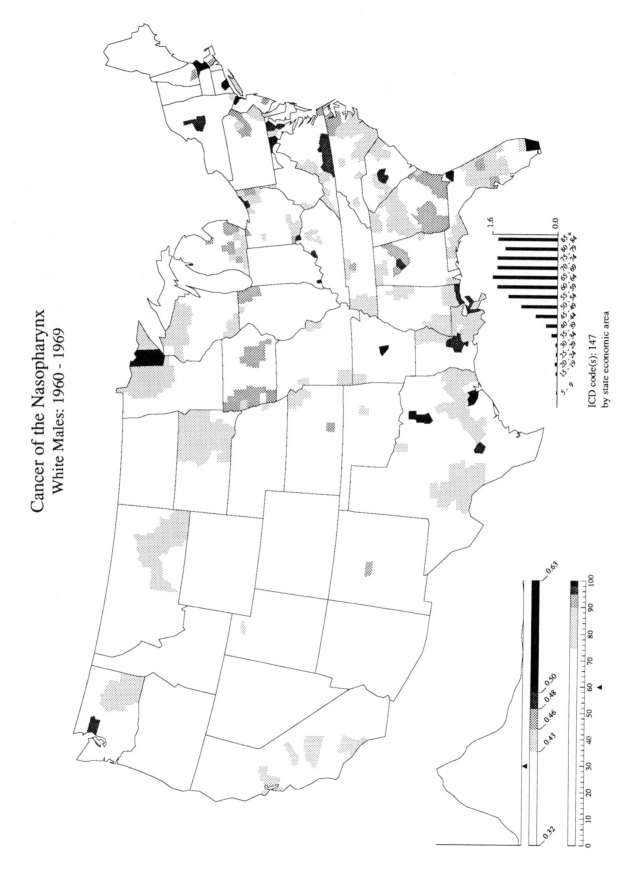

Cancer of the Nasopharynx
White Males: 1960 - 1969

ICD code(s): 147
by state economic area

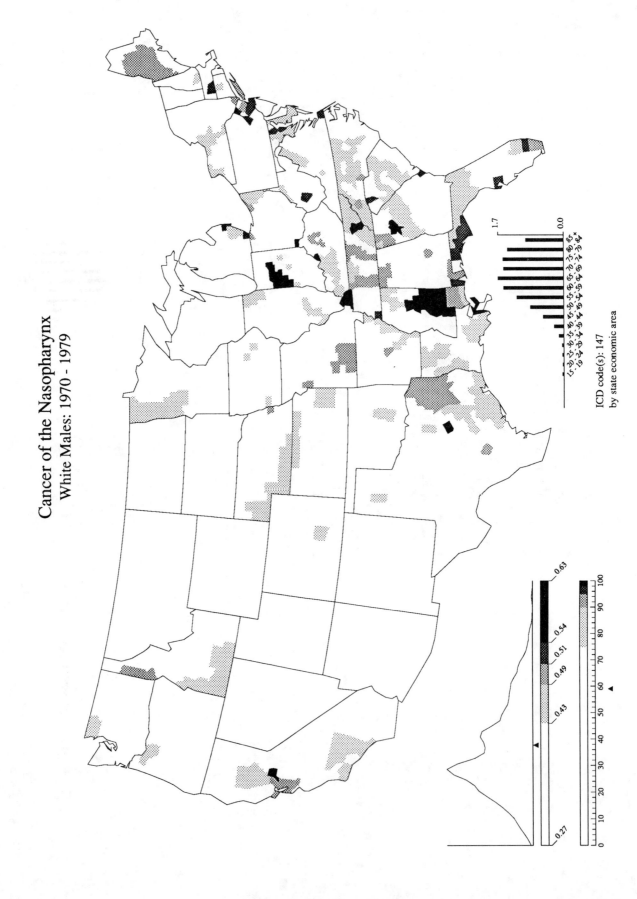

Cancer of the Nasopharynx
White Males: 1970 - 1979

ICD code(s): 147
by state economic area

Cancer of the Nasopharynx
White Males: Relative Change

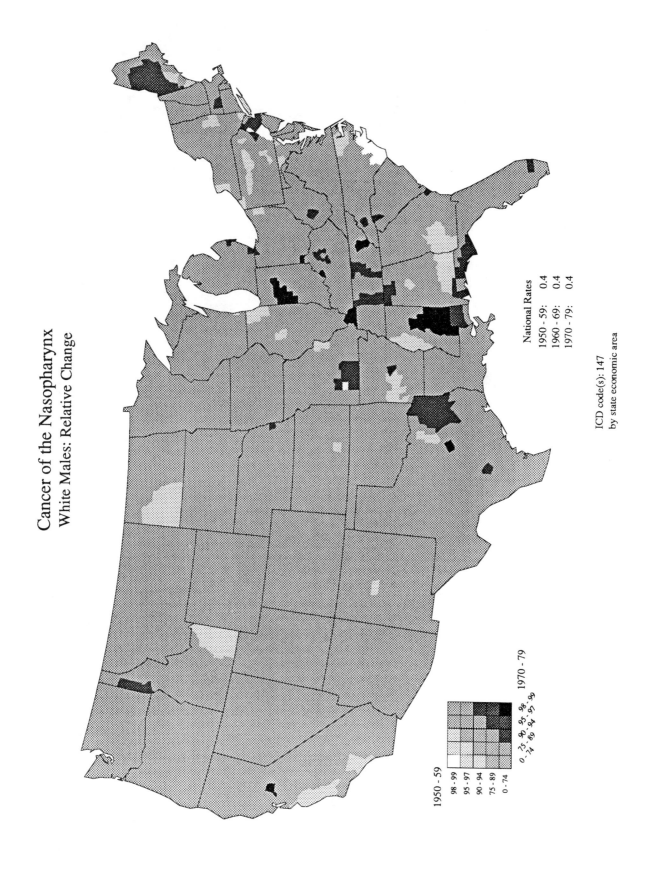

National Rates

1950 - 59:   0.4
1960 - 69:   0.4
1970 - 79:   0.4

ICD code(s): 147
by state economic area

1950 - 59

98 - 99
95 - 97
90 - 94
75 - 89
0 - 74

0 - 75 - 90 - 95 - 98 - 99
74 - 89 - 94 - 97 - 99

1970 - 79

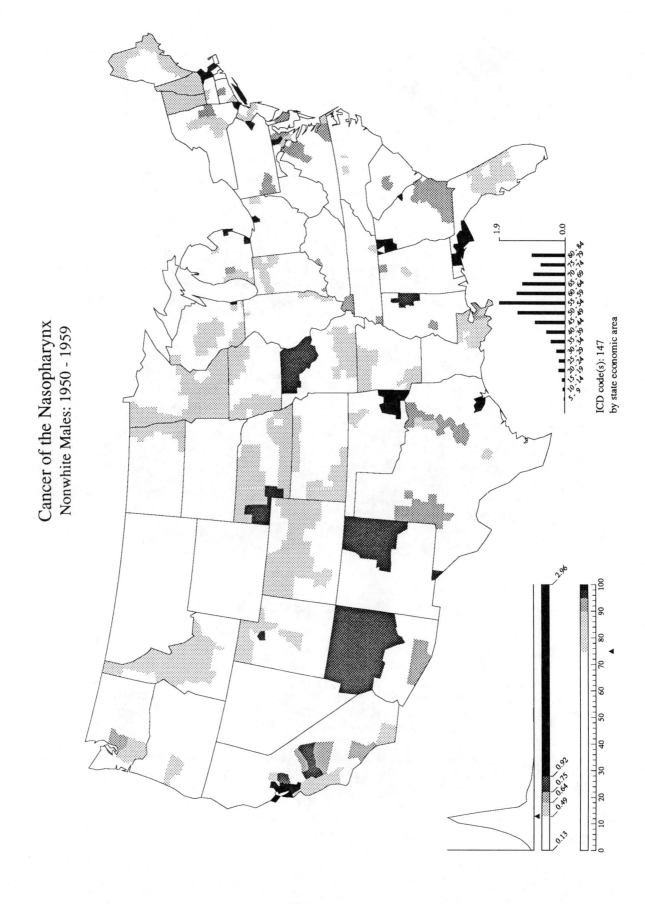

Cancer of the Nasopharynx
Nonwhite Males: 1950 - 1959

ICD code(s): 147
by state economic area

Cancer of the Nasopharynx
Nonwhite Males: 1960 - 1969

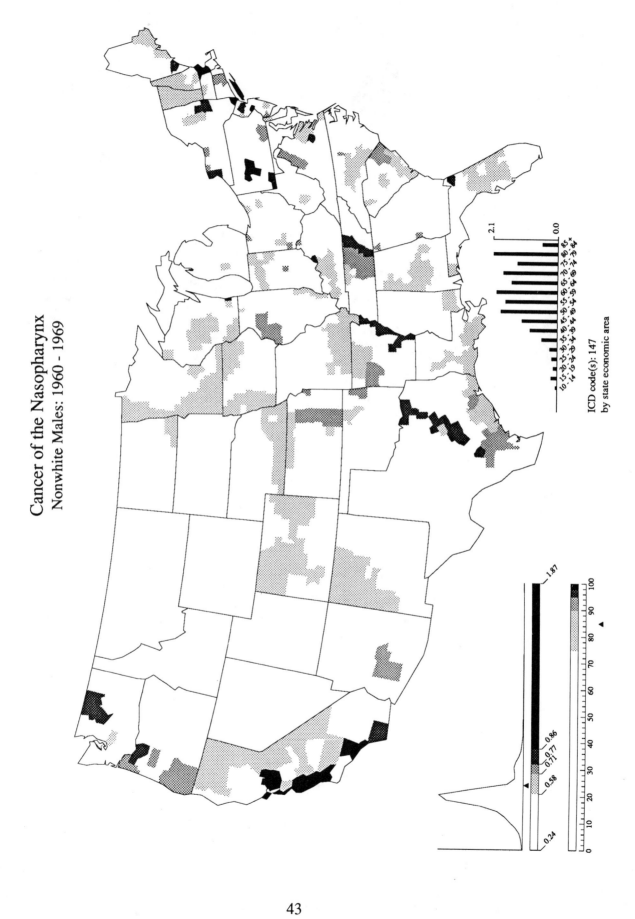

ICD code(s): 147
by state economic area

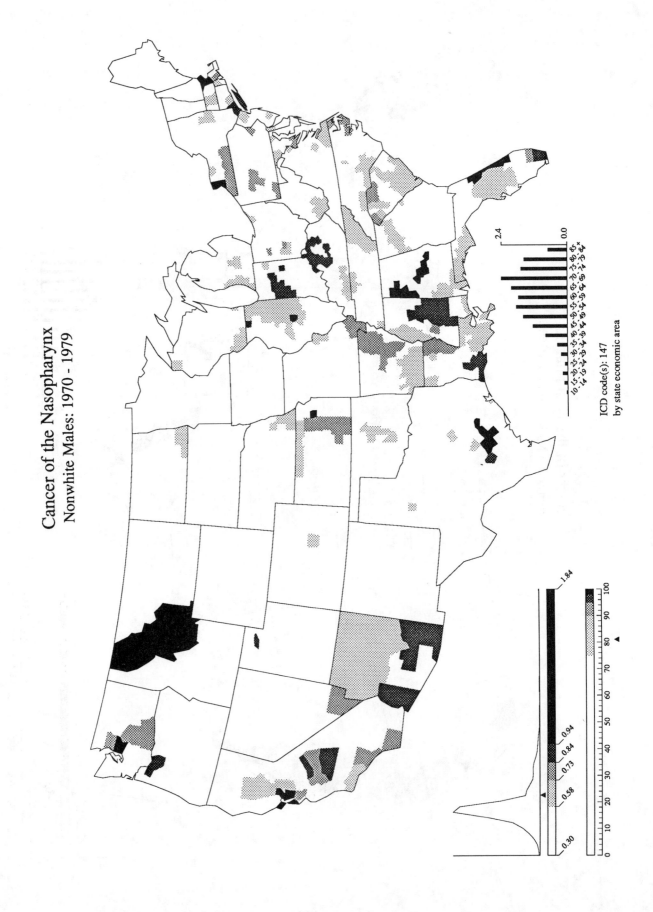

Cancer of the Nasopharynx
Nonwhite Males: 1970 - 1979

ICD code(s): 147
by state economic area

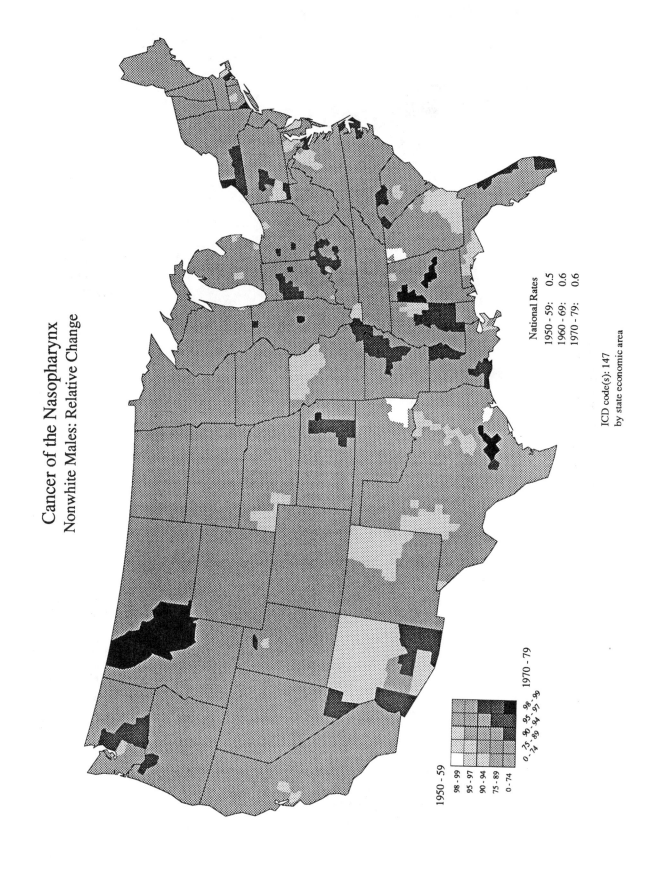

Cancer of the Nasopharynx
Nonwhite Males: Relative Change

National Rates

1950 - 59:	0.5
1960 - 69:	0.6
1970 - 79:	0.6

ICD code(s): 147
by state economic area

1950 - 59

98 - 99
95 - 97
90 - 94
75 - 89
0 - 74

1970 - 79

0 - 74 75 - 89 90 - 94 95 - 97 98 - 99

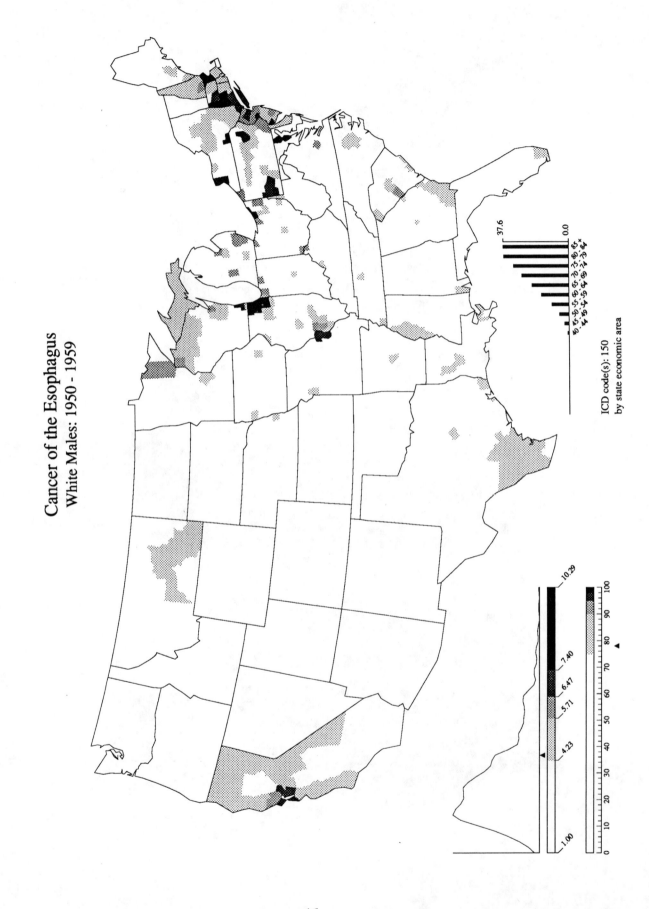

Cancer of the Esophagus
White Males: 1950 - 1959

ICD code(s): 150
by state economic area

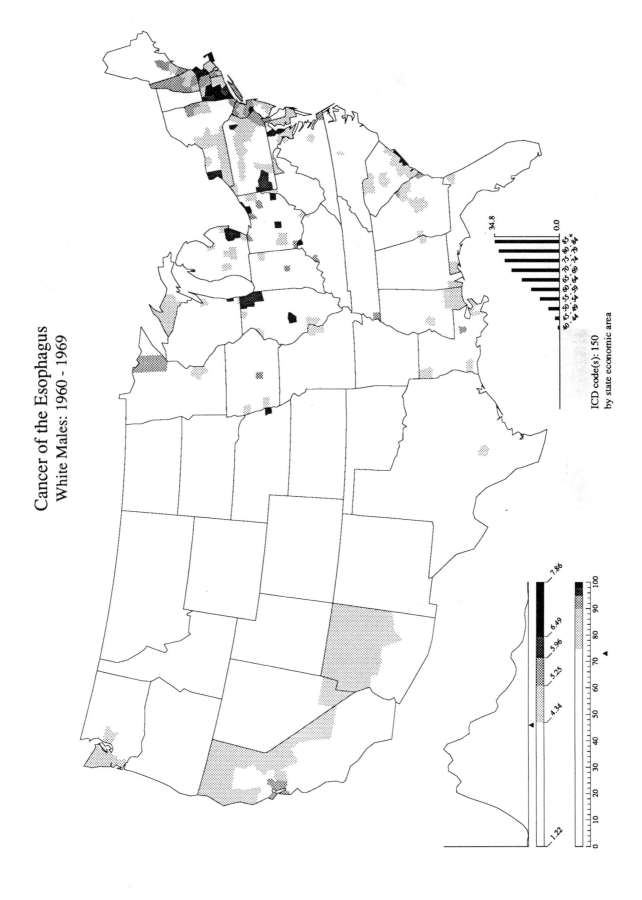

Cancer of the Esophagus
White Males: 1960 - 1969

ICD code(s): 150
by state economic area

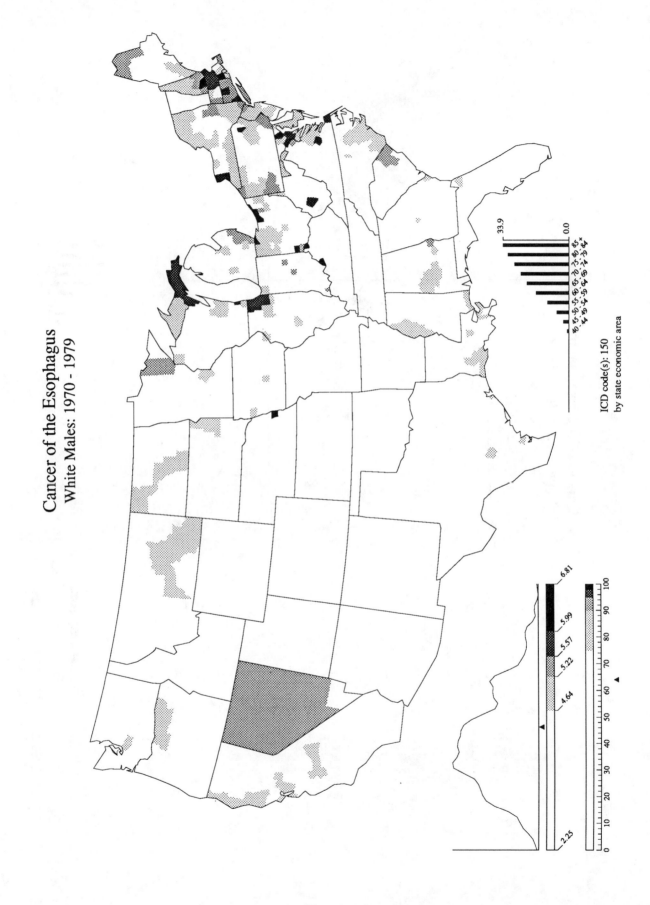

Cancer of the Esophagus
White Males: 1970 - 1979

ICD code(s): 150
by state economic area

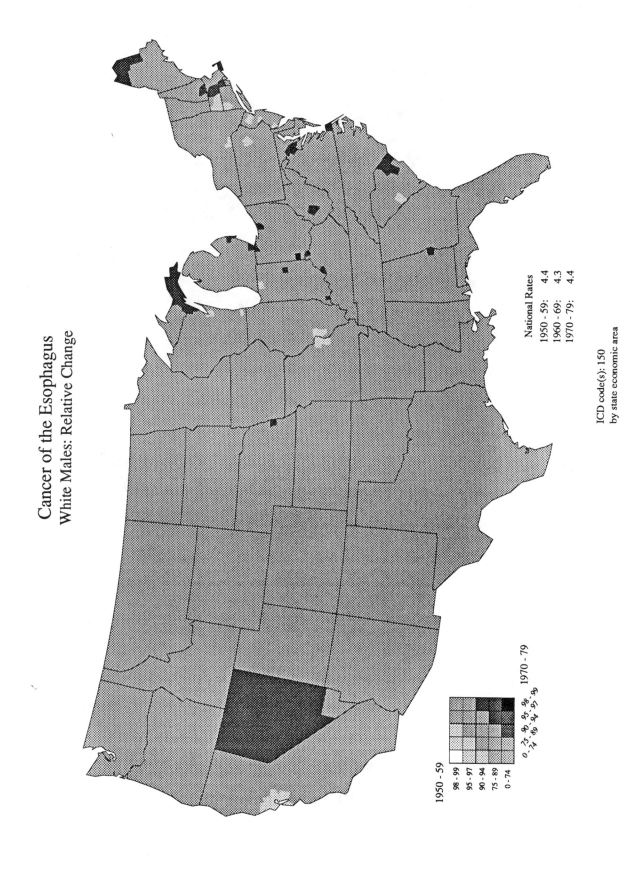

Cancer of the Esophagus
White Males: Relative Change

National Rates

1950 - 59:	4.4
1960 - 69:	4.3
1970 - 79:	4.4

ICD code(s): 150
by state economic area

1950 - 59

98 - 99
95 - 97
90 - 94
75 - 89
0 - 74

1970 - 79
0 - 74 75 - 89 90 - 94 95 - 97 98 - 99

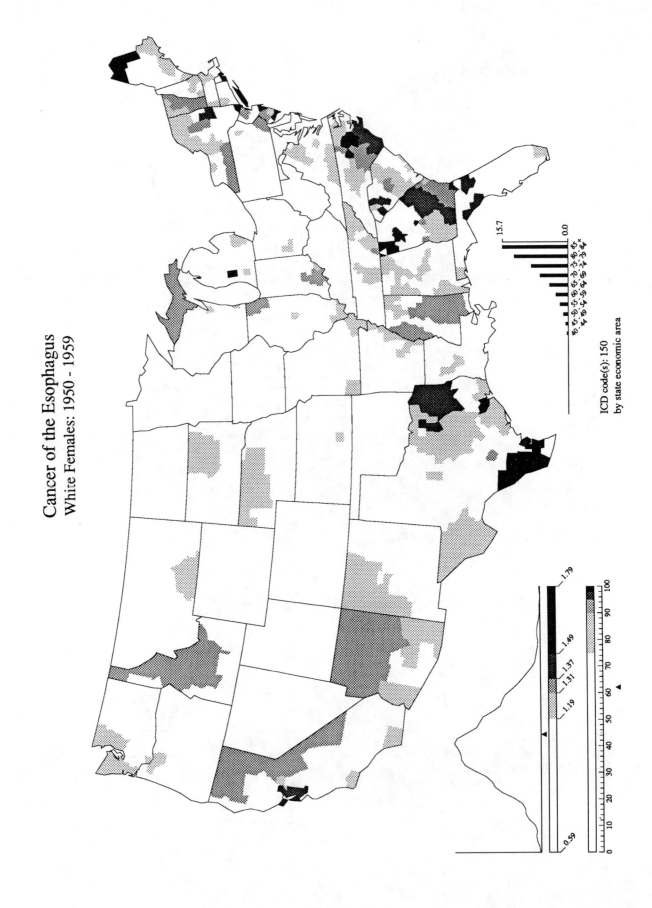

Cancer of the Esophagus
White Females: 1950 - 1959

ICD code(s): 150
by state economic area

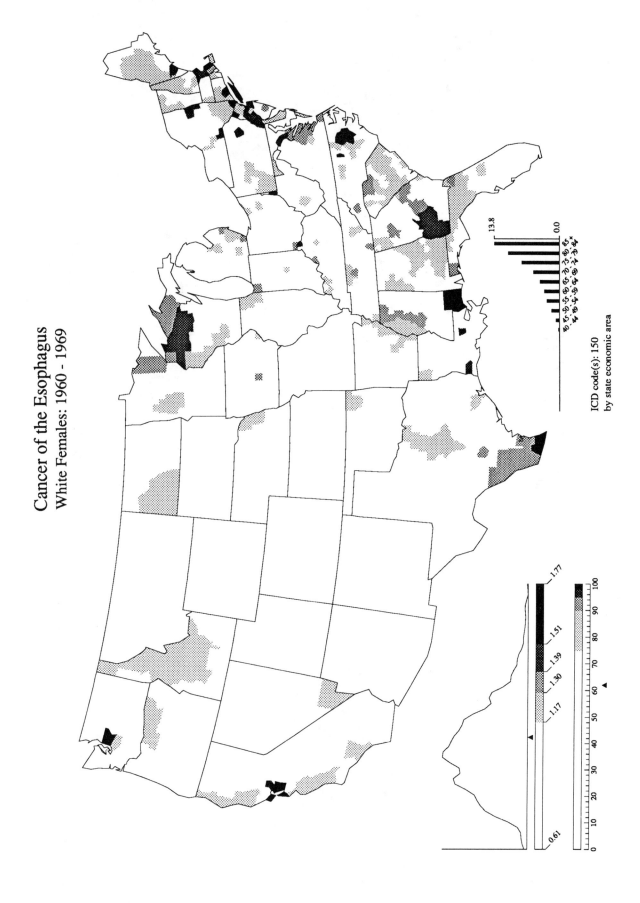

Cancer of the Esophagus
White Females: 1960 - 1969

ICD code(s): 150
by state economic area

51

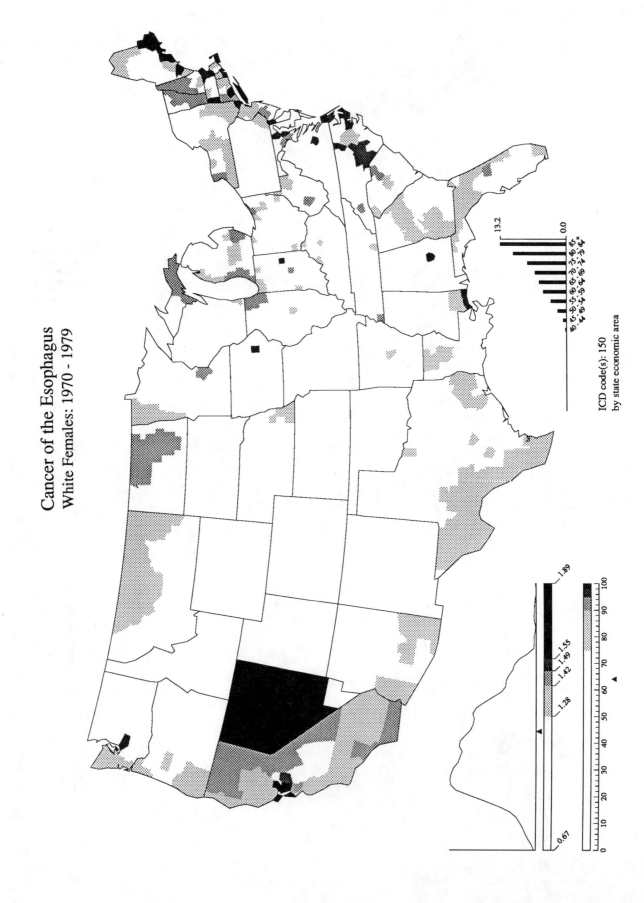

Cancer of the Esophagus
White Females: 1970 - 1979

ICD code(s): 150
by state economic area

Cancer of the Esophagus
White Females: Relative Change

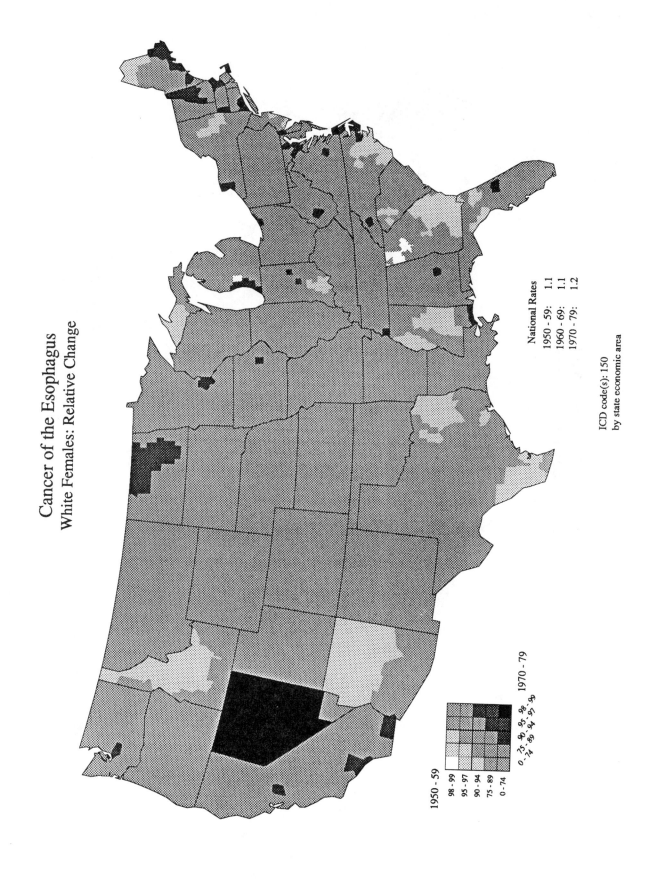

National Rates

1950 - 59:   1.1
1960 - 69:   1.1
1970 - 79:   1.2

ICD code(s): 150
by state economic area

1950 - 59
98 - 99
95 - 97
90 - 94
75 - 89
0 - 74

1970 - 79
0 - 74 75 - 89 90 - 94 95 - 97 98 - 99

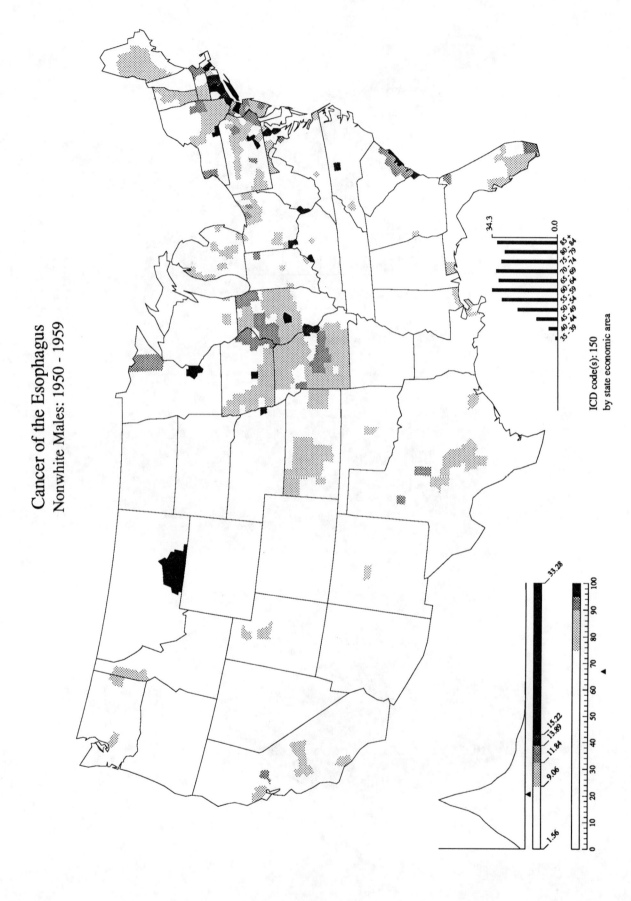

Cancer of the Esophagus
Nonwhite Males: 1950 - 1959

ICD code(s): 150
by state economic area

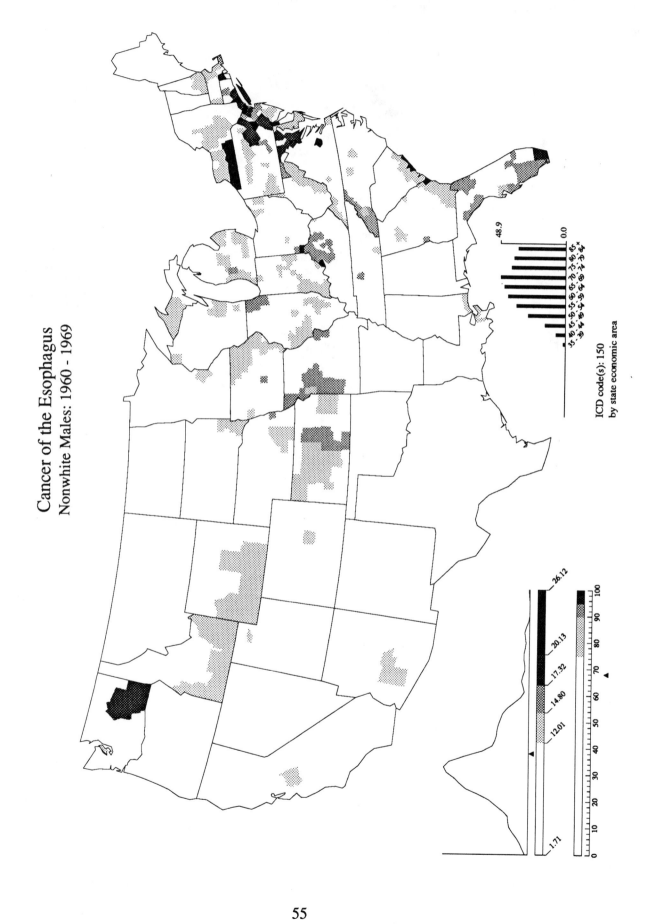

Cancer of the Esophagus
Nonwhite Males: 1960 - 1969

ICD code(s): 150
by state economic area

55

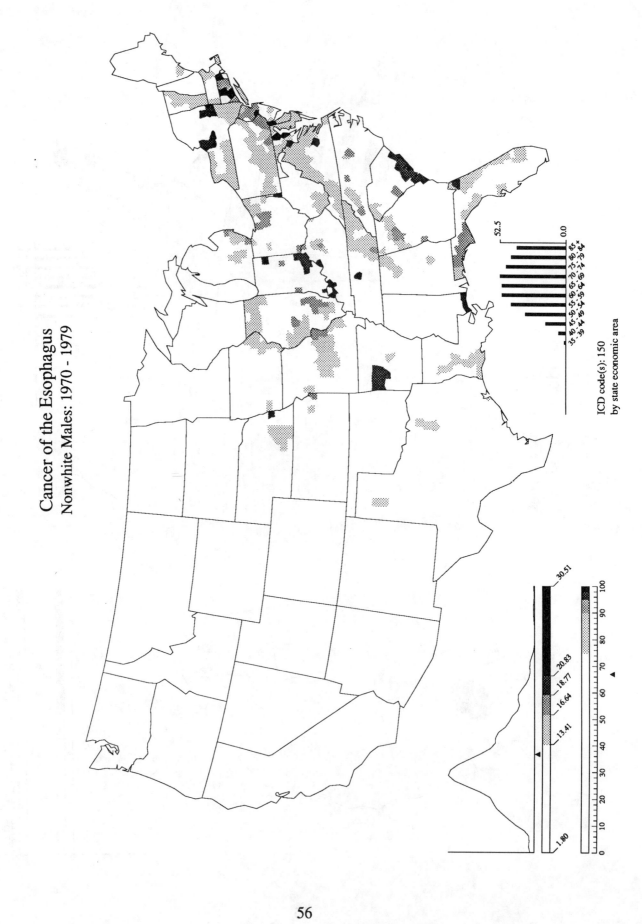

Cancer of the Esophagus
Nonwhite Males: 1970 - 1979

ICD code(s): 150
by state economic area

52.5

0.0

85-
80-84
75-79
70-74
65-69
60-64
55-59
50-54
45-49
40-44
35-39

30.51

20.83
18.77
16.64
13.41

1.80

0 10 20 30 40 50 60 70 80 90 100

Cancer of the Esophagus
Nonwhite Males: Relative Change

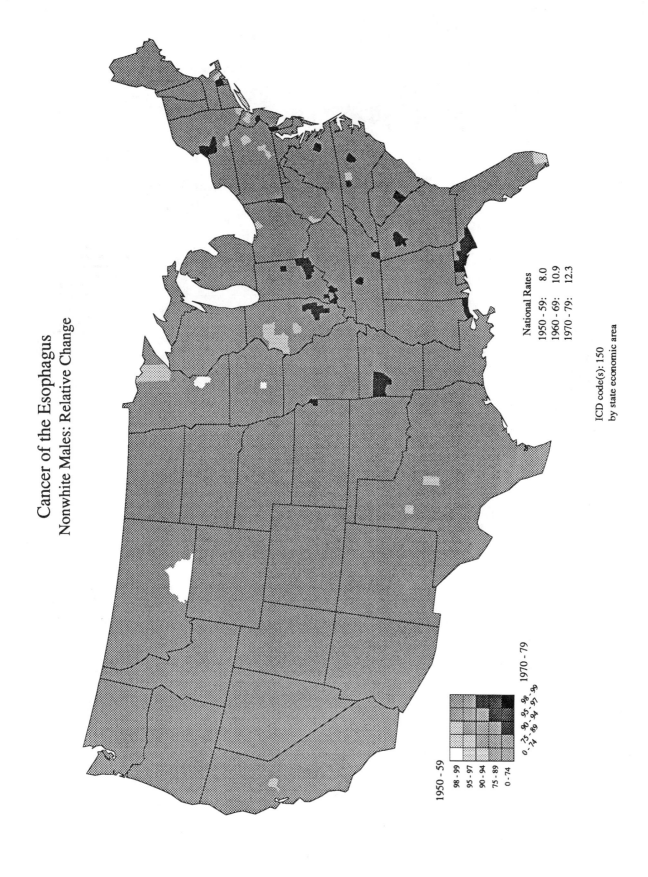

National Rates

1950 - 59:   8.0
1960 - 69:   10.9
1970 - 79:   12.3

ICD code(s): 150
by state economic area

1950 - 59

98 - 99
95 - 97
90 - 94
75 - 89
0 - 74

0 - 74 89 94 97 99 99
        75 90 95 98 99   1970 - 79

Cancer of the Esophagus
Nonwhite Females: 1950 - 1959

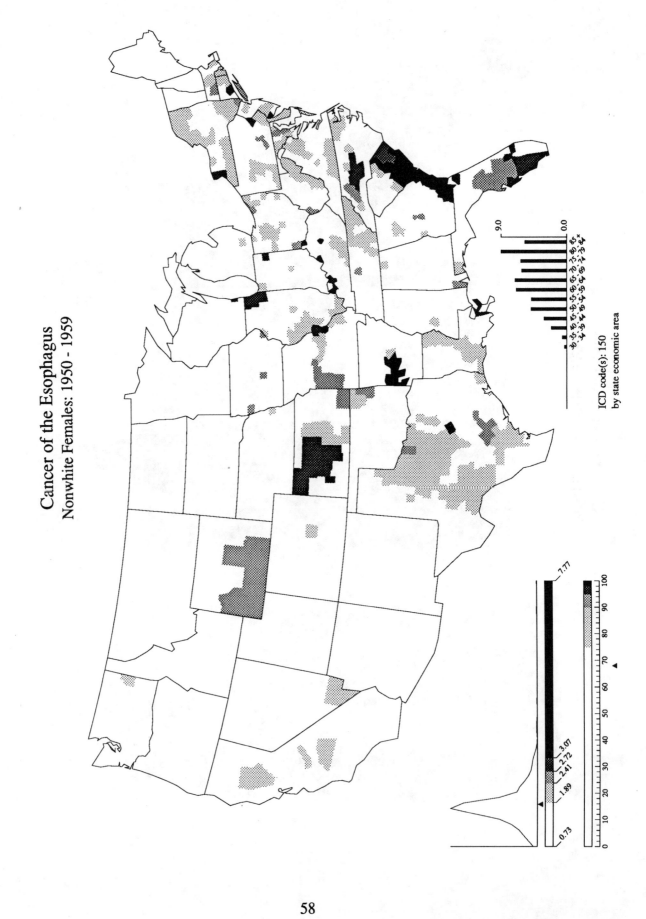

ICD code(s): 150
by state economic area

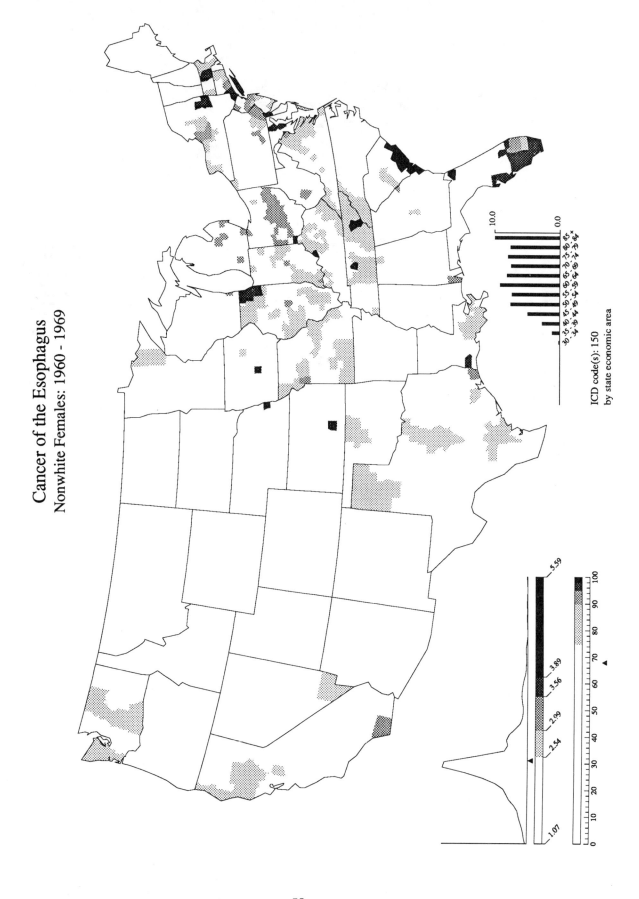

Cancer of the Esophagus
Nonwhite Females: 1960 - 1969

ICD code(s): 150
by state economic area

59

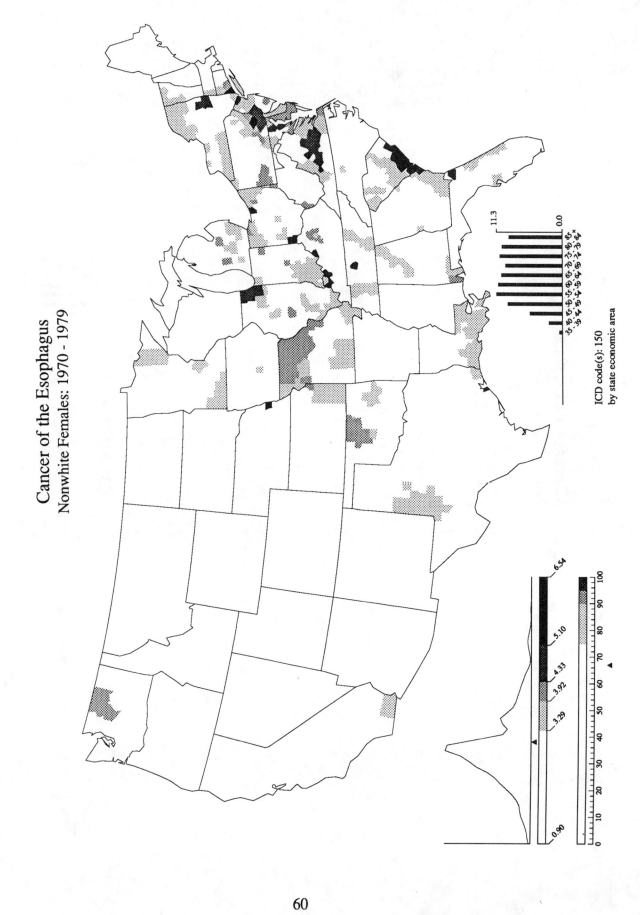

Cancer of the Esophagus
Nonwhite Females: 1970 - 1979

ICD code(s): 150
by state economic area

60

Cancer of the Esophagus
Nonwhite Females: Relative Change

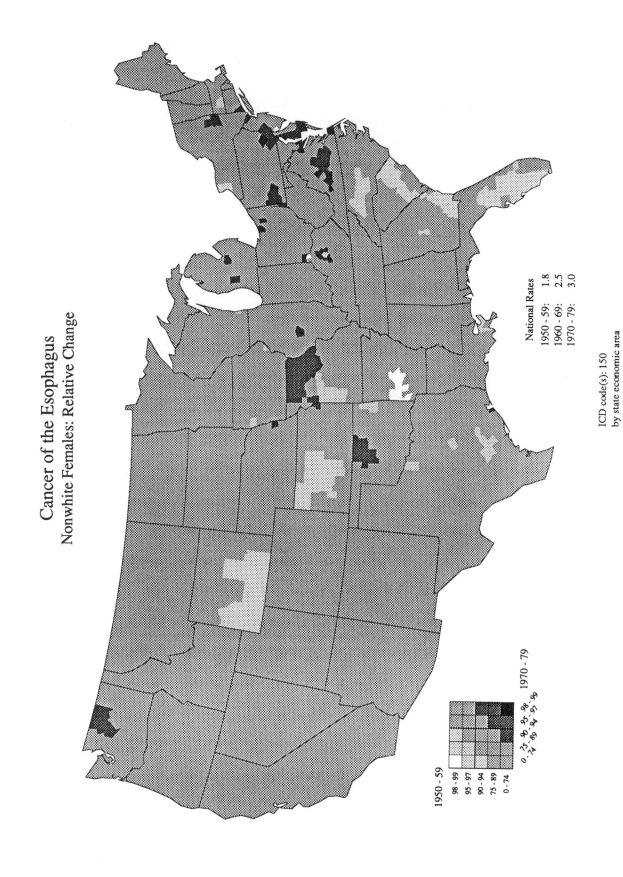

National Rates

1950 - 59:	1.8
1960 - 69:	2.5
1970 - 79:	3.0

ICD code(s): 150
by state economic area

1950 - 59
98 - 99
95 - 97
90 - 94
75 - 89
0 - 74

1970 - 79
0 - 74 89 94 97 99
75 90 95 98

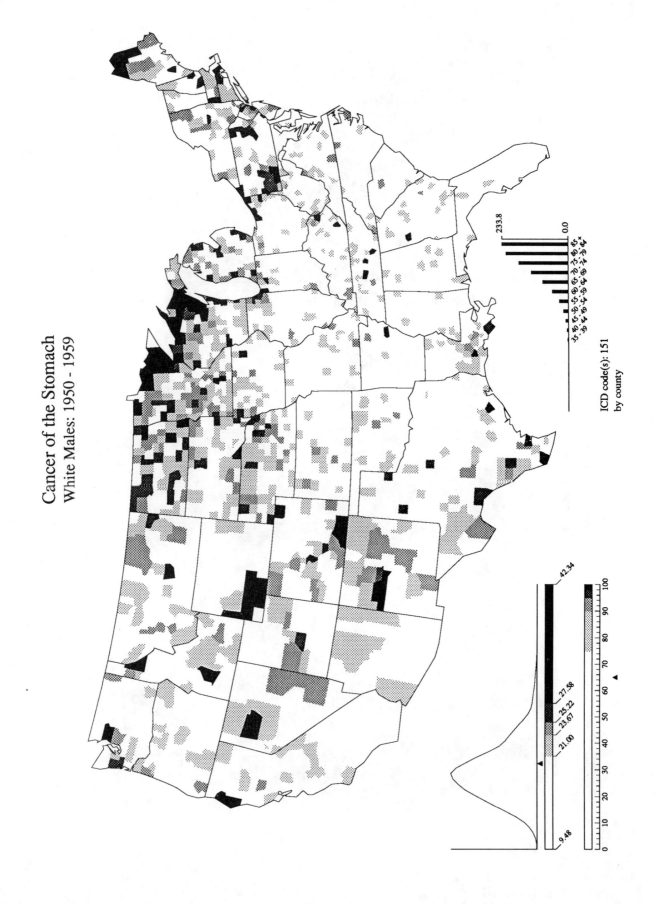

Cancer of the Stomach
White Males: 1950 - 1959

ICD code(s): 151
by county

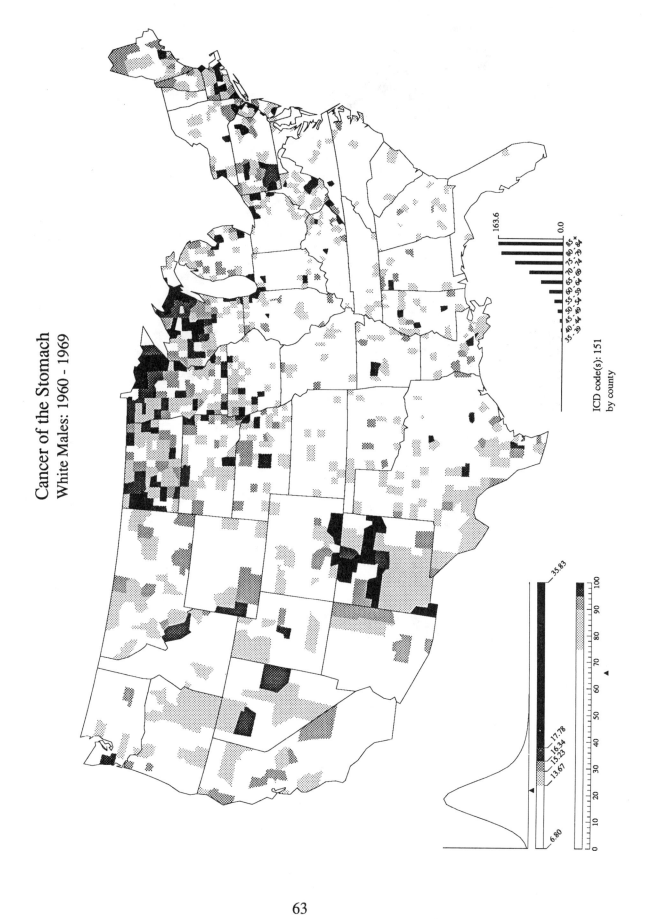

Cancer of the Stomach
White Males: 1960 - 1969

163.6

0.0

85
80
75
70
65
60
55
50
45
40
84+
79
74
69
64
59
54
49
44
39

ICD code(s): 151
by county

35.83

17.78
16.34
15.23
13.67

6.80

0 10 20 30 40 50 60 70 80 90 100

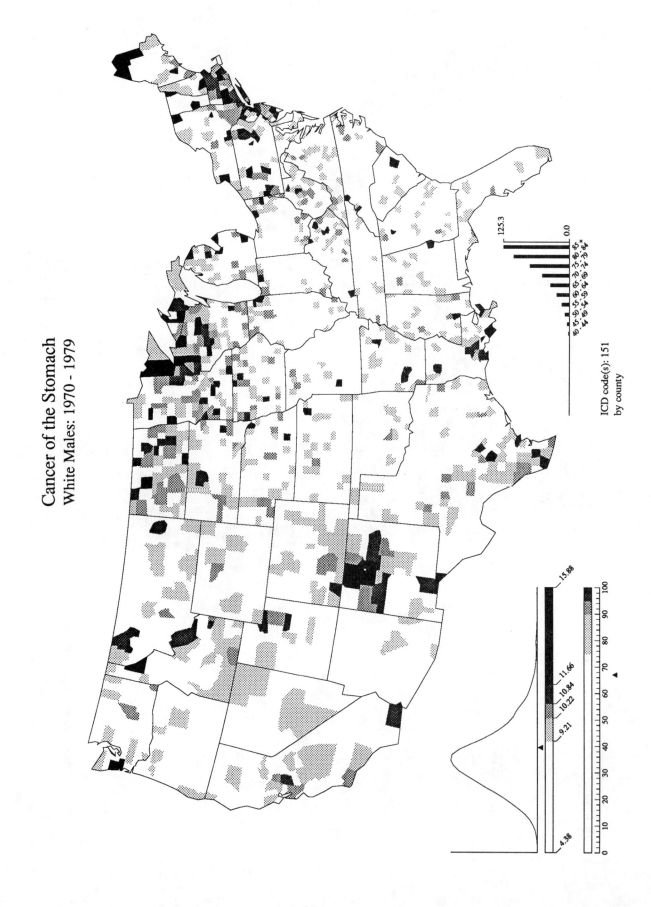

Cancer of the Stomach
White Males: 1970 - 1979

ICD code(s): 151
by county

Cancer of the Stomach
White Males: Relative Change

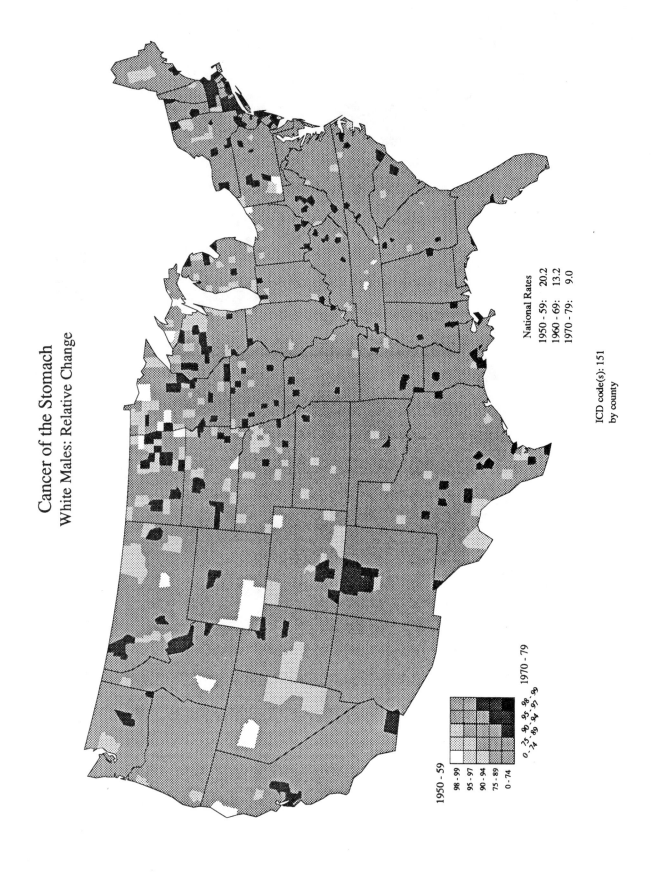

National Rates

1950 - 59: 20.2
1960 - 69: 13.2
1970 - 79:   9.0

ICD code(s): 151
by county

1950 - 59

98 - 99
95 - 97
90 - 94
75 - 89
0 - 74

1970 - 79
0 - 75 - 90 - 95 - 98 - 99
74   89   94   97

65

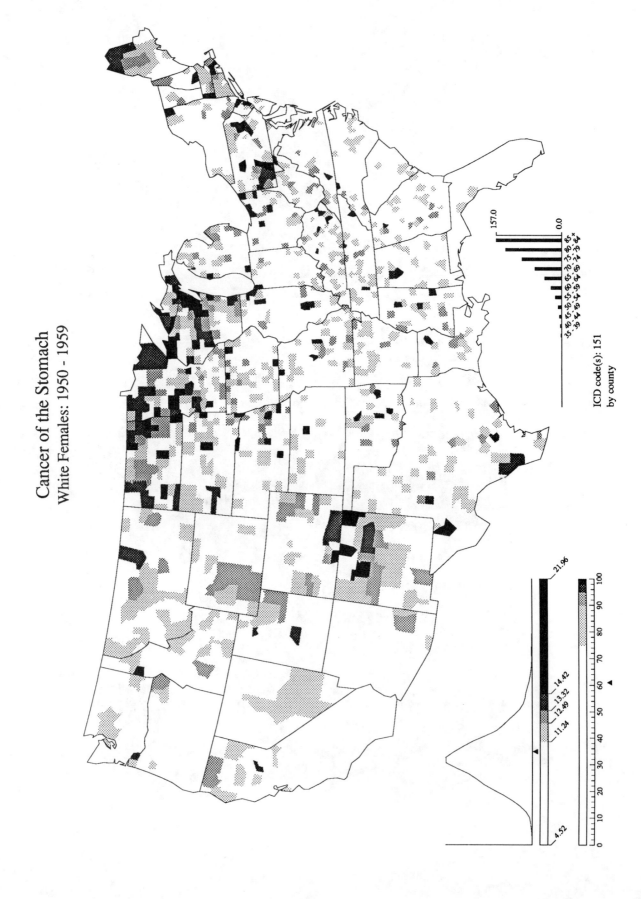

Cancer of the Stomach
White Females: 1950 - 1959

ICD code(s): 151
by county

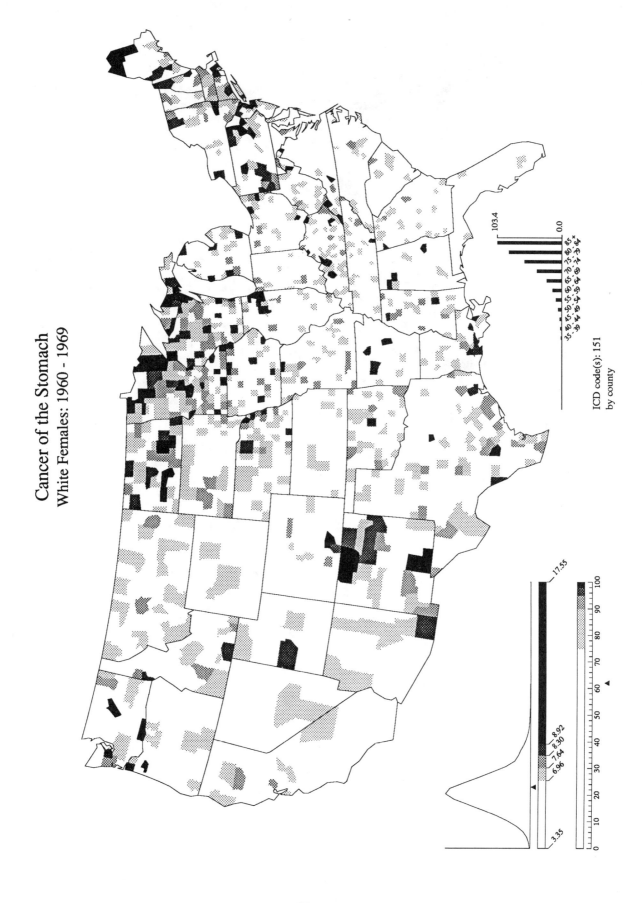

Cancer of the Stomach
White Females: 1960 - 1969

ICD code(s): 151
by county

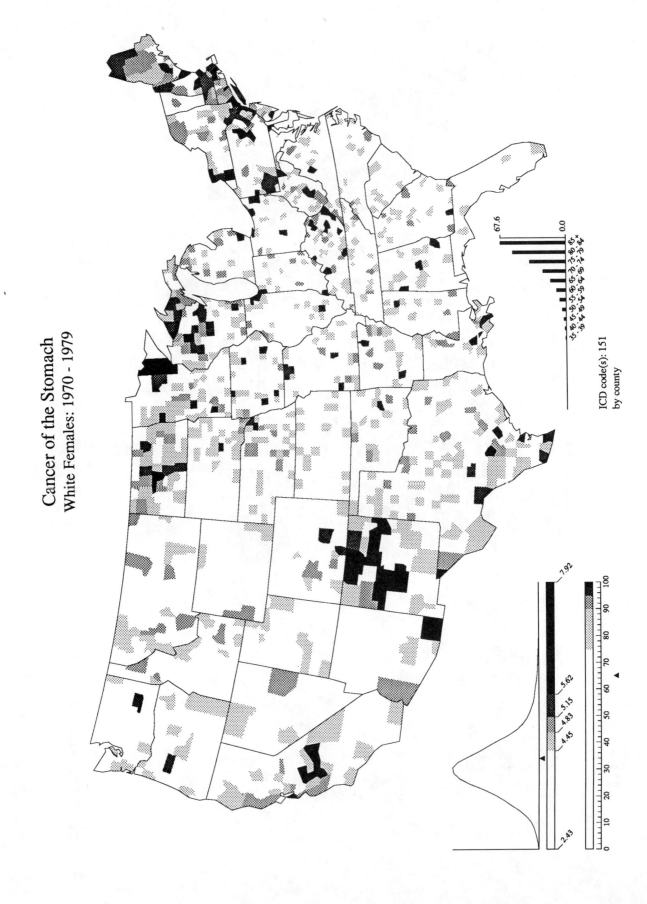

Cancer of the Stomach
White Females: 1970 - 1979

ICD code(s): 151
by county

Cancer of the Stomach
White Females: Relative Change

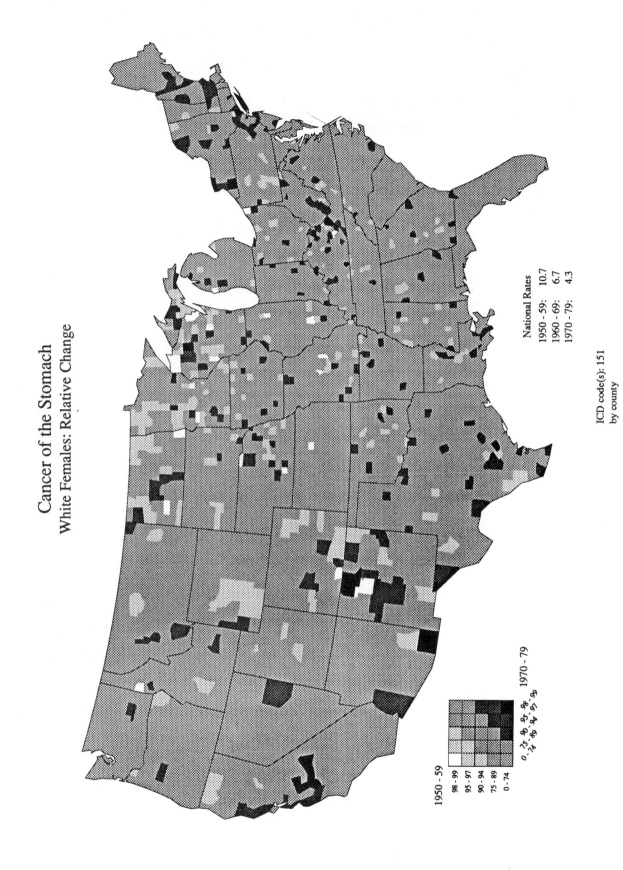

National Rates

1950 - 59: 10.7
1960 - 69:   6.7
1970 - 79:   4.3

ICD code(s): 151
by county

1950 - 59

98 - 99
95 - 97
90 - 94
75 - 89
0 - 74

1970 - 79

0 - 74 75 - 89 90 - 94 95 - 97 98 - 99

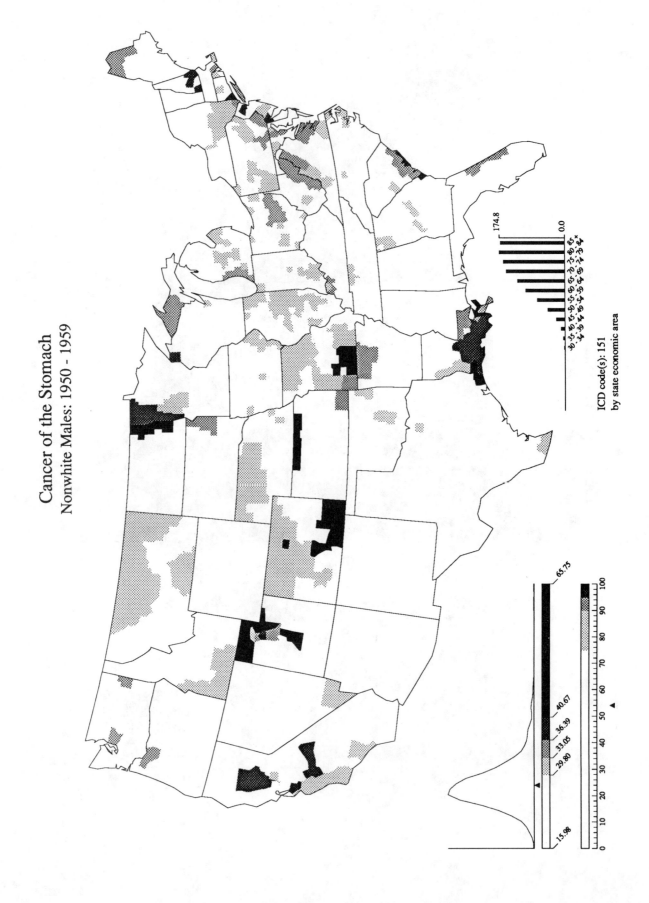

Cancer of the Stomach
Nonwhite Males: 1950 - 1959

ICD code(s): 151
by state economic area

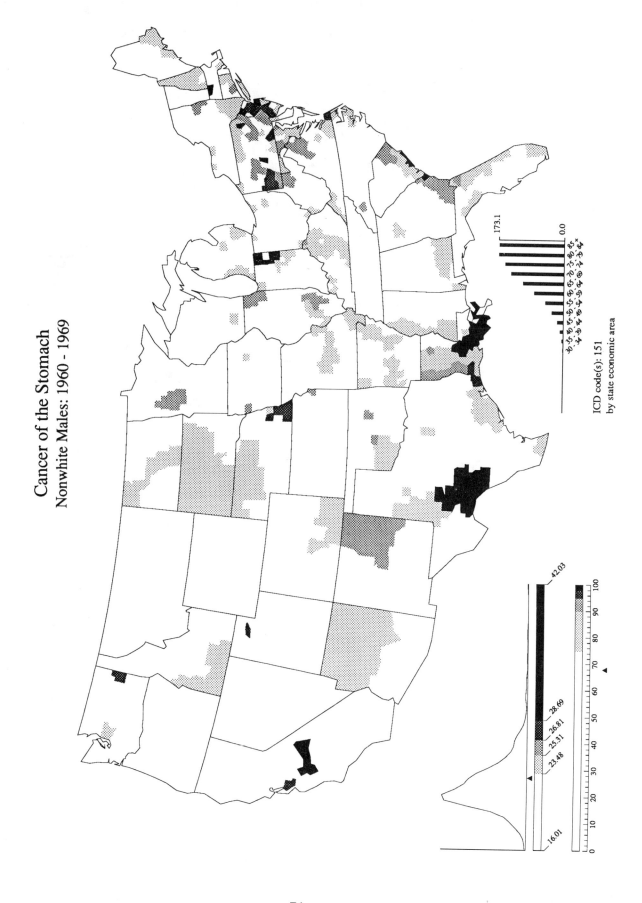

Cancer of the Stomach
Nonwhite Males: 1960 - 1969

ICD code(s): 151
by state economic area

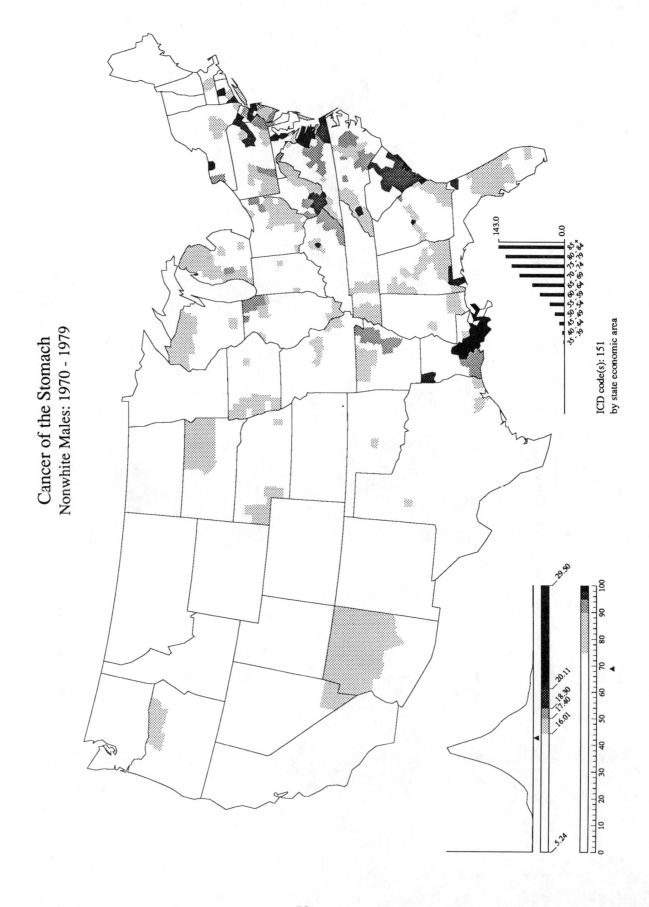

Cancer of the Stomach
Nonwhite Males: 1970 - 1979

ICD code(s): 151
by state economic area

Cancer of the Stomach
Nonwhite Males: Relative Change

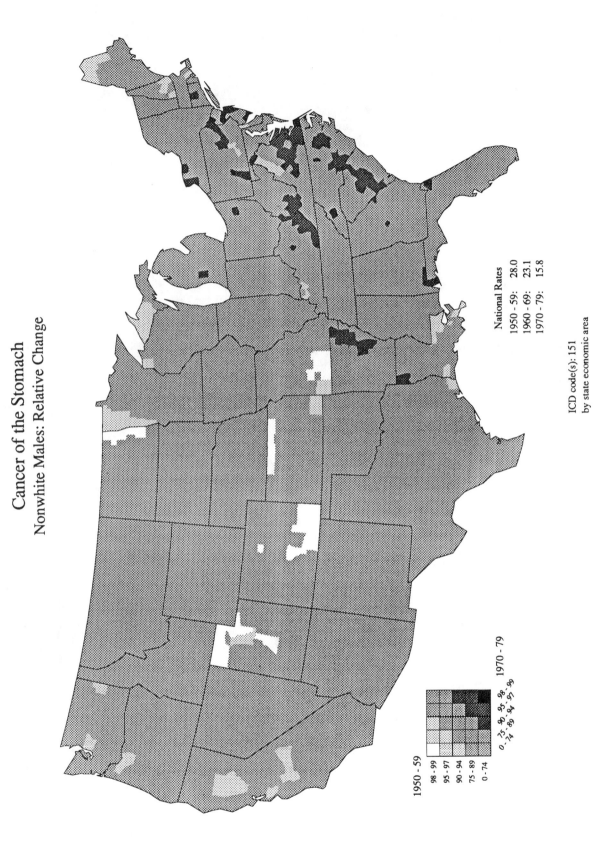

National Rates

1950 - 59:   28.0
1960 - 69:   23.1
1970 - 79:   15.8

ICD code(s): 151
by state economic area

1950 - 59
98 - 99
95 - 97
90 - 94
75 - 89
0 - 74

1970 - 79
0 - 74 75 - 89 90 - 94 95 - 97 98 - 99

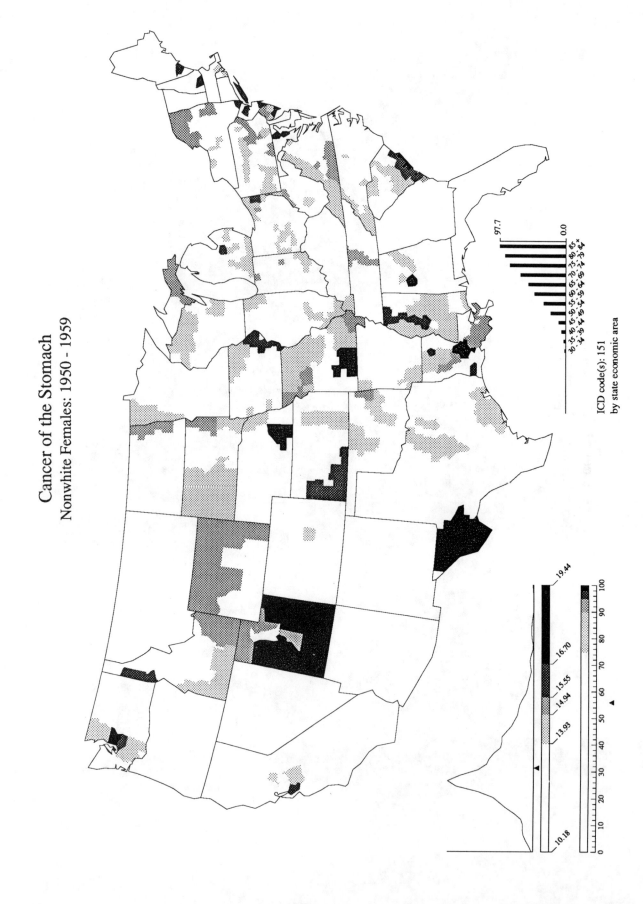

Cancer of the Stomach
Nonwhite Females: 1950 - 1959

ICD code(s): 151
by state economic area

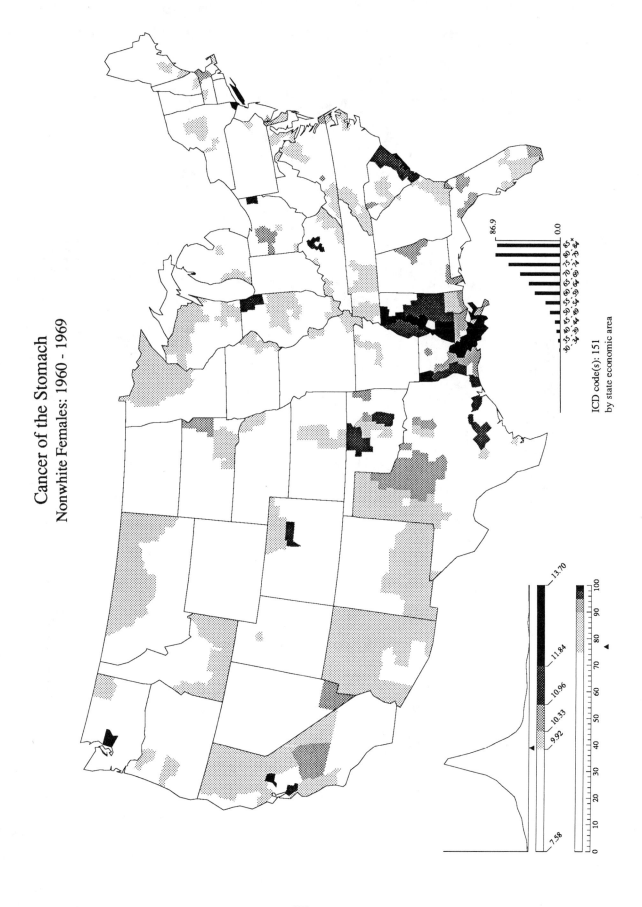

Cancer of the Stomach
Nonwhite Females: 1960 - 1969

ICD code(s): 151
by state economic area

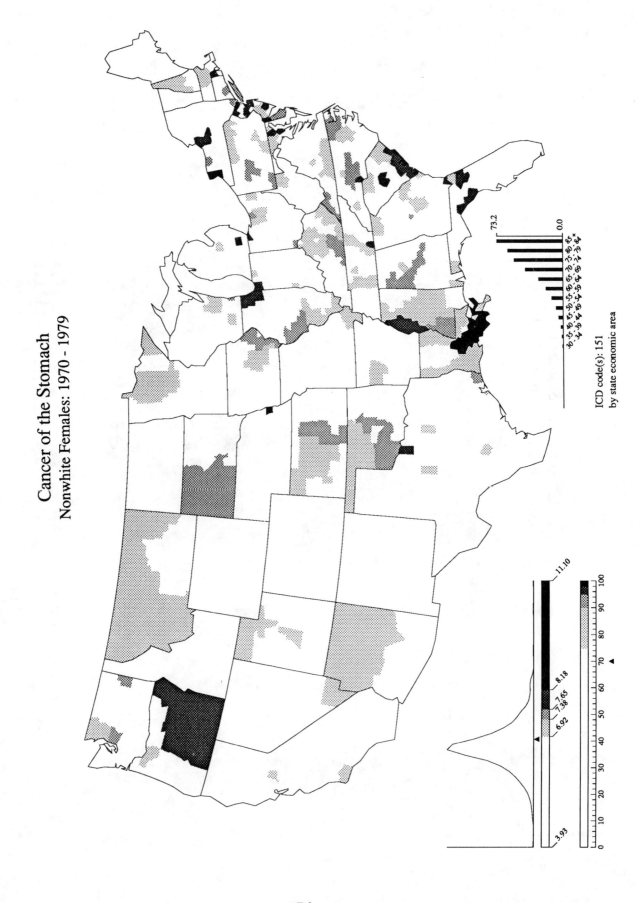

Cancer of the Stomach
Nonwhite Females: 1970 - 1979

ICD code(s): 151
by state economic area

Cancer of the Stomach
Nonwhite Females: Relative Change

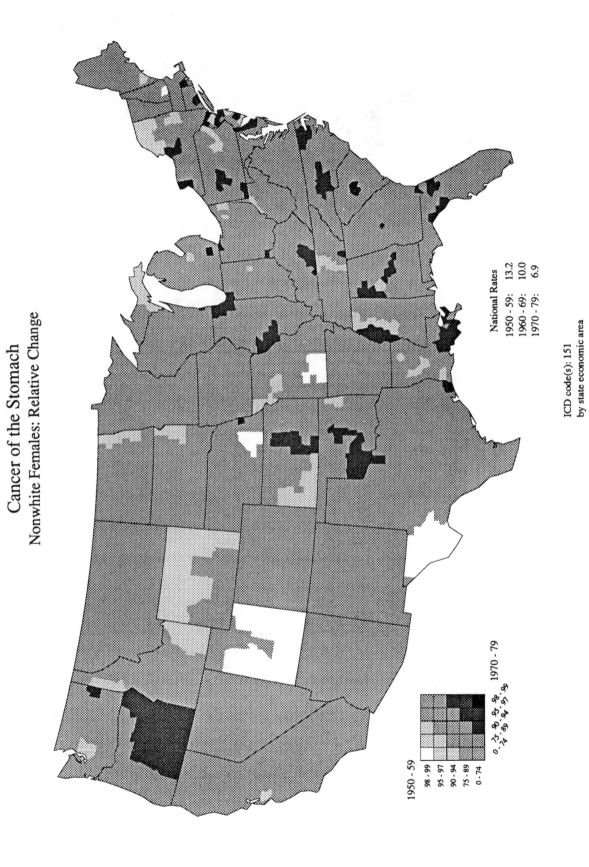

National Rates

1950 - 59: 13.2
1960 - 69: 10.0
1970 - 79:   6.9

ICD code(s): 151
by state economic area

1950 - 59

98 - 99
95 - 97
90 - 94
75 - 89
0 - 74

1970 - 79

0 - 74 75 - 89 90 - 94 95 - 97 98 - 99

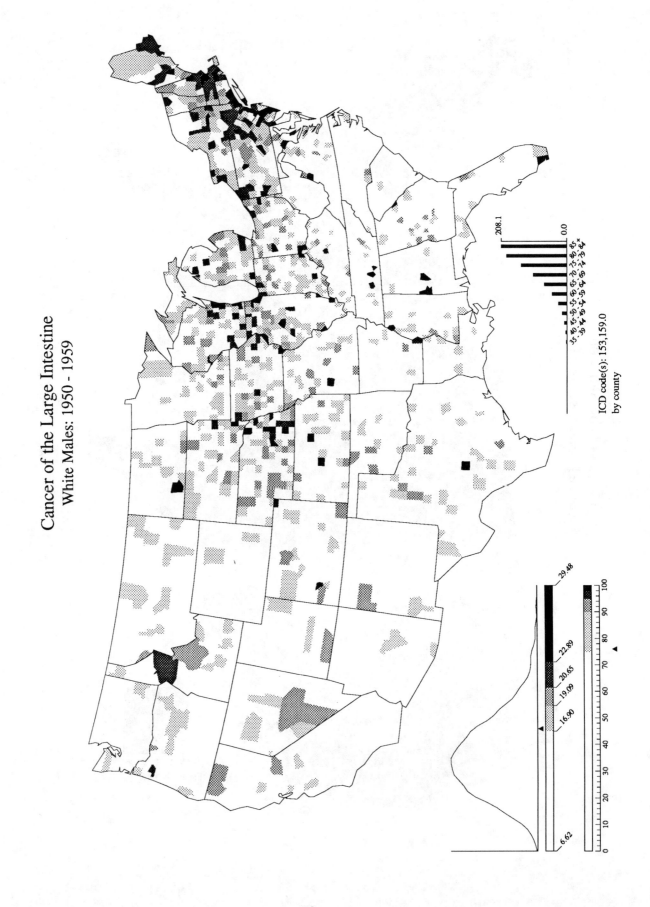

Cancer of the Large Intestine
White Males: 1950 - 1959

ICD code(s): 153,159.0
by county

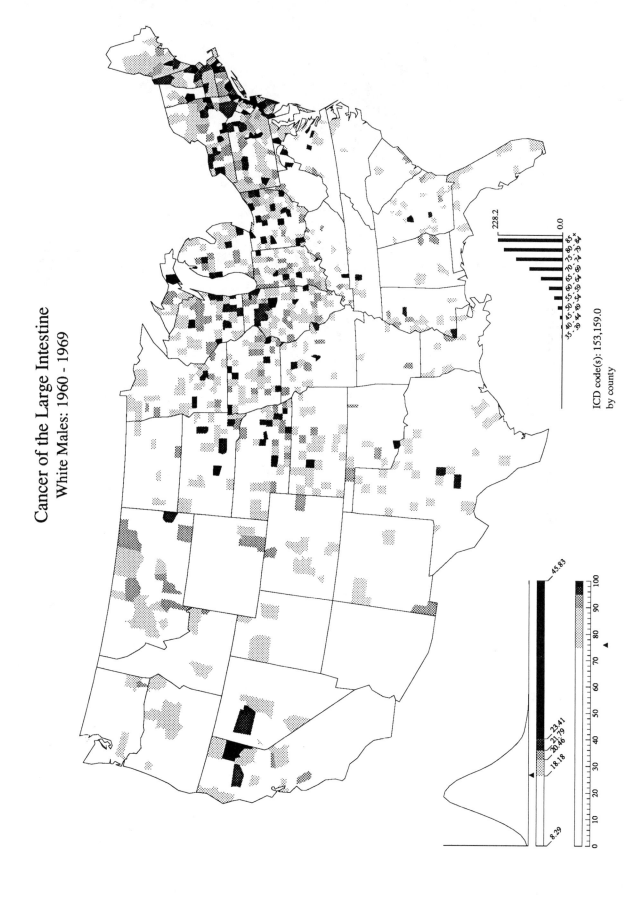

Cancer of the Large Intestine
White Males: 1960 - 1969

ICD code(s): 153,159.0
by county

79

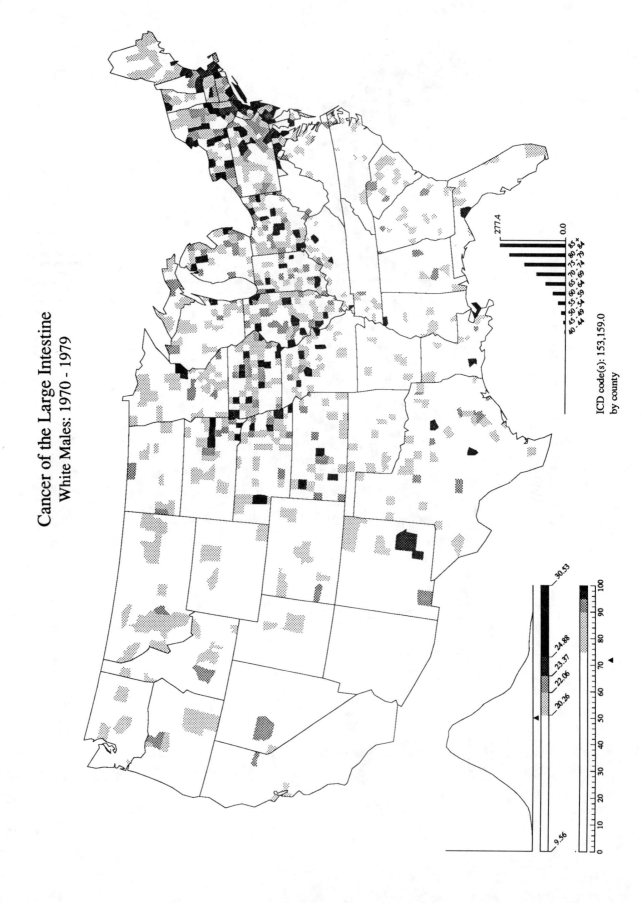

Cancer of the Large Intestine
White Males: 1970 - 1979

ICD code(s): 153,159.0
by county

Cancer of the Large Intestine
White Males: Relative Change

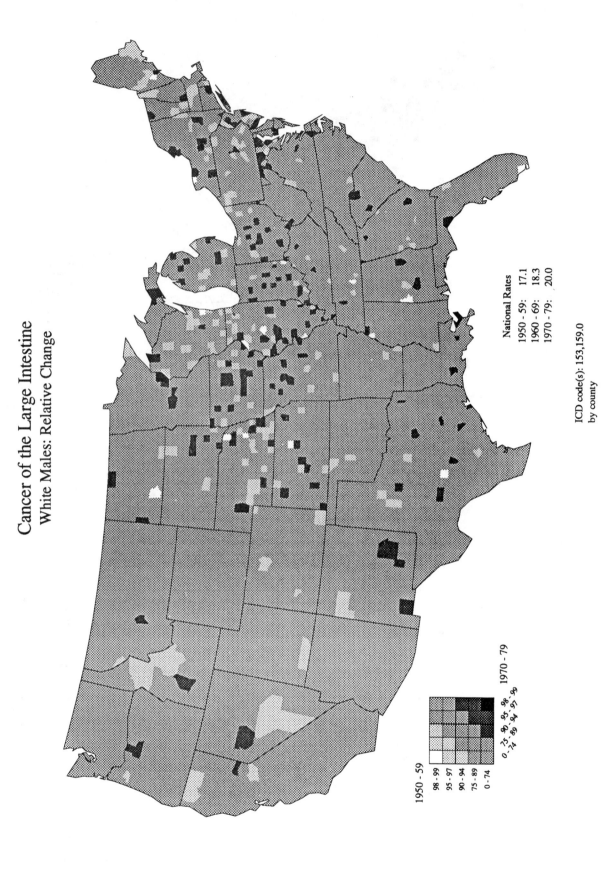

National Rates

1950 - 59: 17.1
1960 - 69: 18.3
1970 - 79: 20.0

ICD code(s): 153,159.0
by county

1950 - 59

98 - 99
95 - 97
90 - 94
75 - 89
0 - 74

0 - 74 75 - 89 90 - 94 95 - 97 98 - 99

1970 - 79

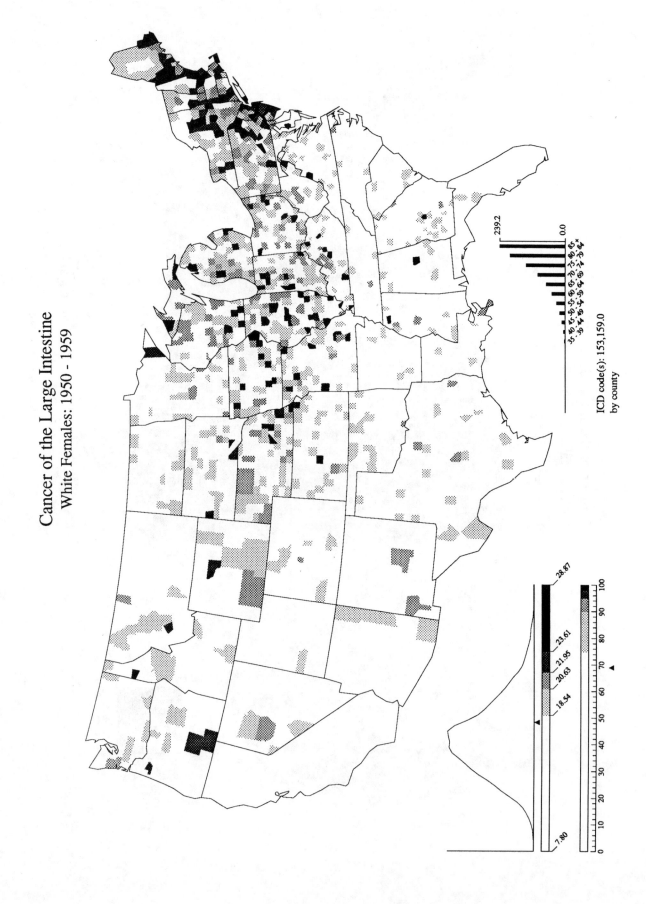

Cancer of the Large Intestine
White Females: 1950 - 1959

ICD code(s): 153,159.0
by county

82

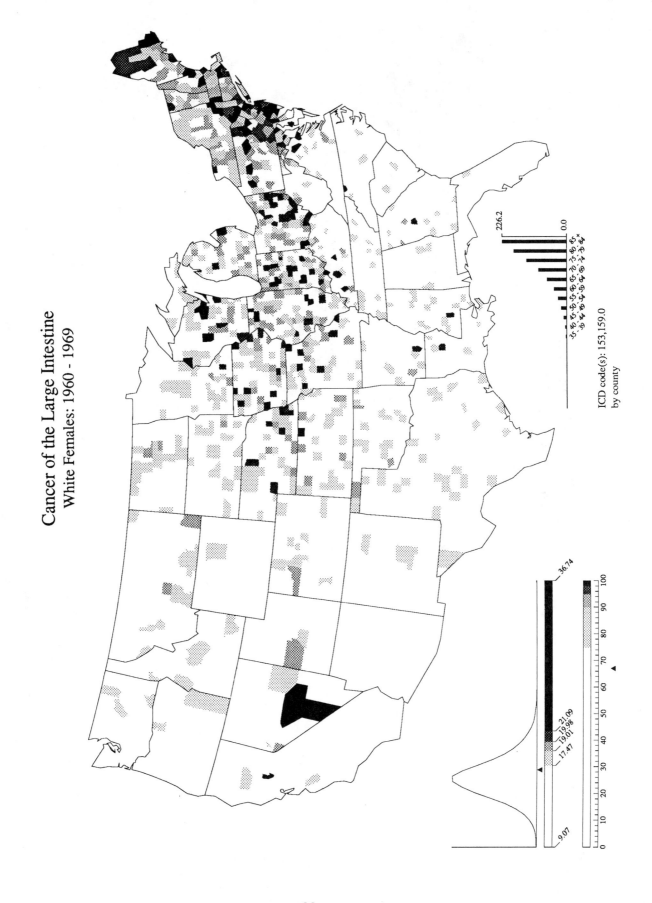

Cancer of the Large Intestine
White Females: 1960 - 1969

ICD code(s): 153,159.0
by county

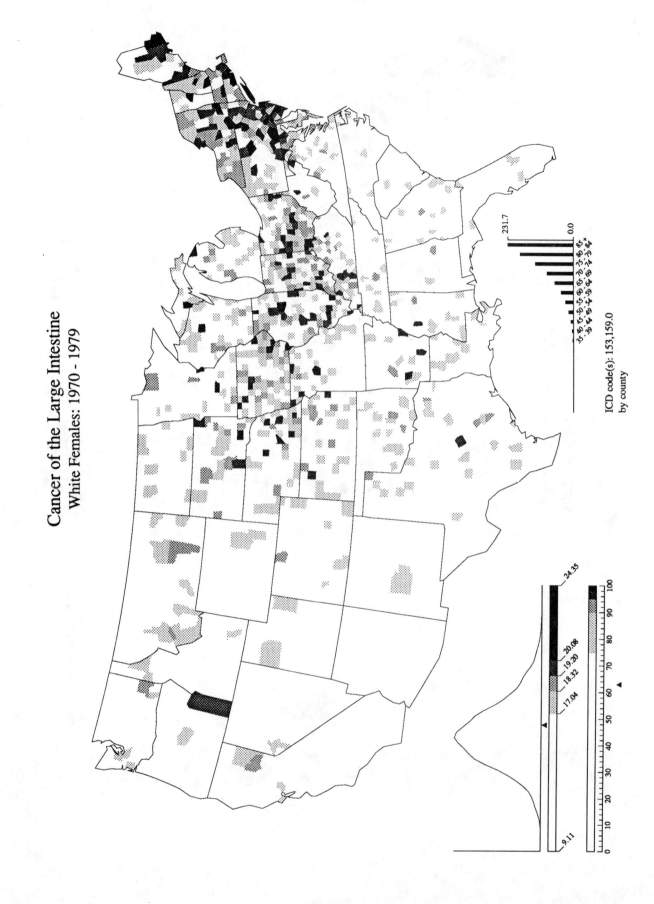

Cancer of the Large Intestine
White Females: 1970 - 1979

ICD code(s): 153,159.0
by county

84

Cancer of the Large Intestine
White Females: Relative Change

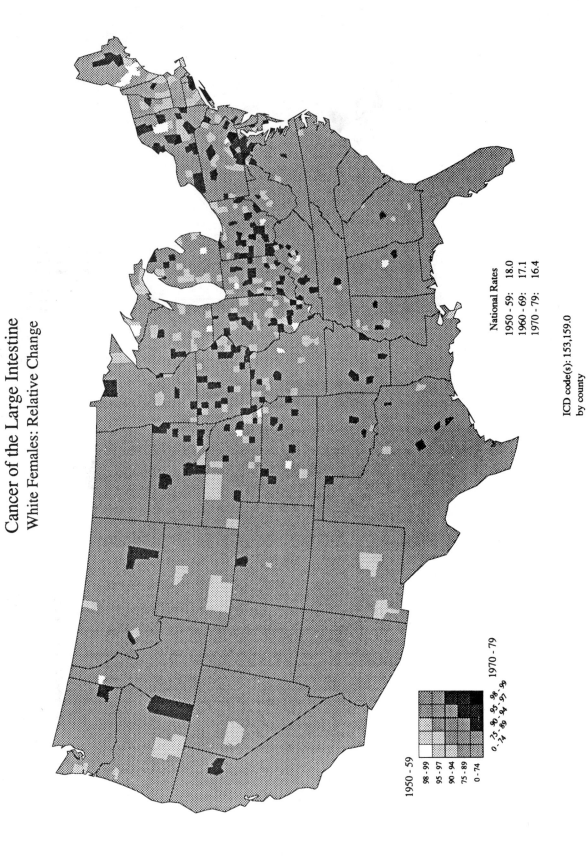

National Rates

1950 - 59: 18.0
1960 - 69: 17.1
1970 - 79: 16.4

ICD code(s): 153,159.0
by county

1950 - 59

98 - 99
95 - 97
90 - 94
75 - 89
0 - 74

0 - 74 89 94 97 99
   75 90 95 98

1970 - 79

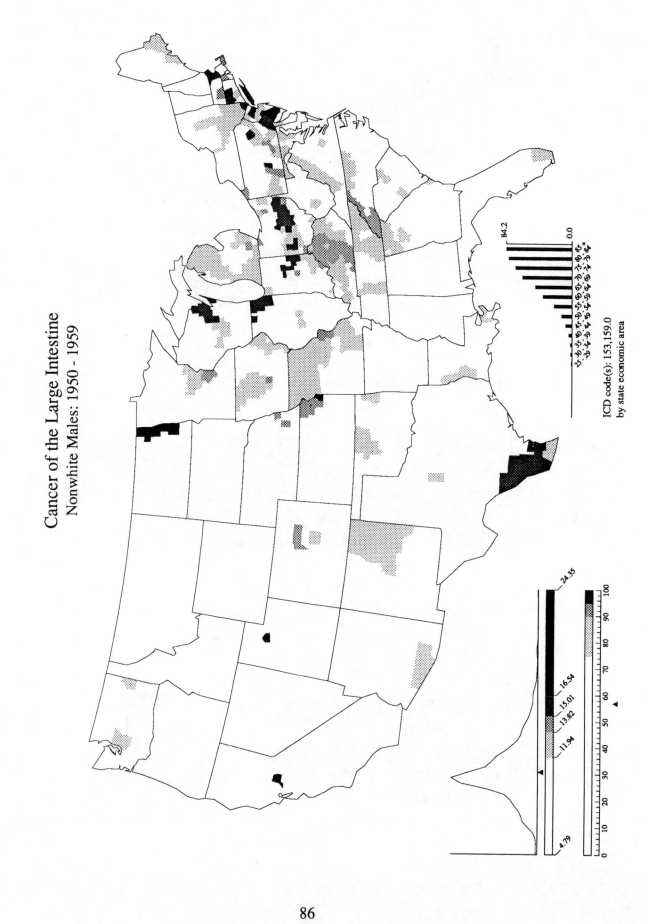

Cancer of the Large Intestine
Nonwhite Males: 1950 - 1959

ICD code(s): 153,159.0
by state economic area

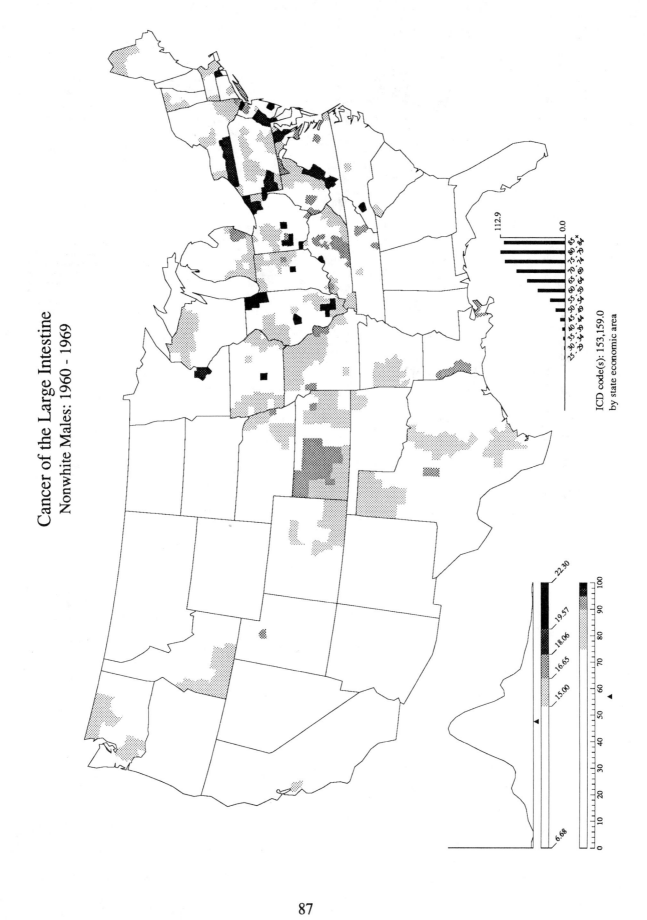

Cancer of the Large Intestine
Nonwhite Males: 1960 - 1969

ICD code(s): 153,159.0
by state economic area

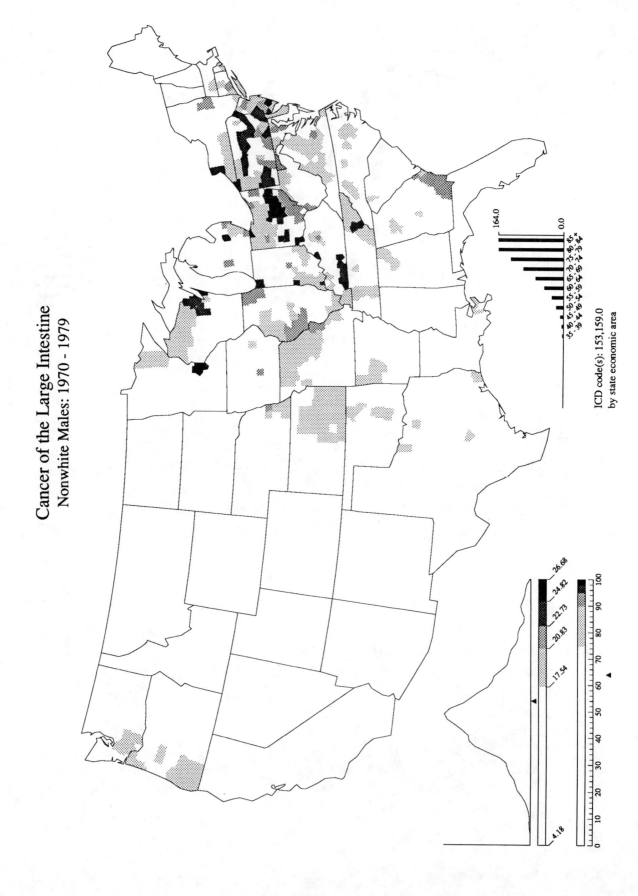

Cancer of the Large Intestine
Nonwhite Males: 1970 - 1979

164.0

0.0

ICD code(s): 153,159.0
by state economic area

26.68 24.82 22.73 20.83 17.54 4.18

Cancer of the Large Intestine
Nonwhite Males: Relative Change

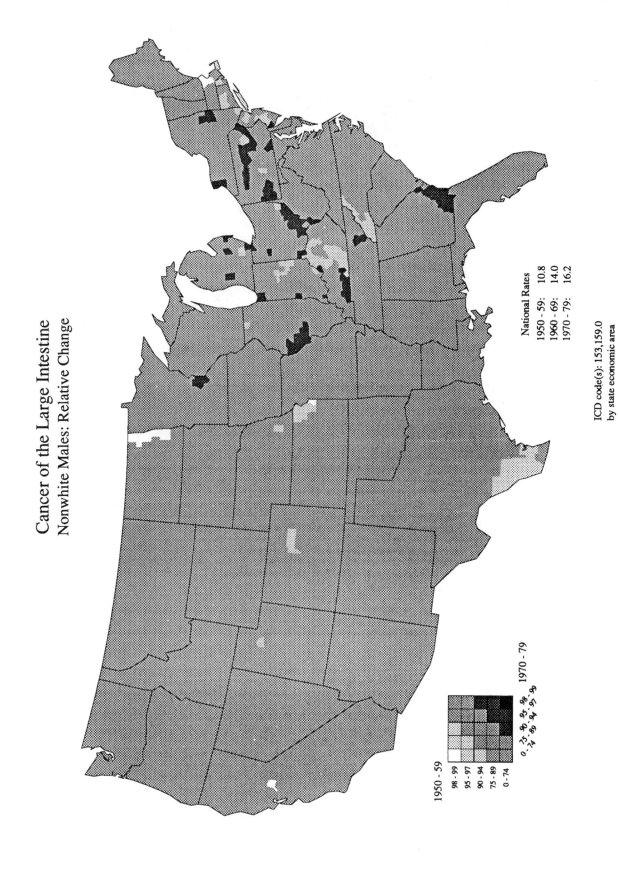

National Rates

1950 - 59: 10.8
1960 - 69: 14.0
1970 - 79: 16.2

ICD code(s): 153,159.0
by state economic area

1950 - 59

98 - 99
95 - 97
90 - 94
75 - 89
0 - 74

1970 - 79

0 - 74 75 - 89 90 - 94 95 - 97 98 - 99

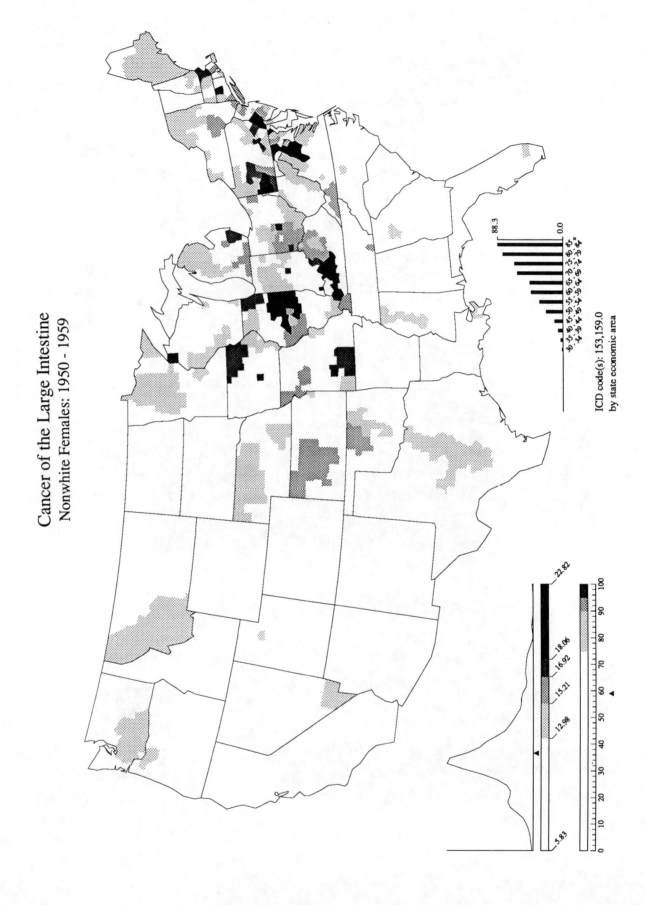

Cancer of the Large Intestine
Nonwhite Females: 1950 - 1959

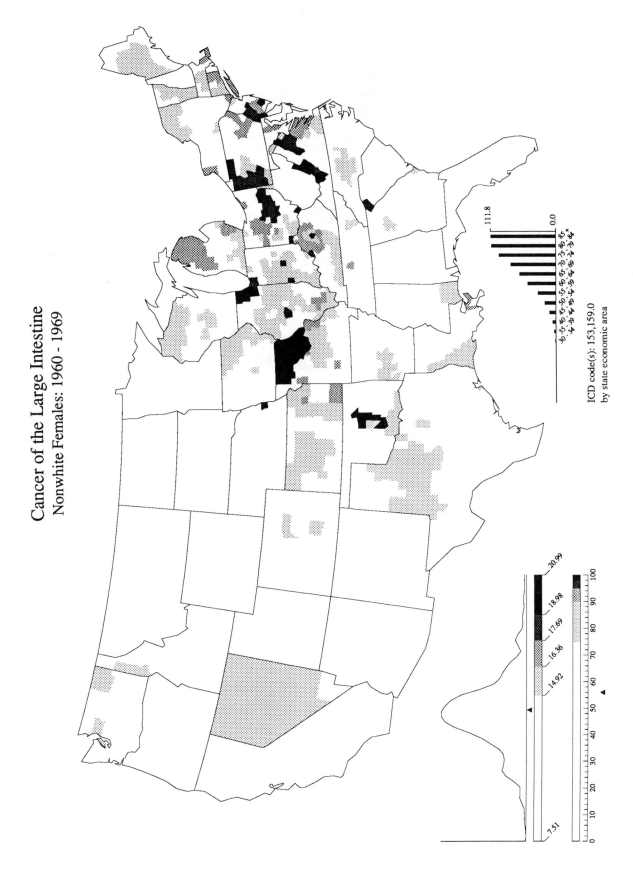

Cancer of the Large Intestine
Nonwhite Females: 1960 - 1969

ICD code(s): 153,159.0
by state economic area

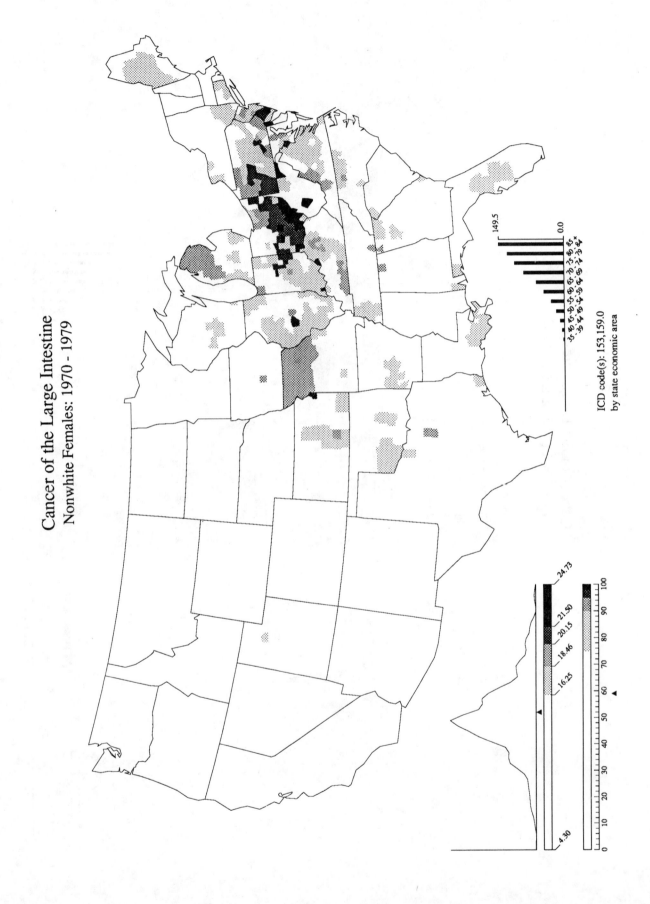

Cancer of the Large Intestine
Nonwhite Females: 1970 - 1979

ICD code(s): 153,159.0
by state economic area

Cancer of the Large Intestine
Nonwhite Females: Relative Change

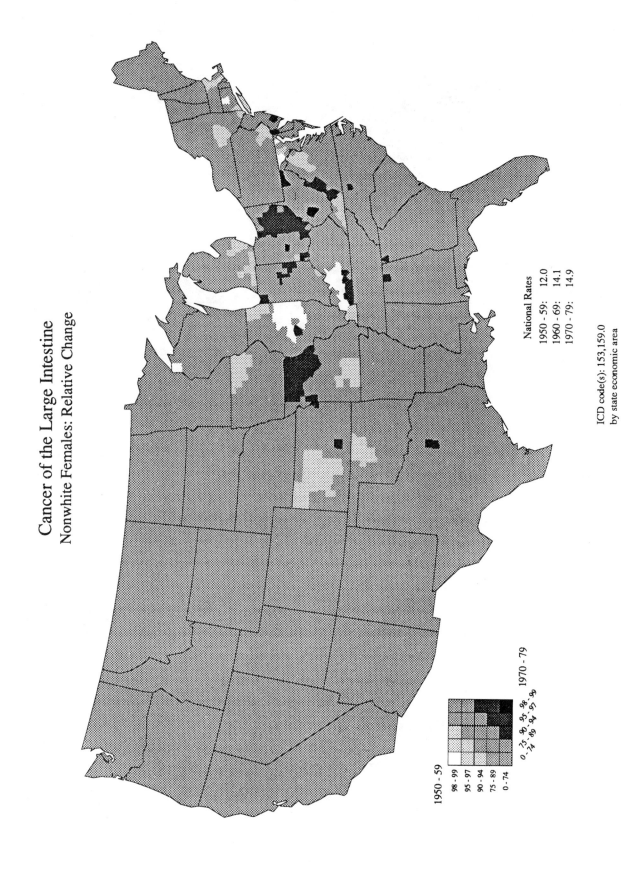

National Rates

1950 - 59:	12.0
1960 - 69:	14.1
1970 - 79:	14.9

ICD code(s): 153,159.0
by state economic area

1950 - 59

98 - 99	
95 - 97	
90 - 94	
75 - 89	
0 - 74	

1970 - 79

0 - 74 75 - 89 90 - 94 95 - 97 98 - 99

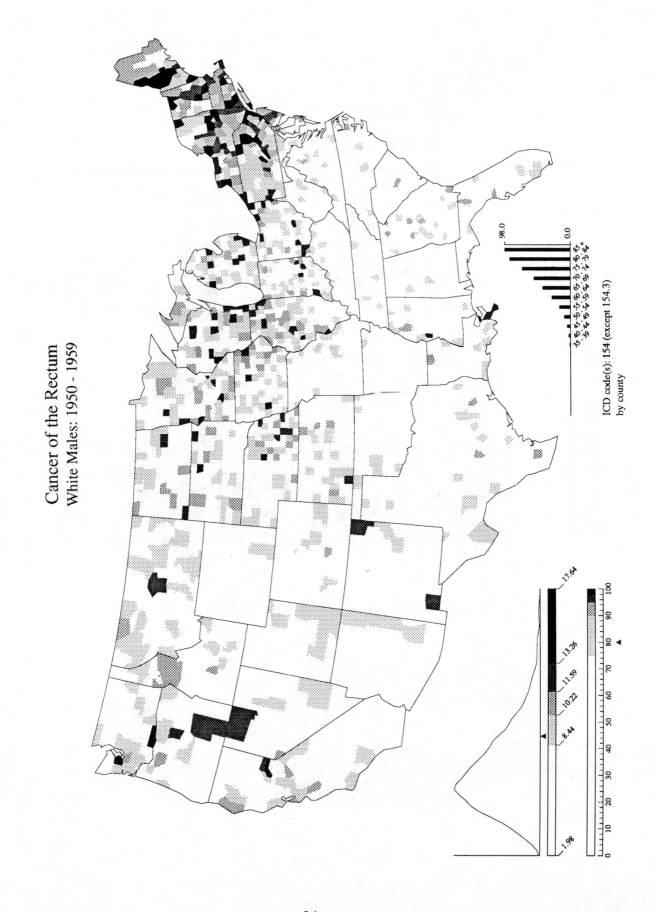

Cancer of the Rectum
White Males: 1950 - 1959

ICD code(s): 154 (except 154.3)
by county

Cancer of the Rectum
White Males: 1960 - 1969

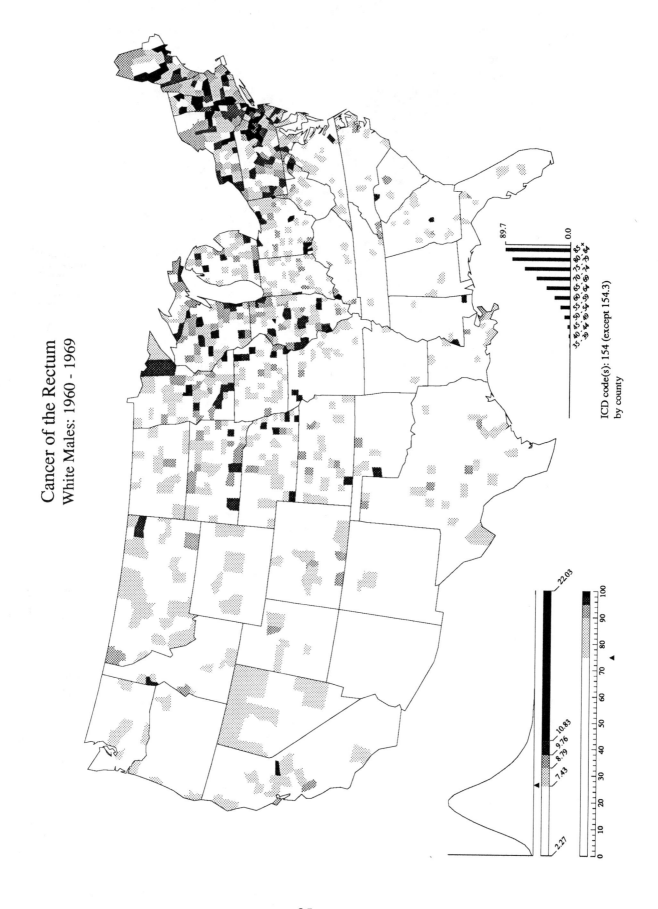

ICD code(s): 154 (except 154.3)
by county

95

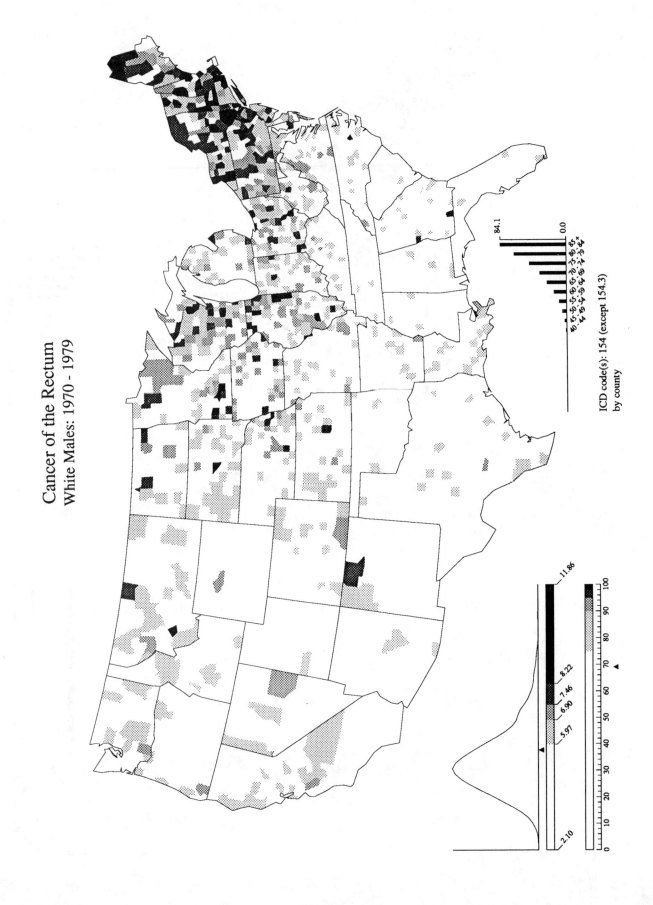

Cancer of the Rectum
White Males: 1970 - 1979

ICD code(s): 154 (except 154.3)
by county

Cancer of the Rectum
White Males: Relative Change

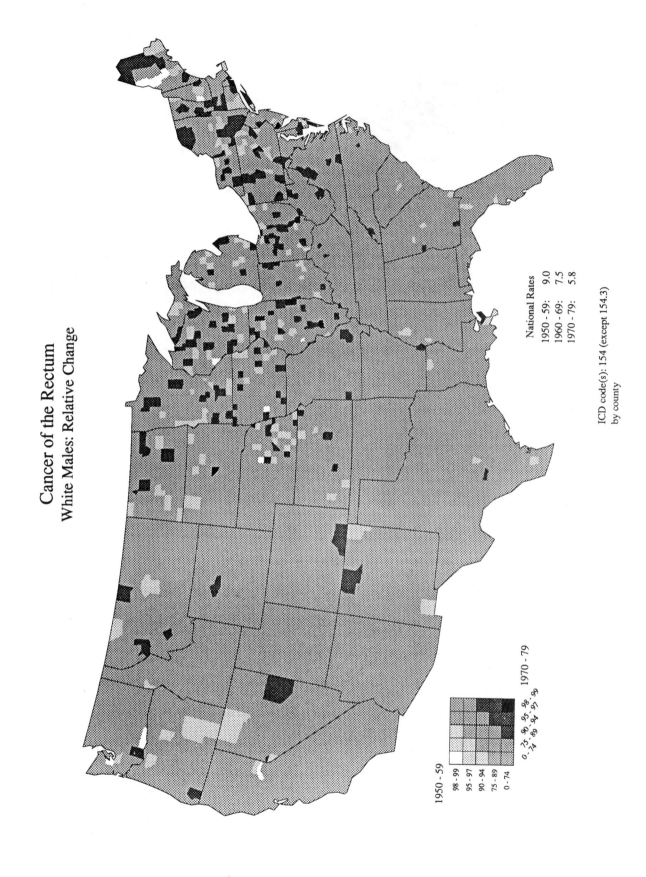

National Rates

1950 - 59:   9.0
1960 - 69:   7.5
1970 - 79:   5.8

ICD code(s): 154 (except 154.3)
by county

1950 - 59
98 - 99
95 - 97
90 - 94
75 - 89
0 - 74

1970 - 79
0 - 74 75 - 89 90 - 94 95 - 97 98 - 99

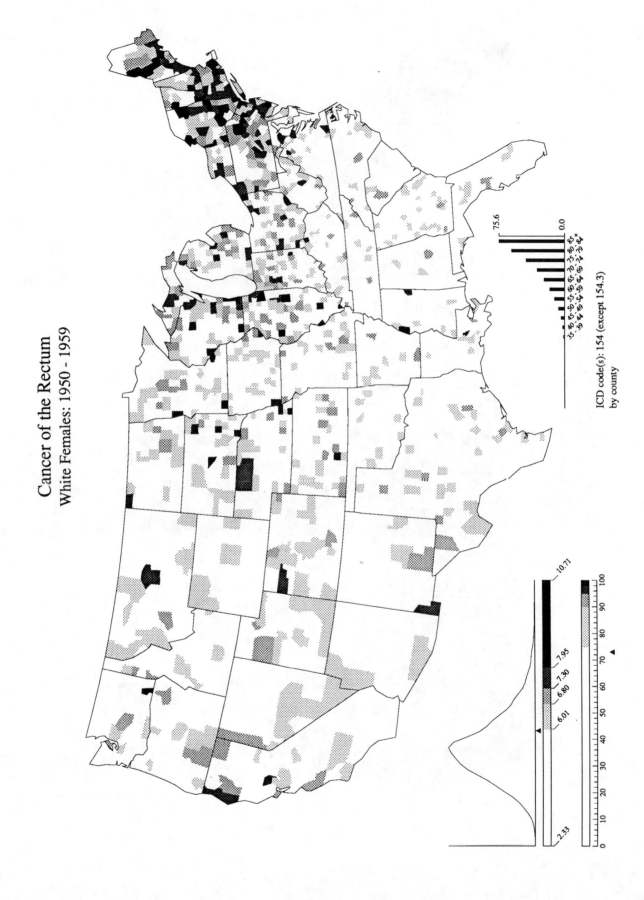

Cancer of the Rectum
White Females: 1950 - 1959

ICD code(s): 154 (except 154.3)
by county

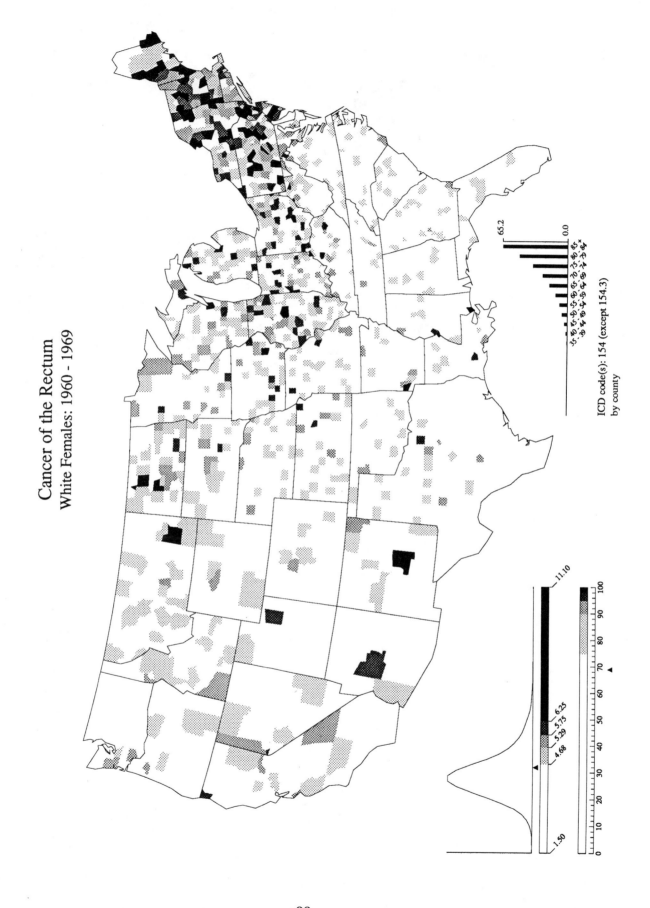

Cancer of the Rectum
White Females: 1960 - 1969

ICD code(s): 154 (except 154.3)
by county

65.2

0.0

35 40 45 50 55 60 65 70 75 80 85
-39 -44 -49 -54 -59 -64 -69 -74 -79 -84 +

11.10

6.25
5.75
5.29
4.68

1.50

0 10 20 30 40 50 60 70 80 90 100

99

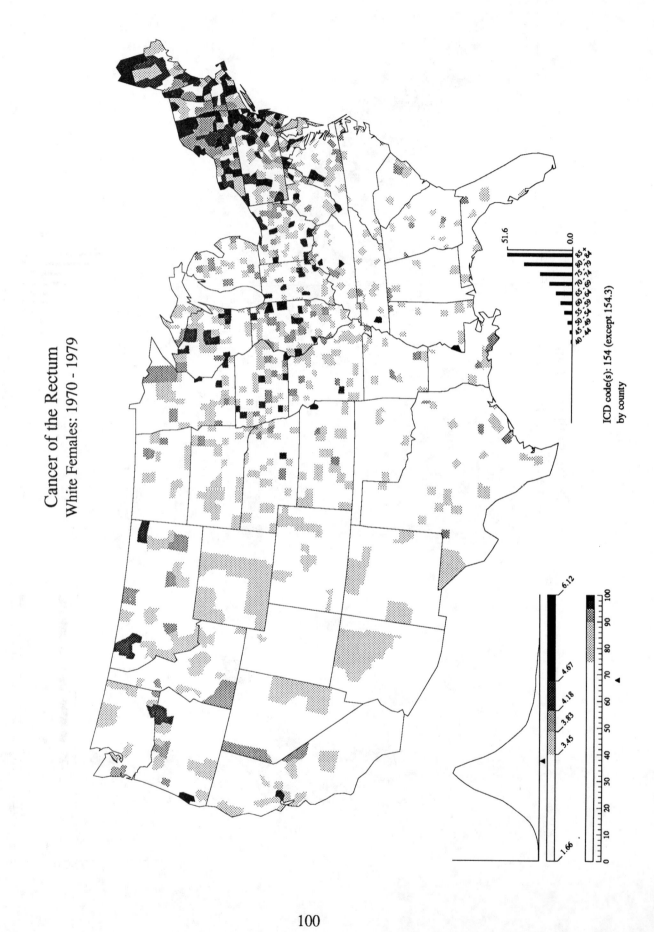

Cancer of the Rectum
White Females: 1970 - 1979

ICD code(s): 154 (except 154.3)
by county

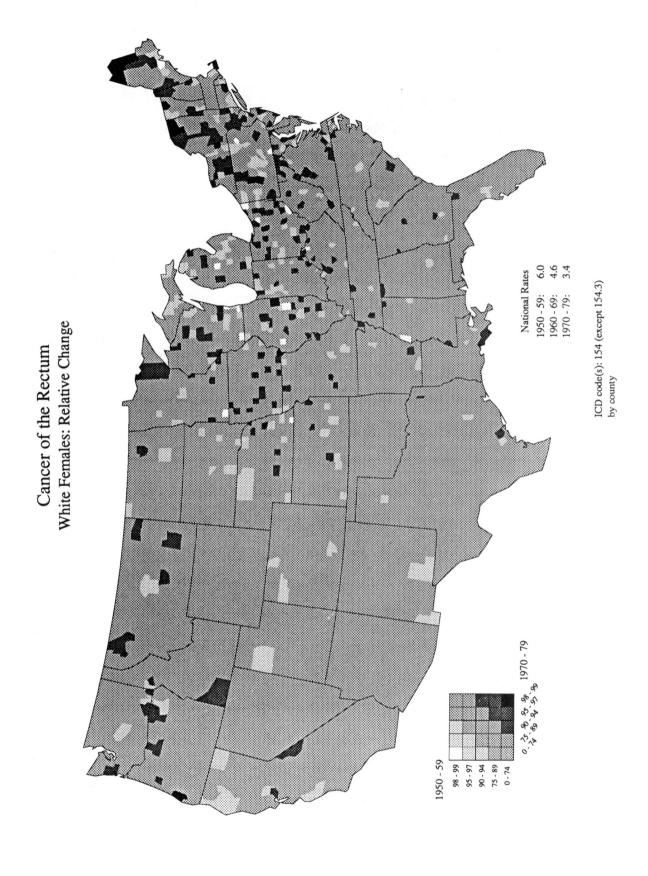

Cancer of the Rectum
White Females: Relative Change

National Rates

1950 - 59:   6.0
1960 - 69:   4.6
1970 - 79:   3.4

ICD code(s): 154 (except 154.3)
by county

1950 - 59

98 - 99
95 - 97
90 - 94
75 - 89
0 - 74

0 - 74 75 - 89 90 - 94 95 - 97 98 - 99   1970 - 79

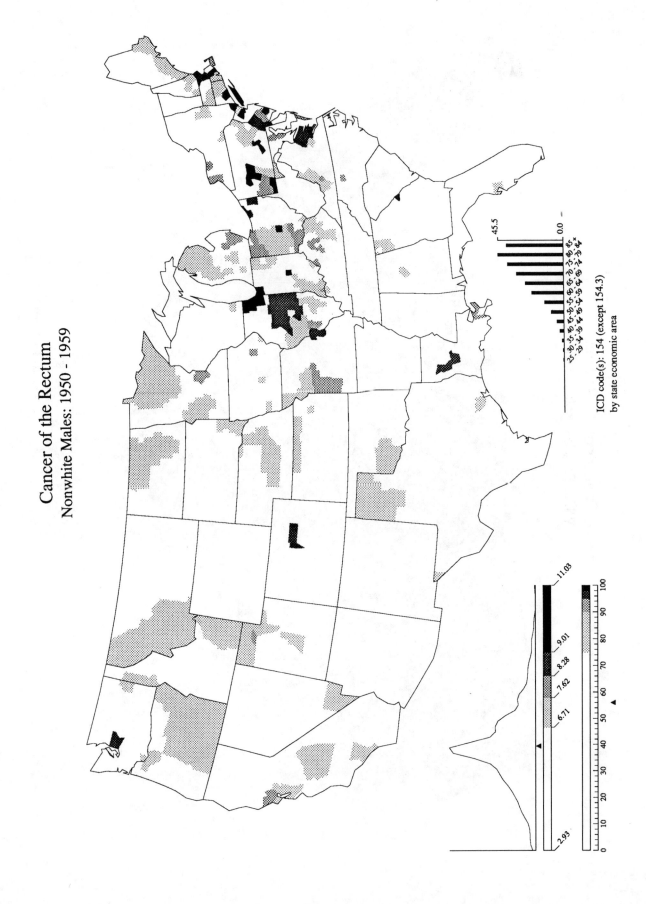

Cancer of the Rectum
Nonwhite Males: 1950 - 1959

ICD code(s): 154 (except 154.3)
by state economic area

Cancer of the Rectum
Nonwhite Males: 1960 - 1969

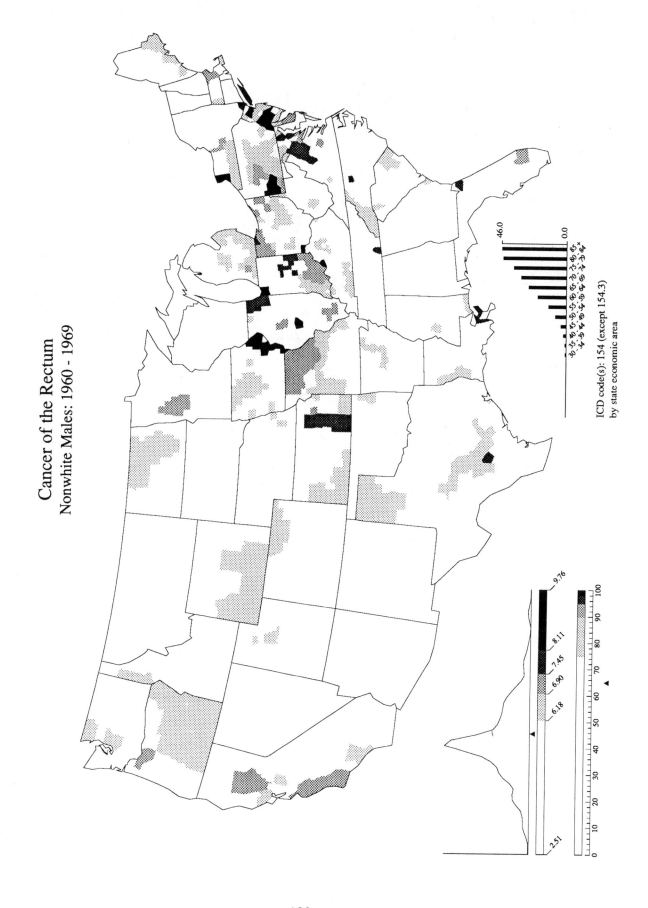

ICD code(s): 154 (except 154.3)
by state economic area

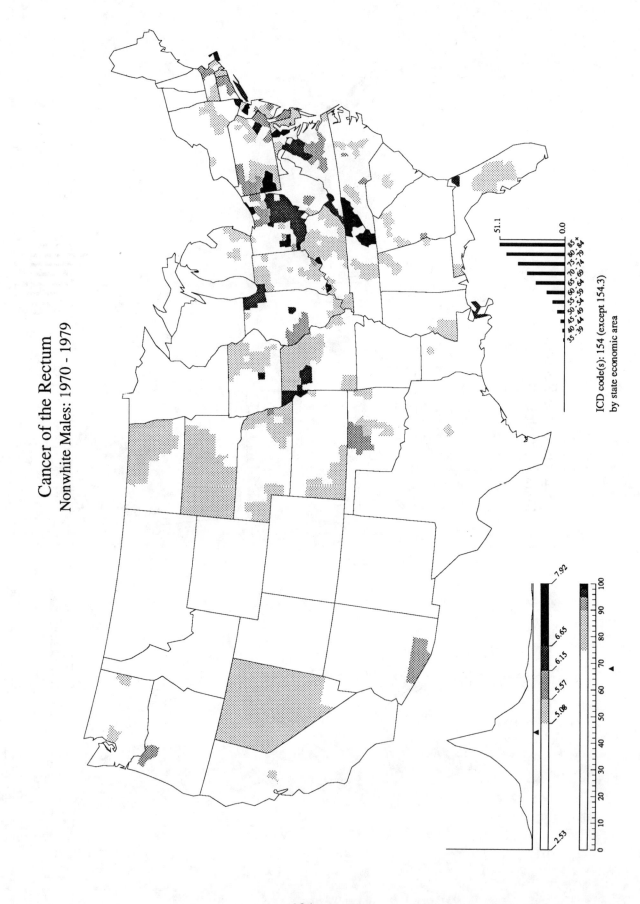

Cancer of the Rectum
Nonwhite Males: 1970 - 1979

ICD code(s): 154 (except 154.3)
by state economic area

Cancer of the Rectum
Nonwhite Males: Relative Change

National Rates

1950 - 59:	6.1
1960 - 69:	5.8
1970 - 79:	5.0

ICD code(s): 154 (except 154.3)
by state economic area

1950 - 59

98 - 99
95 - 97
90 - 94
75 - 89
0 - 74

1970 - 79
98 - 99
95 - 97
90 - 94
75 - 89
0 - 74

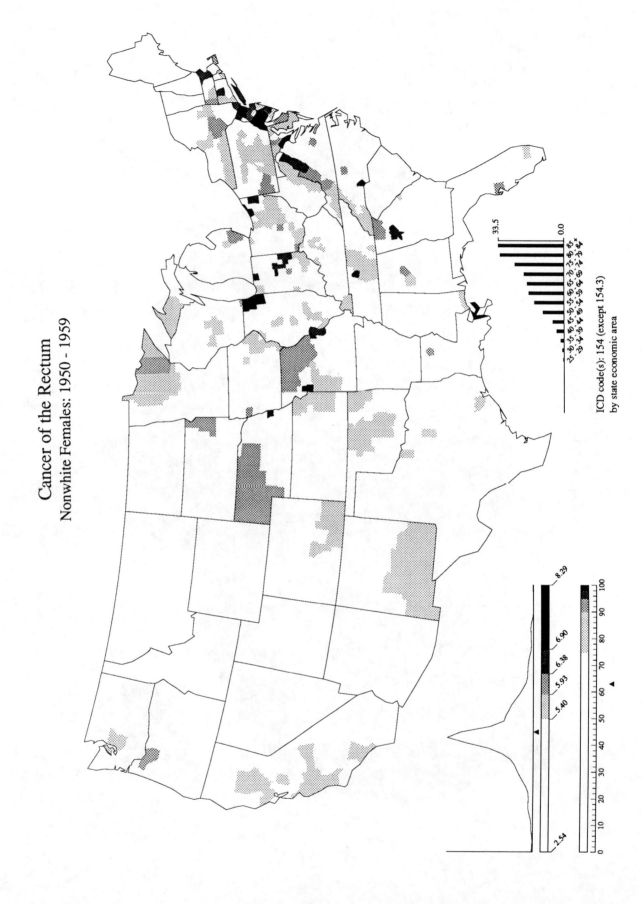

Cancer of the Rectum
Nonwhite Females: 1950 - 1959

ICD code(s): 154 (except 154.3)
by state economic area

Cancer of the Rectum
Nonwhite Females: 1960 - 1969

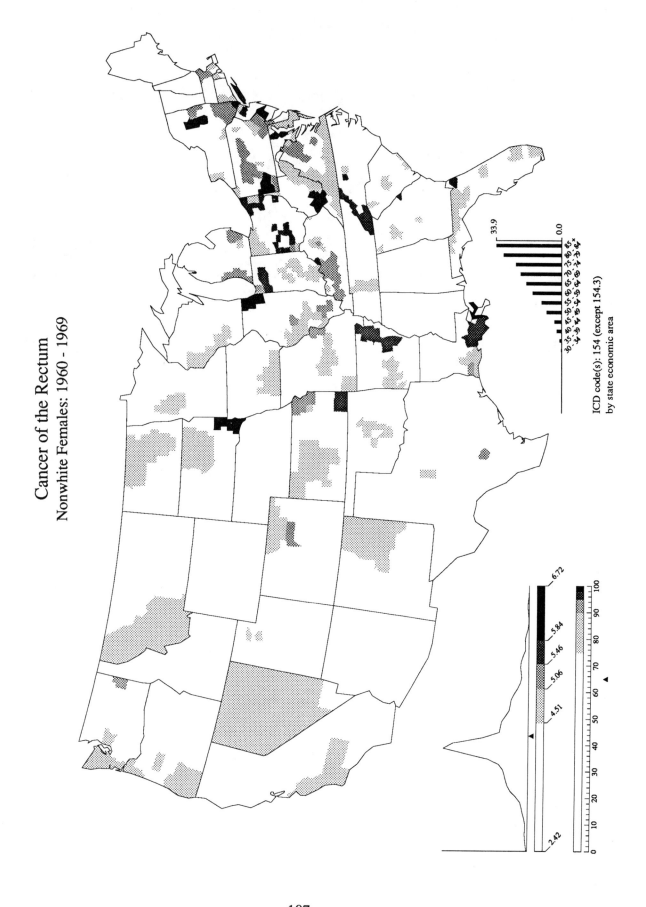

ICD code(s): 154 (except 154.3)
by state economic area

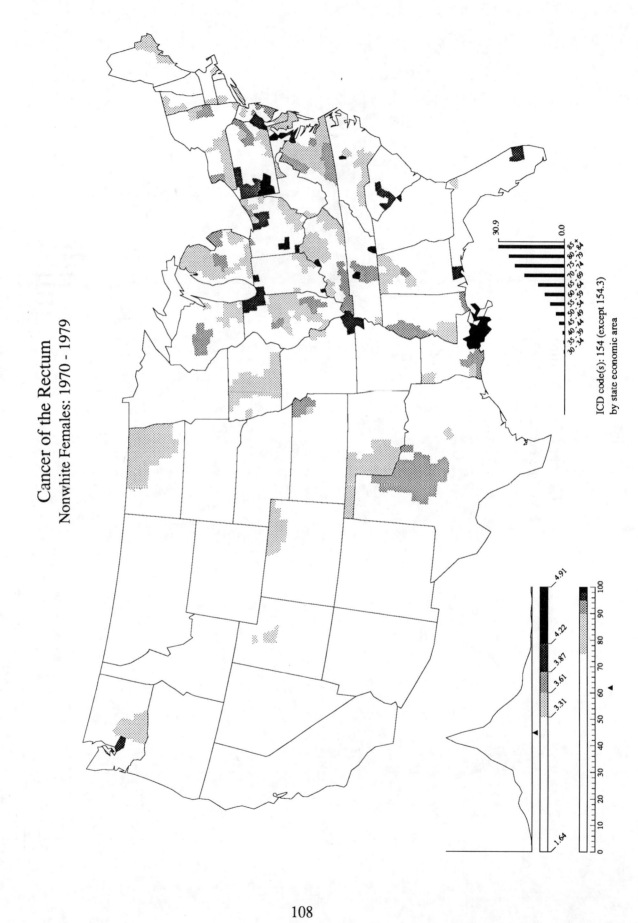

Cancer of the Rectum
Nonwhite Females: 1970 - 1979

ICD code(s): 154 (except 154.3)
by state economic area

Cancer of the Rectum
Nonwhite Females: Relative Change

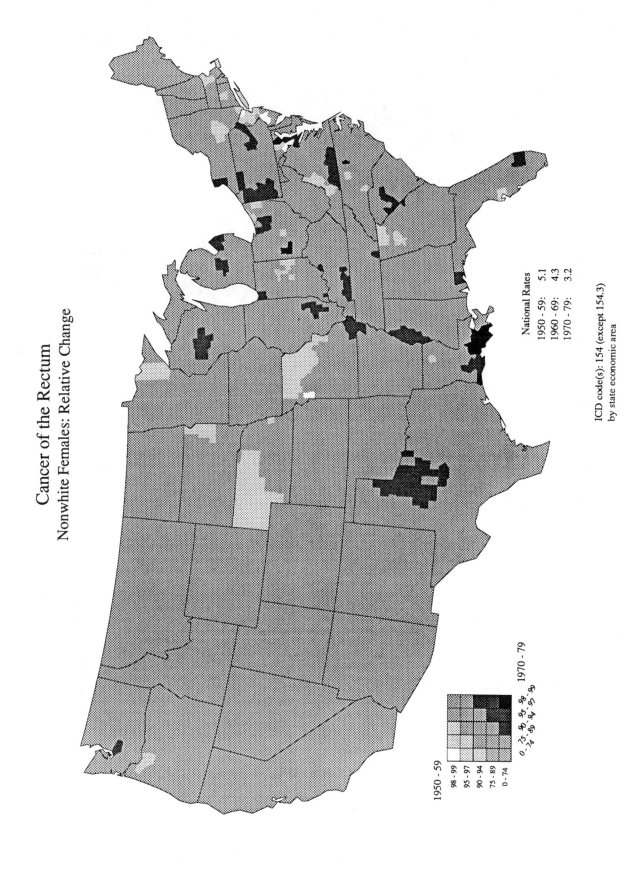

National Rates

1950 - 59:	5.1
1960 - 69:	4.3
1970 - 79:	3.2

ICD code(s): 154 (except 154.3)
by state economic area

1950 - 59

98 - 99
95 - 97
90 - 94
75 - 89
0 - 74

1970 - 79

0 - 74 75 - 89 90 - 94 95 - 97 98 - 99

Cancer of the Liver and Gallbladder including Bile Ducts
White Males: 1950 - 1959

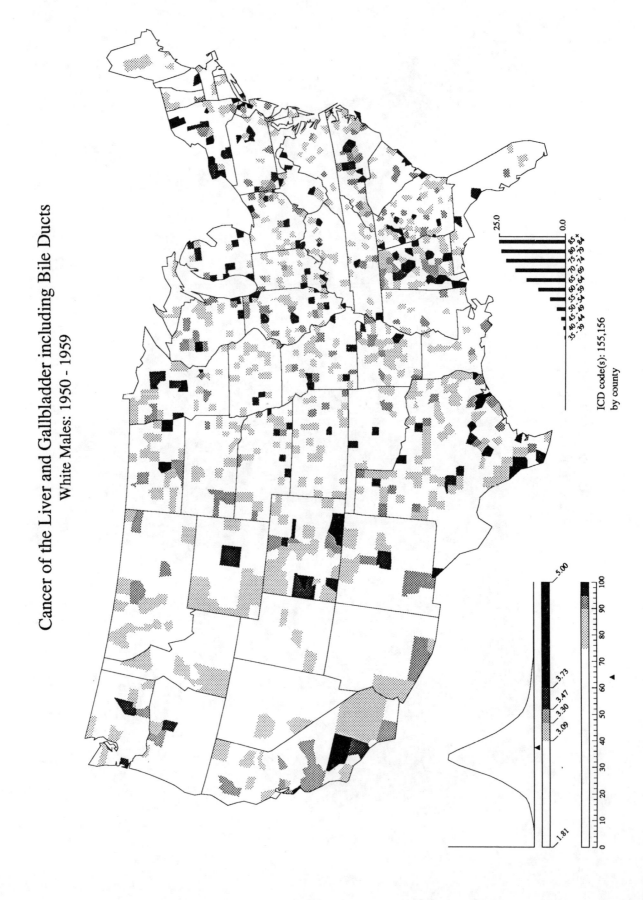

ICD code(s): 155,156
by county

110

Cancer of the Liver and Gallbladder including Bile Ducts
White Males: 1960 - 1969

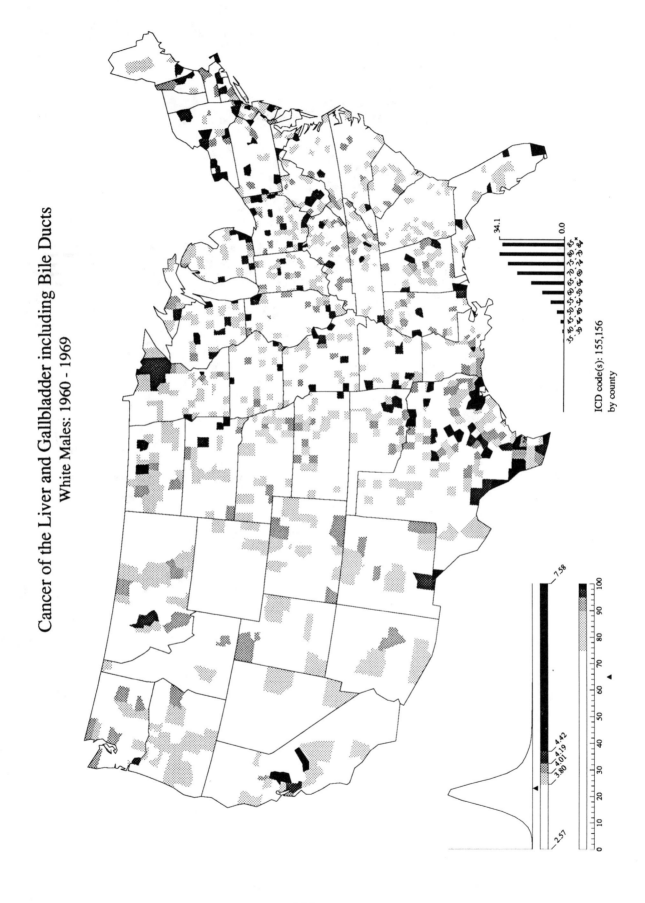

ICD code(s): 155,156
by county

Cancer of the Liver and Gallbladder including Bile Ducts
White Males: 1970 - 1979

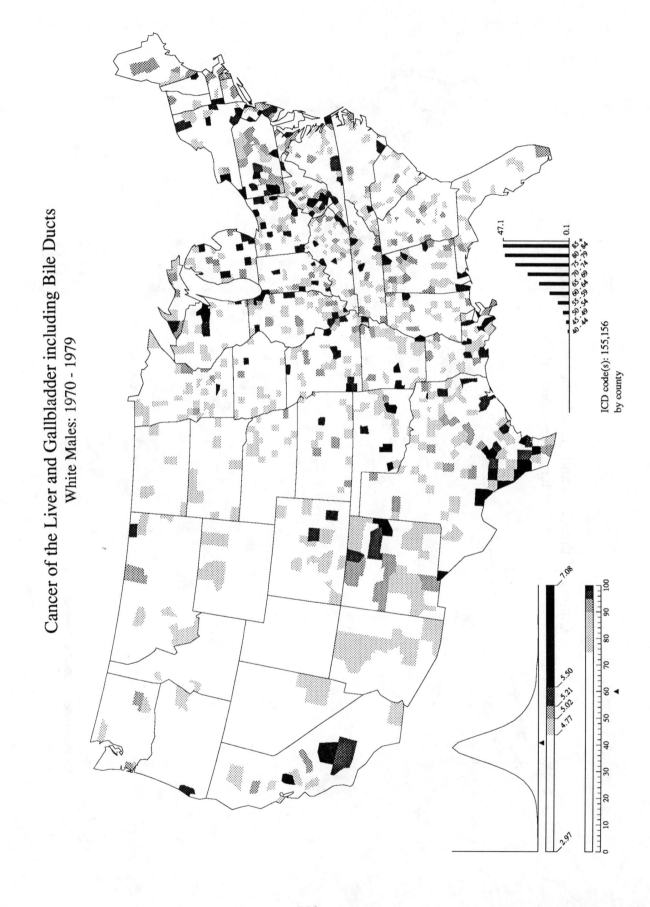

ICD code(s): 155,156
by county

Cancer of the Liver and Gallbladder including Bile Ducts
White Males: Relative Change

National Rates

1950 - 59:	3.0
1960 - 69:	3.7
1970 - 79:	4.6

ICD code(s): 155,156
by county

1950 - 59

| 98 - 99 |
| 95 - 97 |
| 90 - 94 |
| 75 - 89 |
| 0 - 74 |

1970 - 79

0 - 74   75 - 89   90 - 94   95 - 97   98 - 99

Cancer of the Liver and Gallbladder including Bile Ducts
White Females: 1950 - 1959

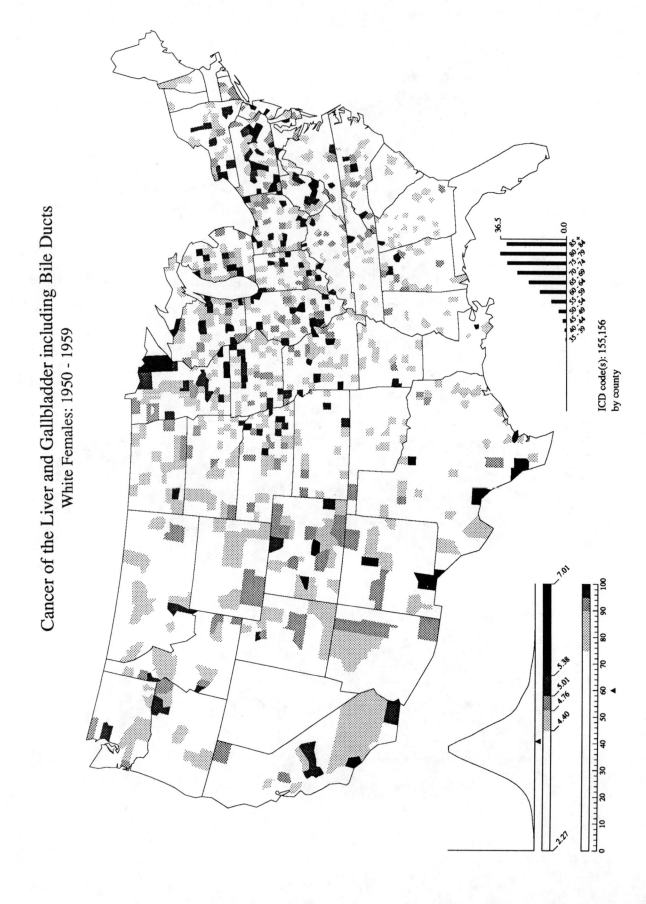

ICD code(s): 155,156
by county

Cancer of the Liver and Gallbladder including Bile Ducts
White Females: 1960 - 1969

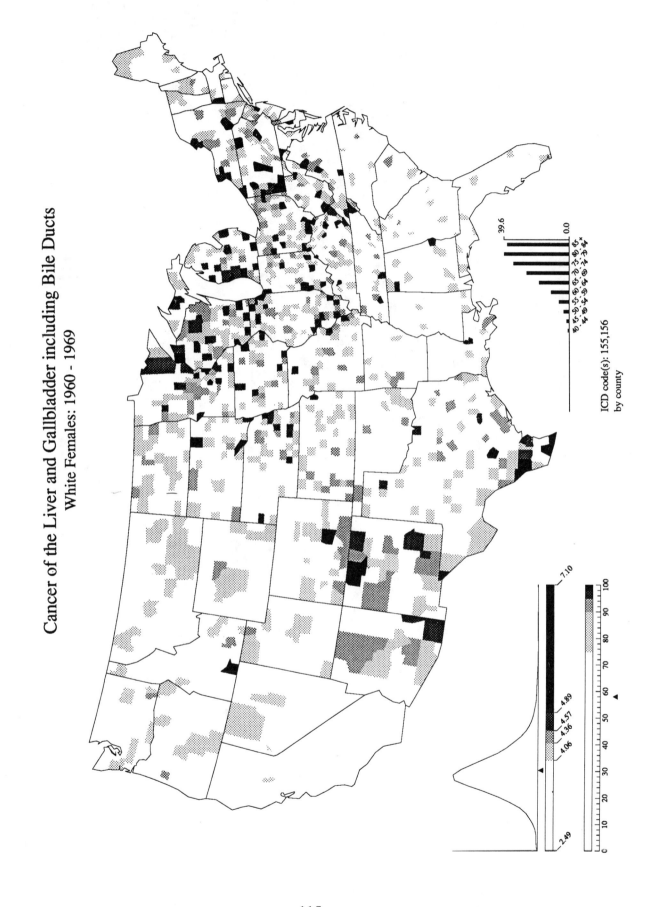

ICD code(s): 155,156
by county

Cancer of the Liver and Gallbladder including Bile Ducts
White Females: 1970 - 1979

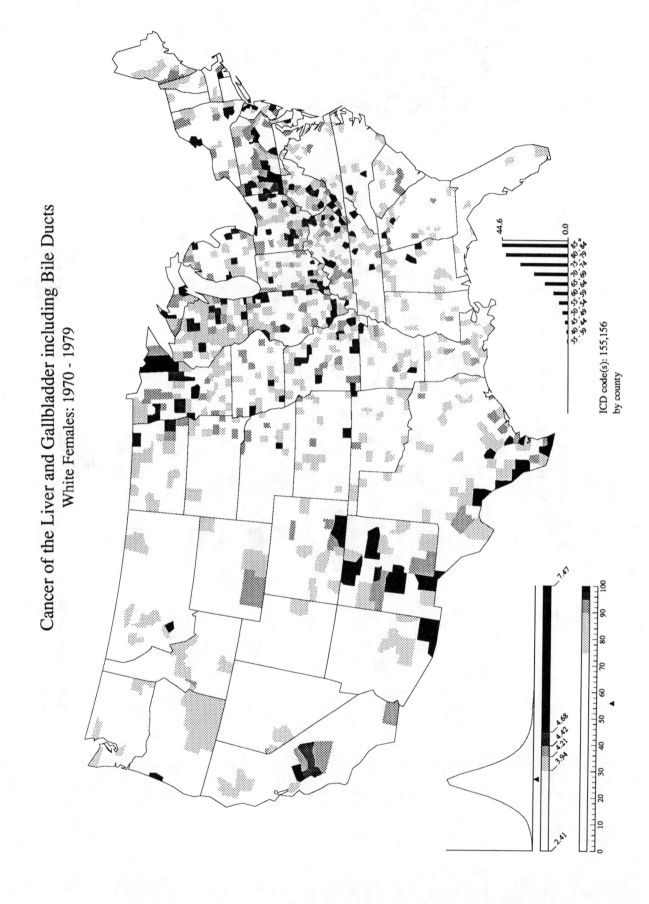

ICD code(s): 155,156
by county

Cancer of the Liver and Gallbladder including Bile Ducts

White Females: Relative Change

National Rates

1950 - 59: 4.2
1960 - 69: 3.9
1970 - 79: 3.8

ICD code(s): 155,156
by county

1950 - 59

98 - 99
95 - 97
90 - 94
75 - 89
0 - 74

1970 - 79

0 - 74 75 - 89 90 - 94 95 - 97 98 - 99

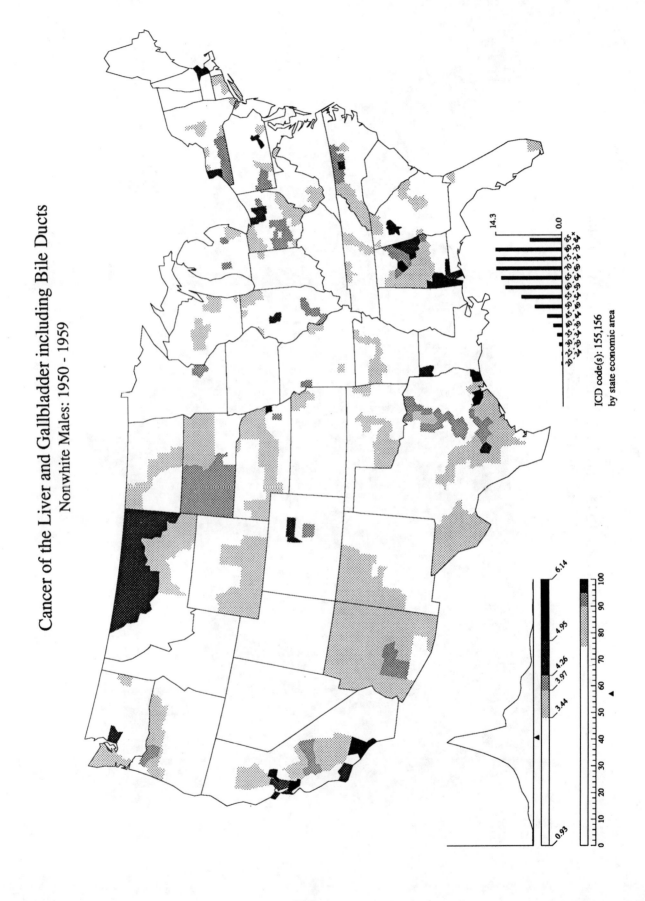

Cancer of the Liver and Gallbladder including Bile Ducts
Nonwhite Males: 1950 - 1959

ICD code(s): 155,156
by state economic area

Cancer of the Liver and Gallbladder including Bile Ducts
Nonwhite Males: 1960 - 1969

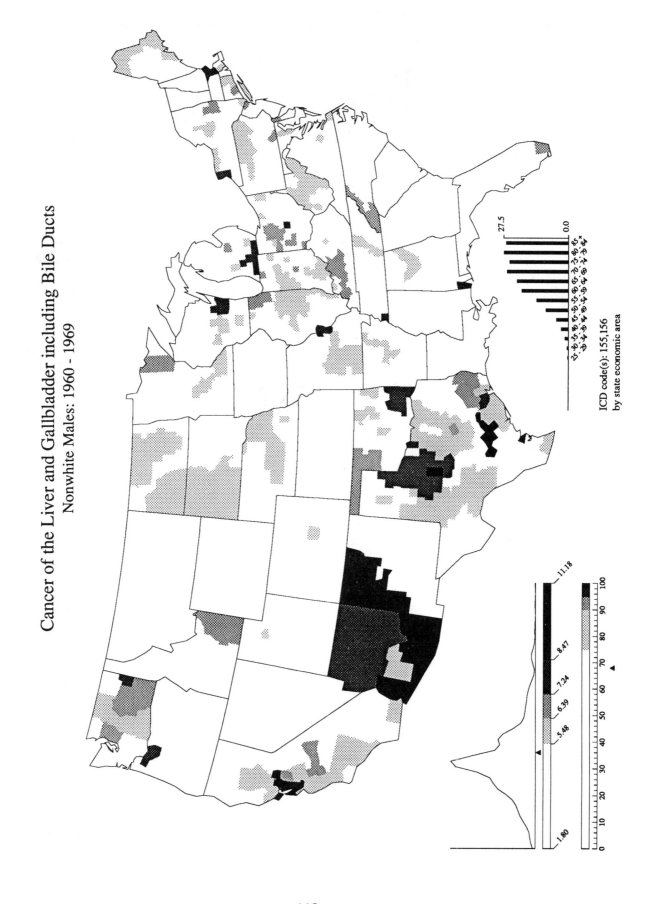

ICD code(s): 155,156
by state economic area

Cancer of the Liver and Gallbladder including Bile Ducts
Nonwhite Males: 1970 - 1979

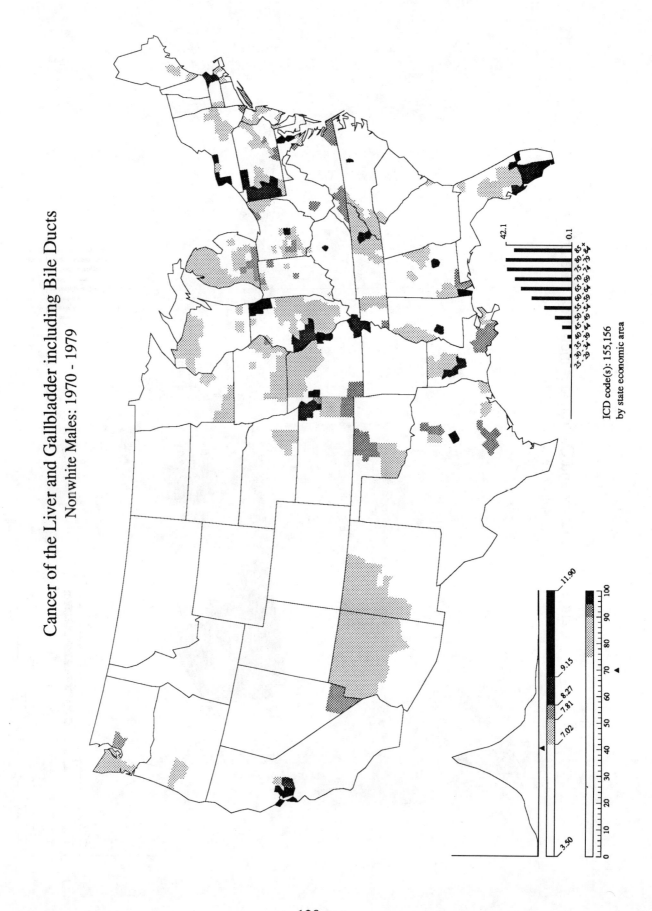

ICD code(s): 155,156
by state economic area

Cancer of the Liver and Gallbladder including Bile Ducts
Nonwhite Males: Relative Change

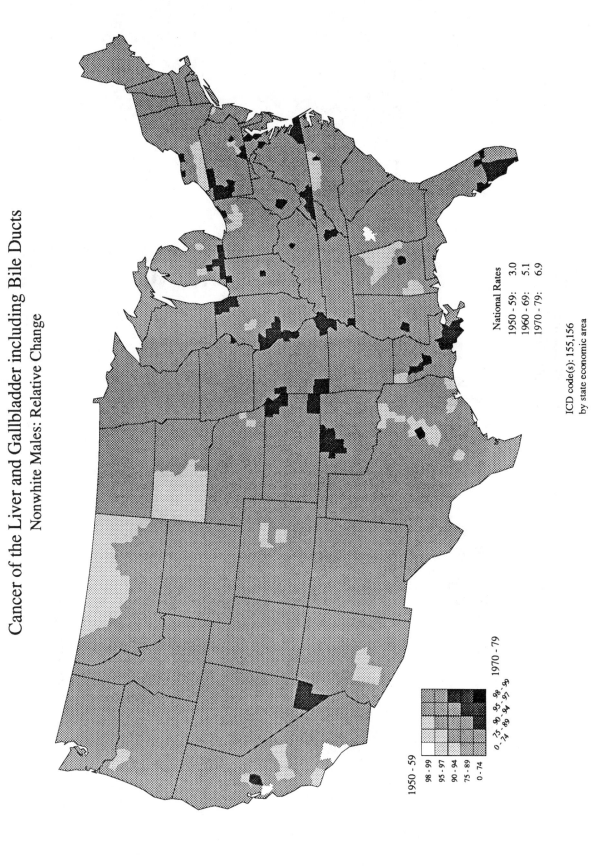

National Rates

1950 - 59:	3.0
1960 - 69:	5.1
1970 - 79:	6.9

ICD code(s): 155,156
by state economic area

1950 - 59

98 - 99
95 - 97
90 - 94
75 - 89
0 - 74

0 - 74 75 - 89 90 - 94 95 - 97 98 - 99

1970 - 79

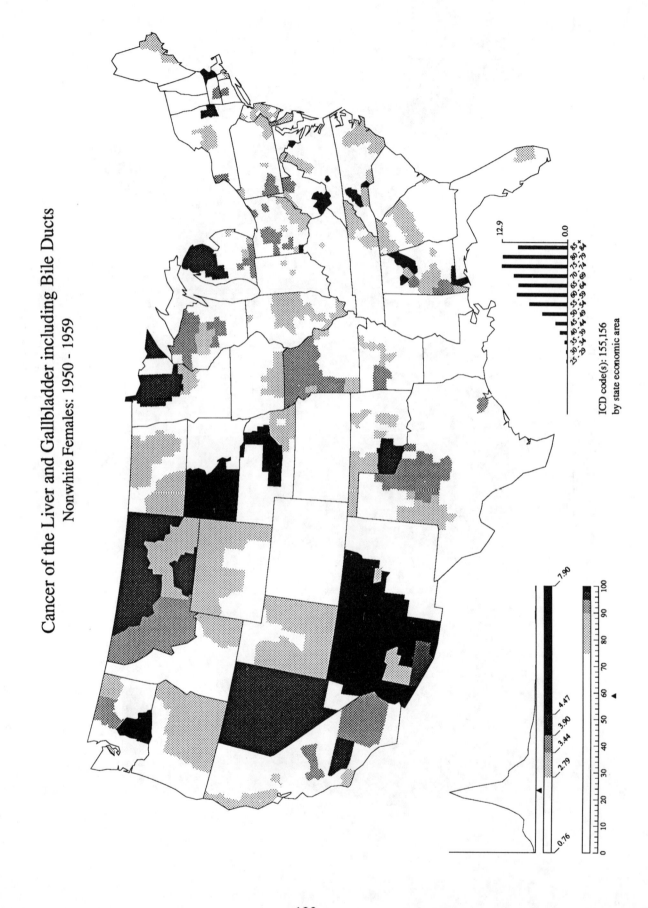

Cancer of the Liver and Gallbladder including Bile Ducts
Nonwhite Females: 1950 - 1959

ICD code(s): 155,156
by state economic area

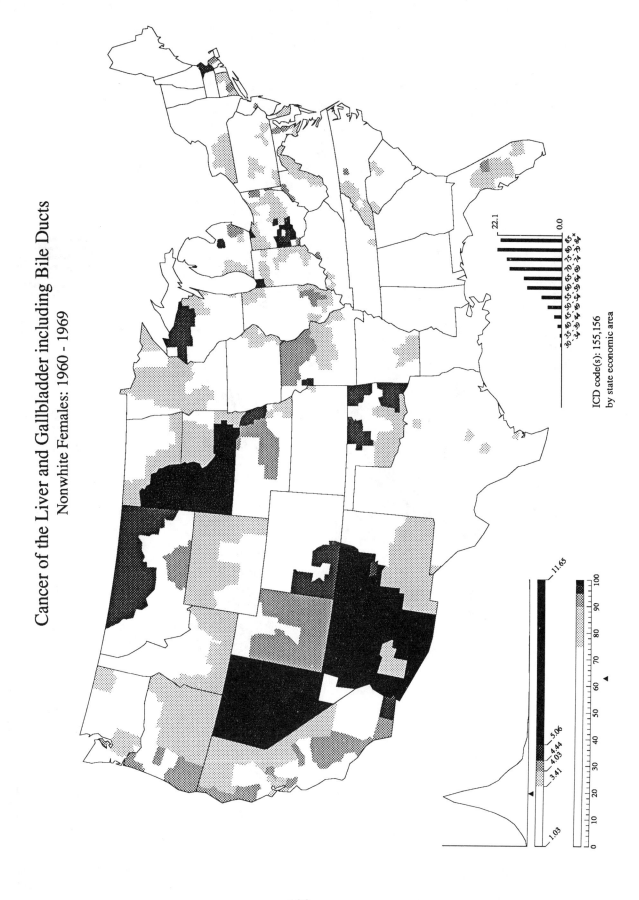

Cancer of the Liver and Gallbladder including Bile Ducts
Nonwhite Females: 1960 - 1969

ICD code(s): 155,156
by state economic area

Cancer of the Liver and Gallbladder including Bile Ducts
Nonwhite Females: 1970 - 1979

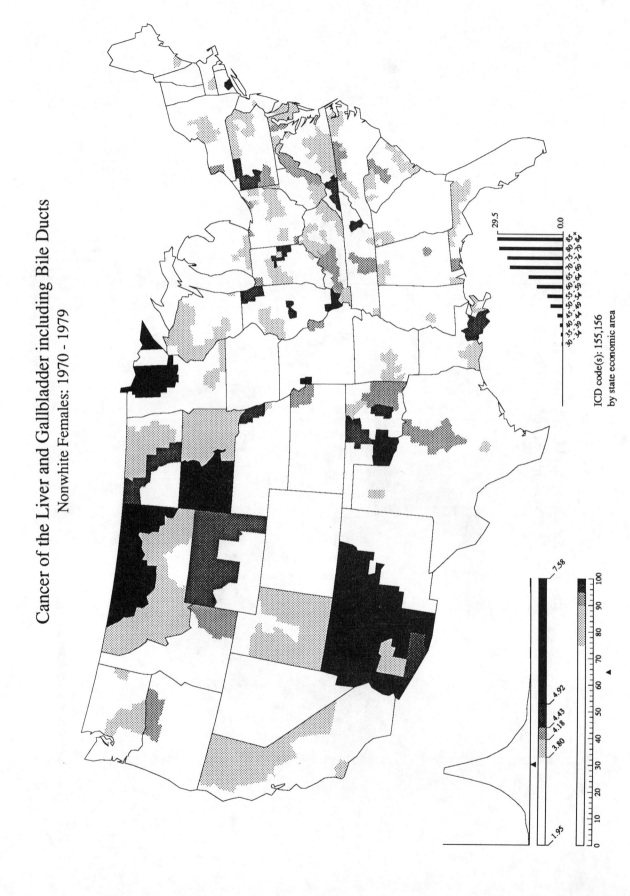

ICD code(s): 155,156
by state economic area

Cancer of the Liver and Gallbladder including Bile Ducts
Nonwhite Females: Relative Change

National Rates

1950 - 59:	2.4
1960 - 69:	3.1
1970 - 79:	3.7

ICD code(s): 155,156
by state economic area

1950 - 59

98 - 99
95 - 97
90 - 94
75 - 89
0 - 74

1970 - 79

0 - 74 75 - 89 90 - 94 95 - 97 98 - 99

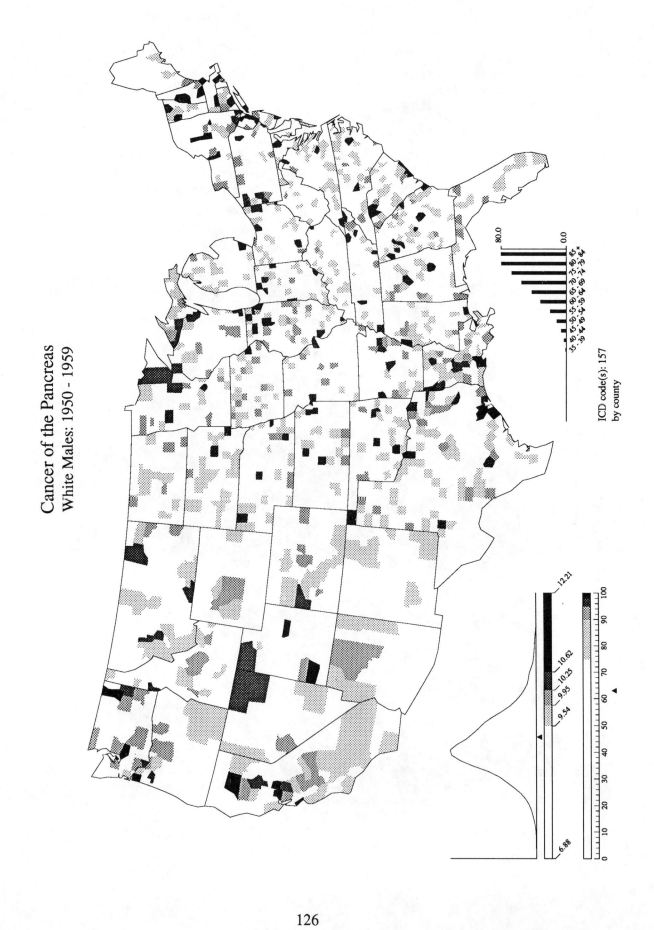

Cancer of the Pancreas
White Males: 1950 - 1959

ICD code(s): 157
by county

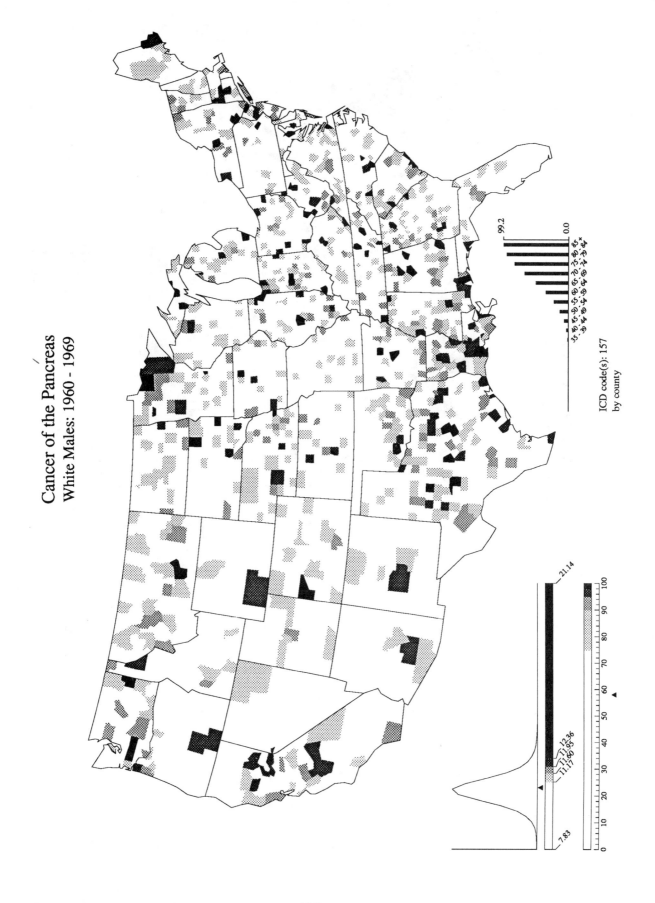

Cancer of the Pancreas
White Males: 1960 - 1969

ICD code(s): 157
by county

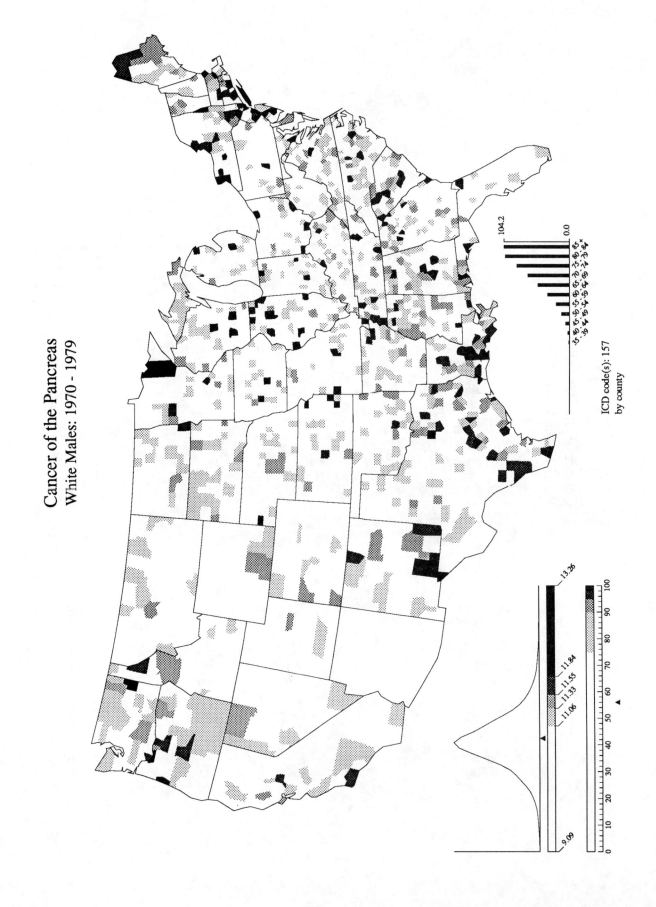

Cancer of the Pancreas
White Males: 1970 - 1979

ICD code(s): 157
by county

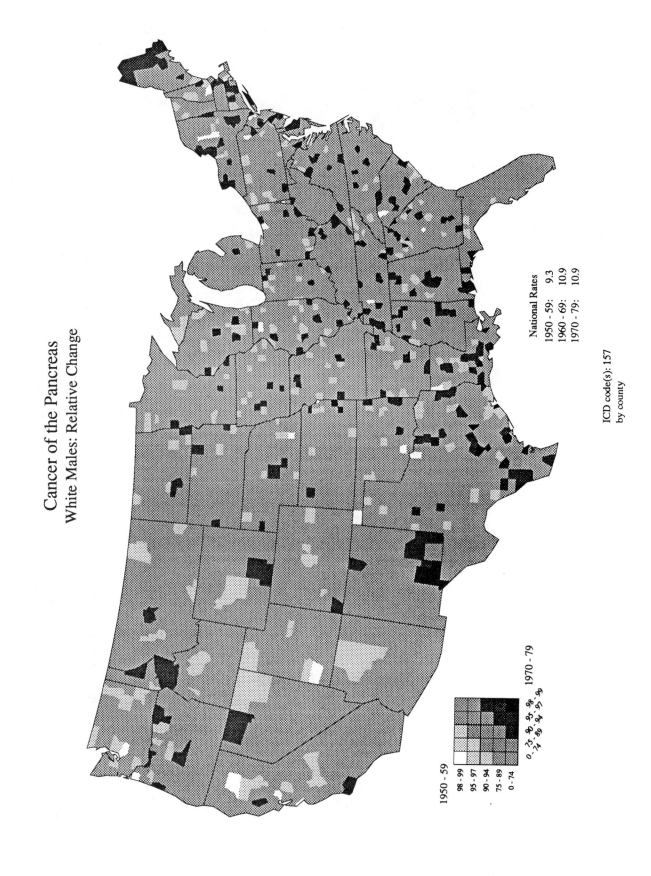

Cancer of the Pancreas
White Males: Relative Change

National Rates

1950 - 59:   9.3
1960 - 69:   10.9
1970 - 79:   10.9

ICD code(s): 157
by county

1950 - 59

98 - 99
95 - 97
90 - 94
75 - 89
0 - 74

1970 - 79

0 - 75 90 95 98 99
  74 89 94 97 99

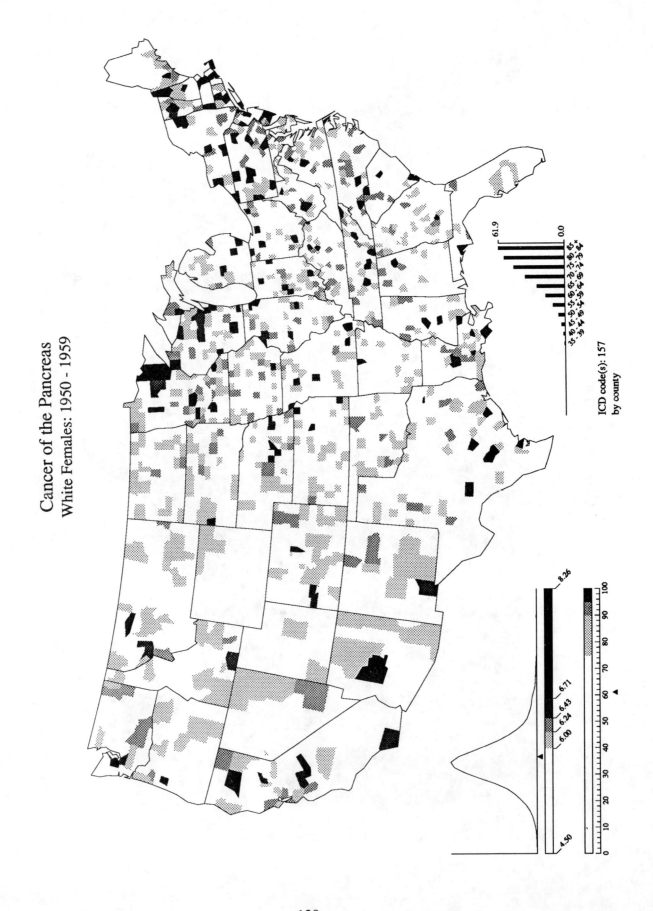

Cancer of the Pancreas
White Females: 1950 - 1959

ICD code(s): 157
by county

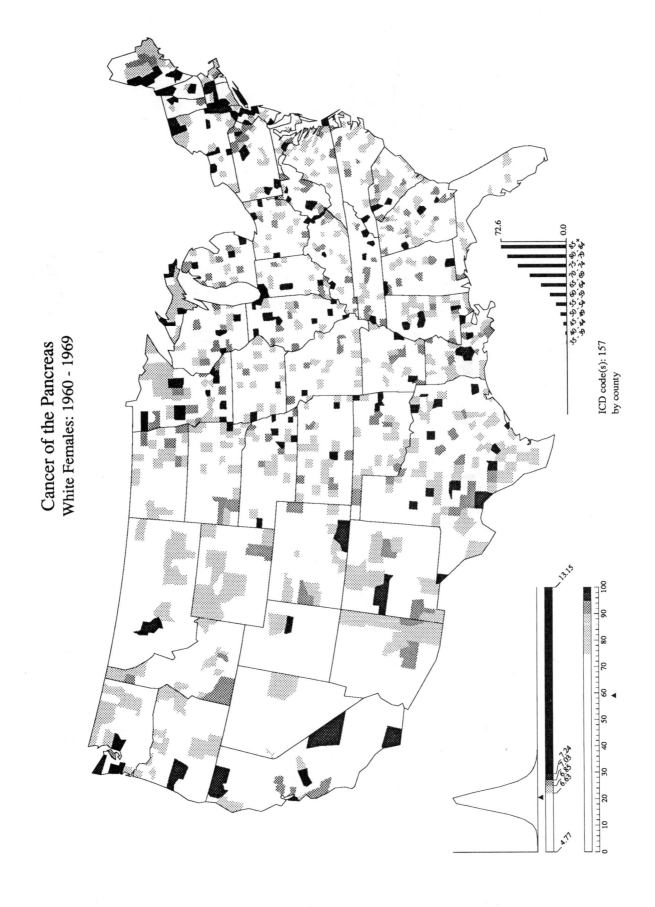

Cancer of the Pancreas
White Females: 1960 - 1969

ICD code(s): 157
by county

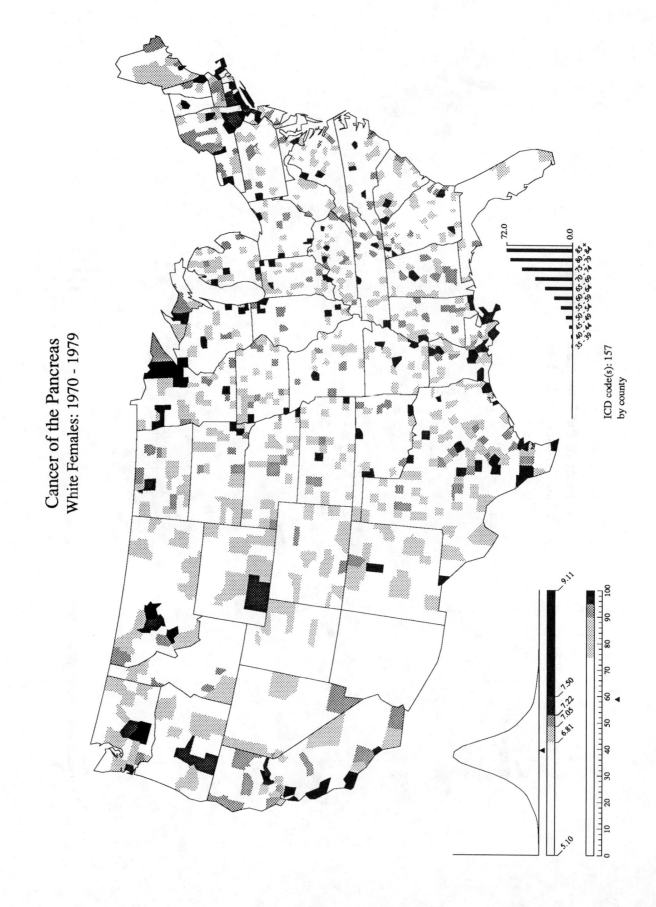

Cancer of the Pancreas
White Females: 1970 - 1979

ICD code(s): 157
by county

Cancer of the Pancreas
White Females: Relative Change

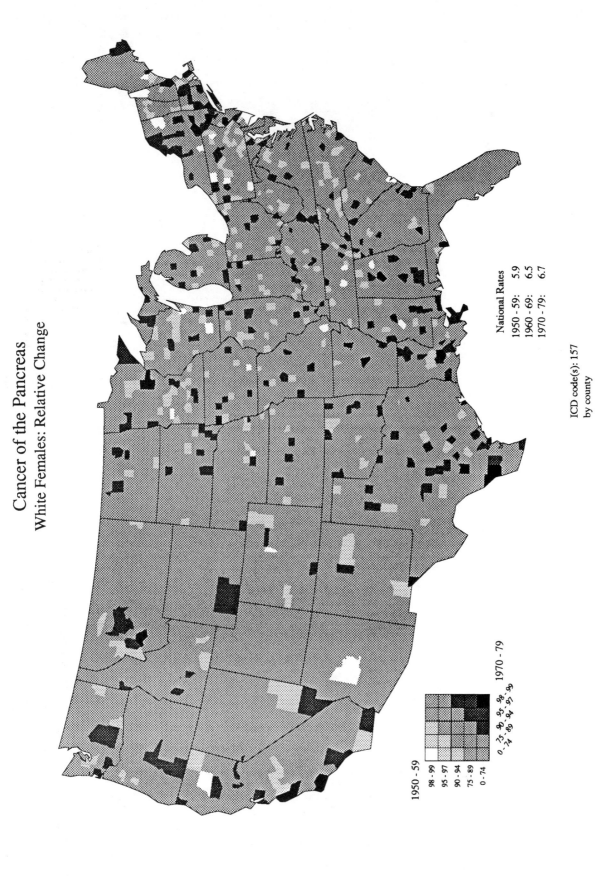

National Rates

1950 - 59: 5.9
1960 - 69: 6.5
1970 - 79: 6.7

ICD code(s): 157
by county

1950 - 59

98 - 99
95 - 97
90 - 94
75 - 89
0 - 74

0 - 75 - 90 - 95 - 98 -
74   89   94   97   99

1970 - 79

Cancer of the Pancreas
Nonwhite Males: 1950 - 1959

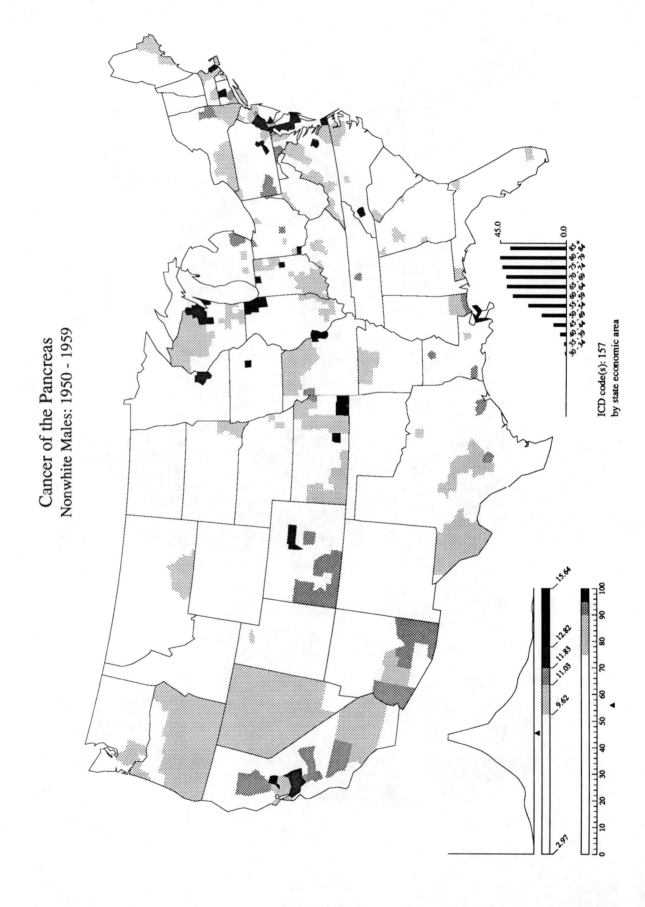

ICD code(s): 157
by state economic area

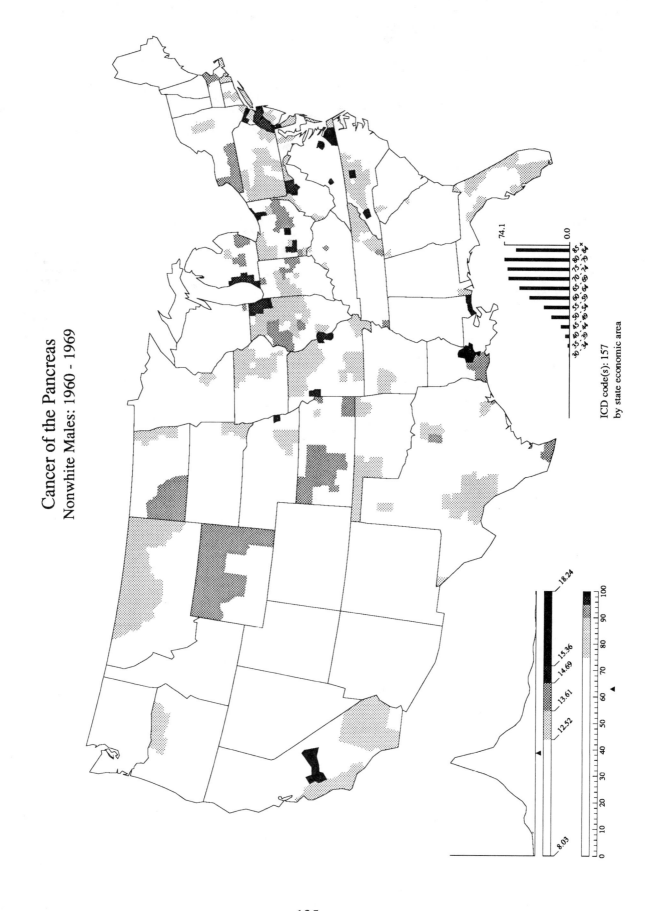

Cancer of the Pancreas
Nonwhite Males: 1960 - 1969

ICD code(s): 157
by state economic area

135

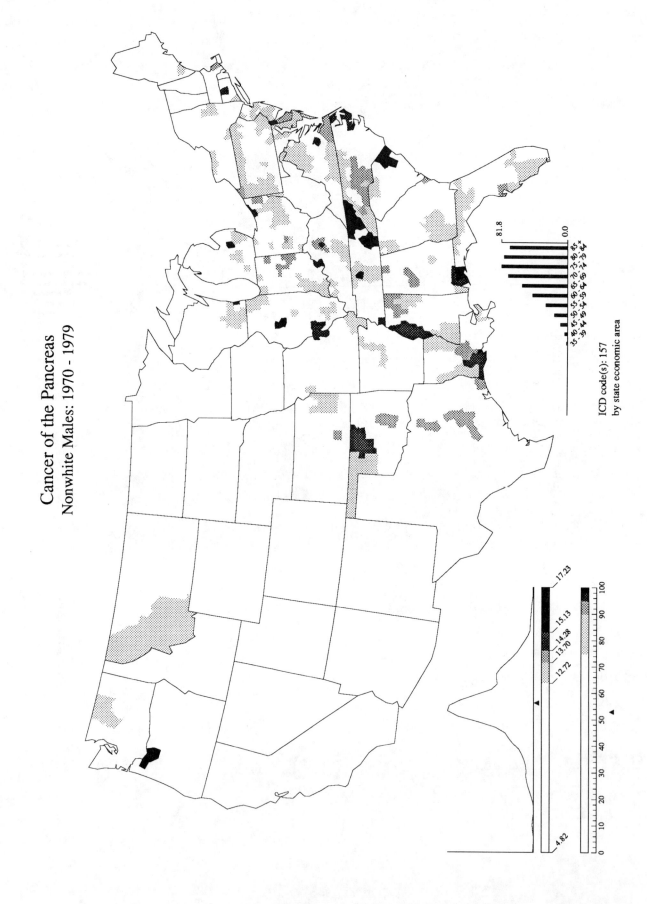

Cancer of the Pancreas
Nonwhite Males: 1970 - 1979

ICD code(s): 157
by state economic area

Cancer of the Pancreas
Nonwhite Males: Relative Change

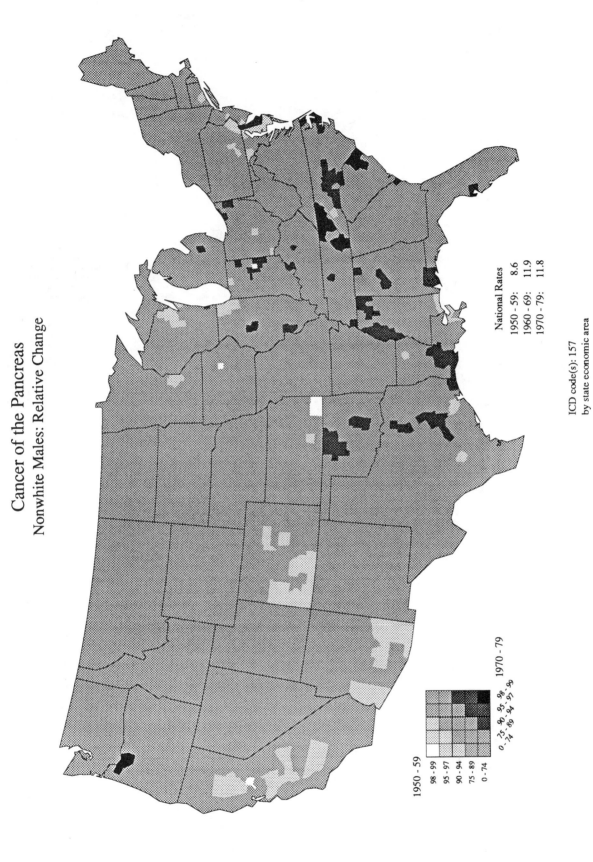

National Rates

1950 - 59: 8.6
1960 - 69: 11.9
1970 - 79: 11.8

ICD code(s): 157
by state economic area

1950 - 59

98 - 99
95 - 97
90 - 94
75 - 89
0 - 74

1970 - 79
98 - 99
95 - 97
90 - 94
75 - 89
0 - 74

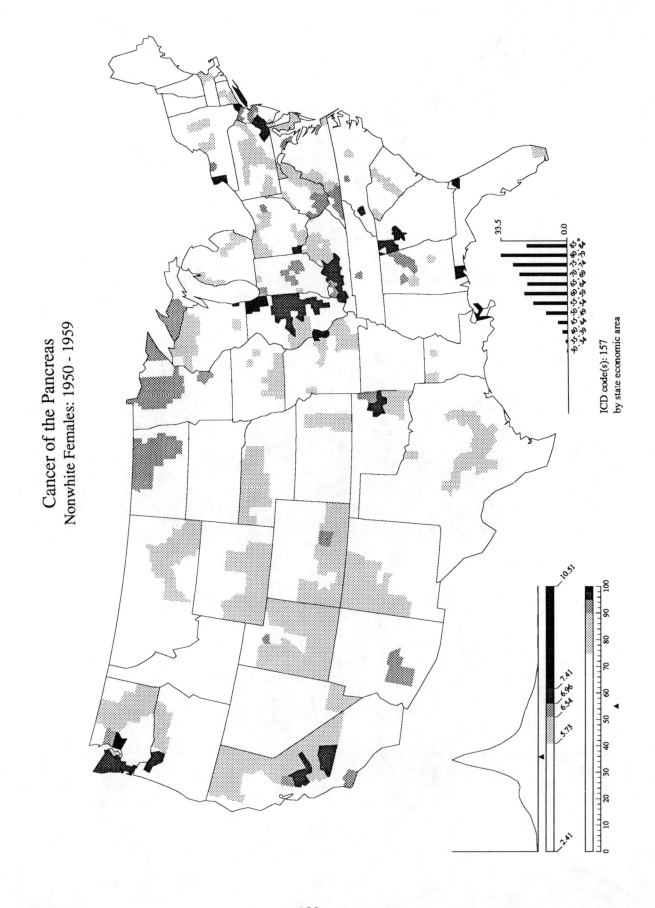

Cancer of the Pancreas
Nonwhite Females: 1950 - 1959

ICD code(s): 157
by state economic area

Cancer of the Pancreas
Nonwhite Females: 1960 - 1969

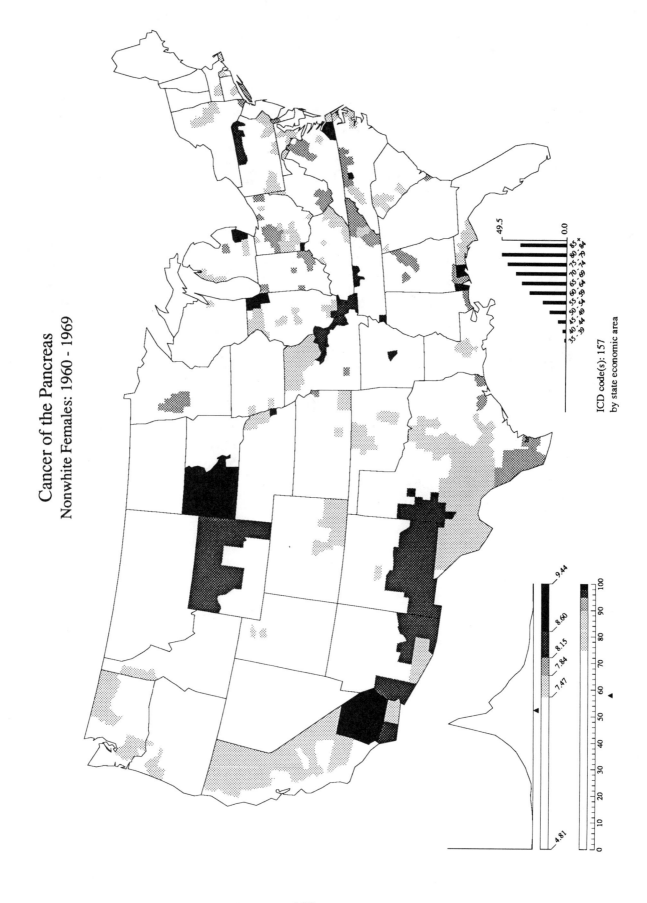

ICD code(s): 157
by state economic area

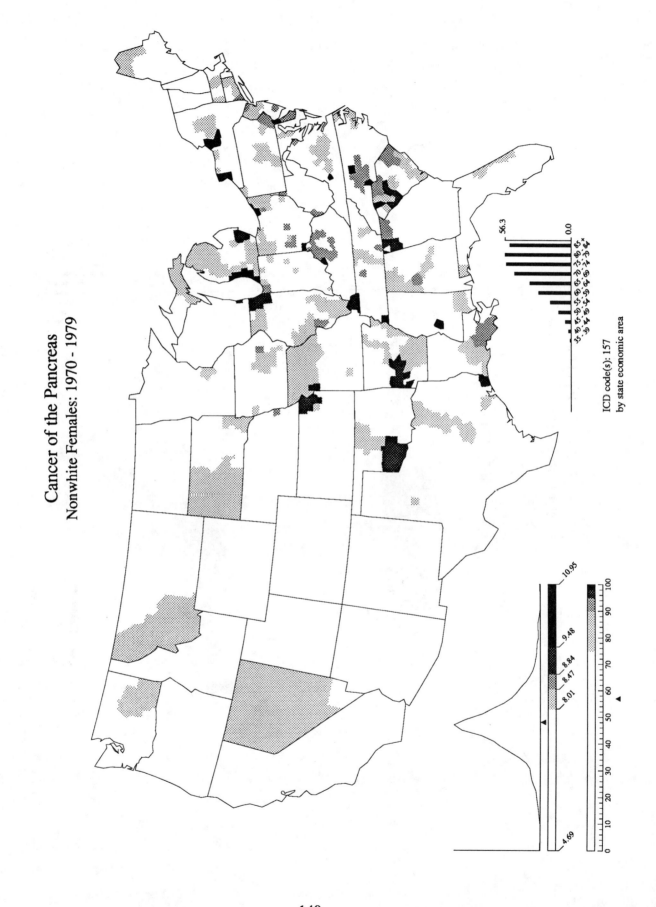

Cancer of the Pancreas
Nonwhite Females: 1970 - 1979

ICD code(s): 157
by state economic area

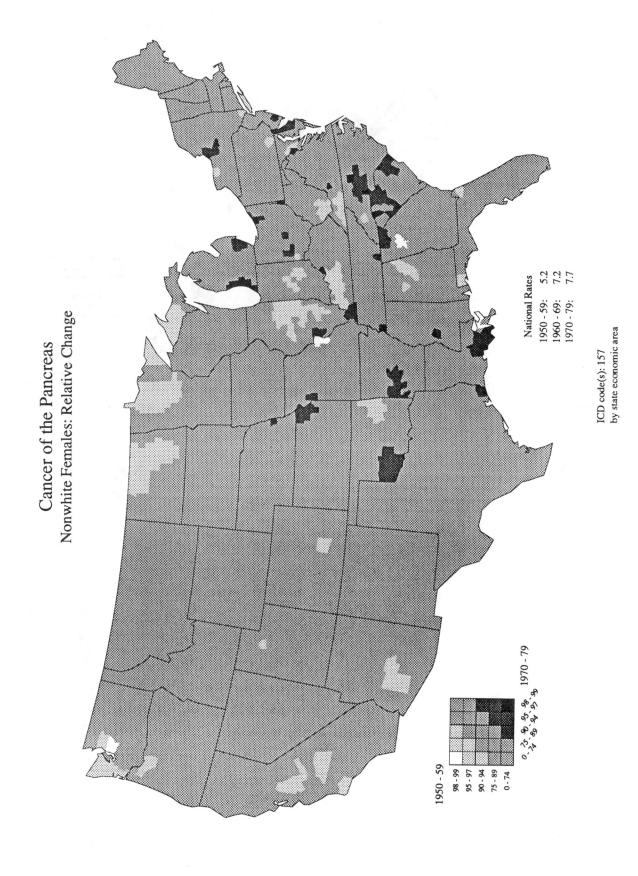

Cancer of the Pancreas
Nonwhite Females: Relative Change

National Rates

1950 - 59: 5.2
1960 - 69: 7.2
1970 - 79: 7.7

ICD code(s): 157
by state economic area

1950 - 59

98 - 99
95 - 97
90 - 94
75 - 89
0 - 74

1970 - 79

0 - 74 75 - 89 90 - 94 95 - 97 98 - 99

141

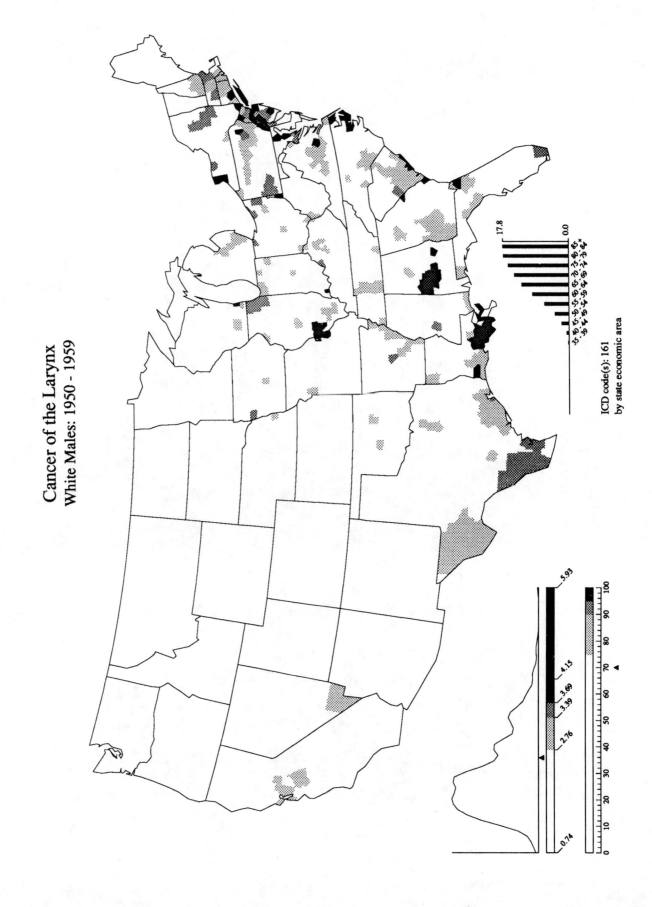

Cancer of the Larynx
White Males: 1950 - 1959

ICD code(s): 161
by state economic area

142

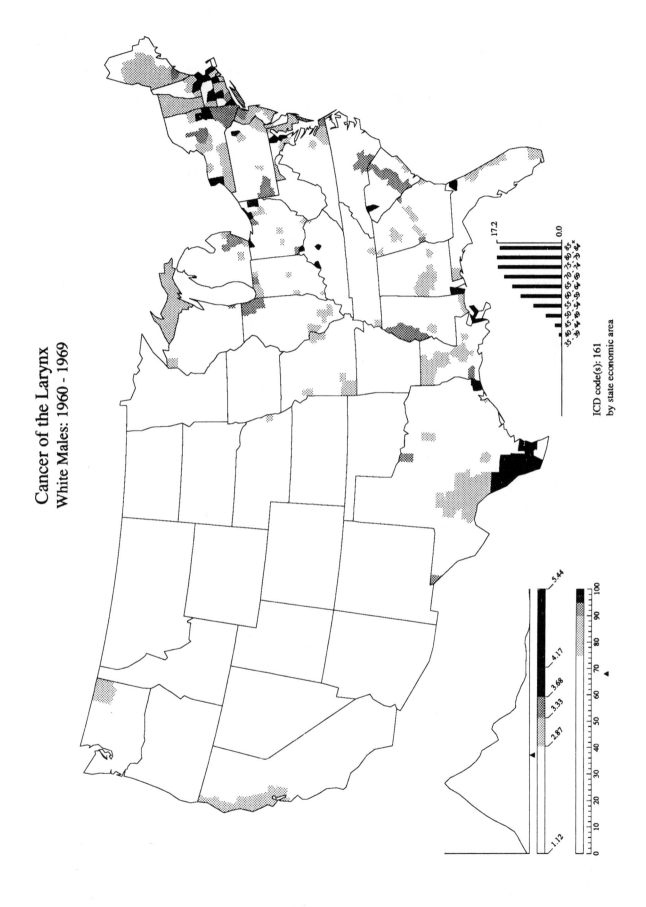

Cancer of the Larynx
White Males: 1960 - 1969

ICD code(s): 161
by state economic area

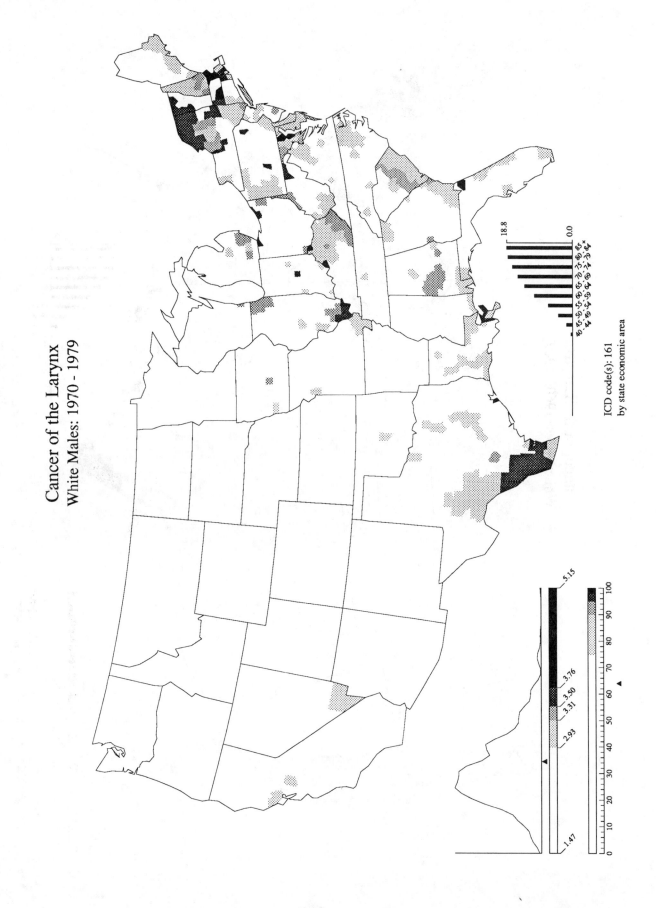

Cancer of the Larynx
White Males: 1970 - 1979

ICD code(s): 161
by state economic area

Cancer of the Larynx
White Males: Relative Change

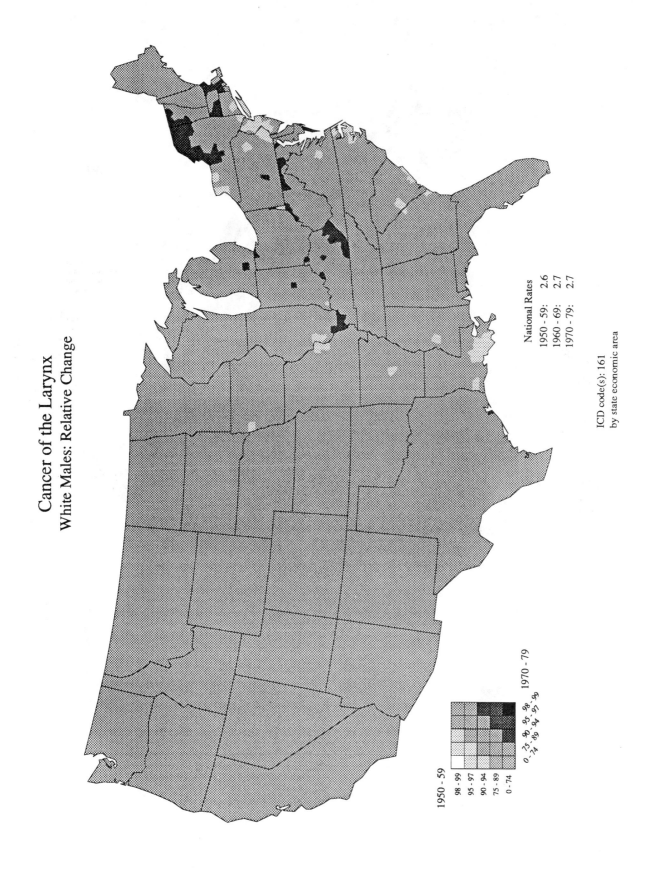

National Rates

1950 - 59:   2.6
1960 - 69:   2.7
1970 - 79:   2.7

ICD code(s): 161
by state economic area

1950 - 59
98 - 99
95 - 97
90 - 94
75 - 89
0 - 74

1970 - 79
98 - 99
95 - 97
90 - 94
75 - 89
0 - 74

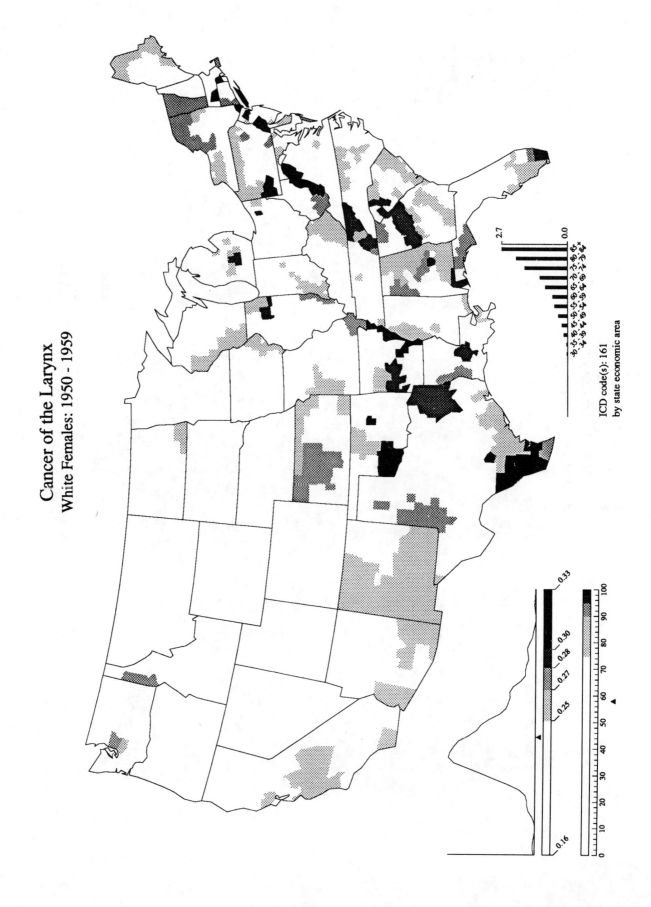

Cancer of the Larynx
White Females: 1950 - 1959

ICD code(s): 161
by state economic area

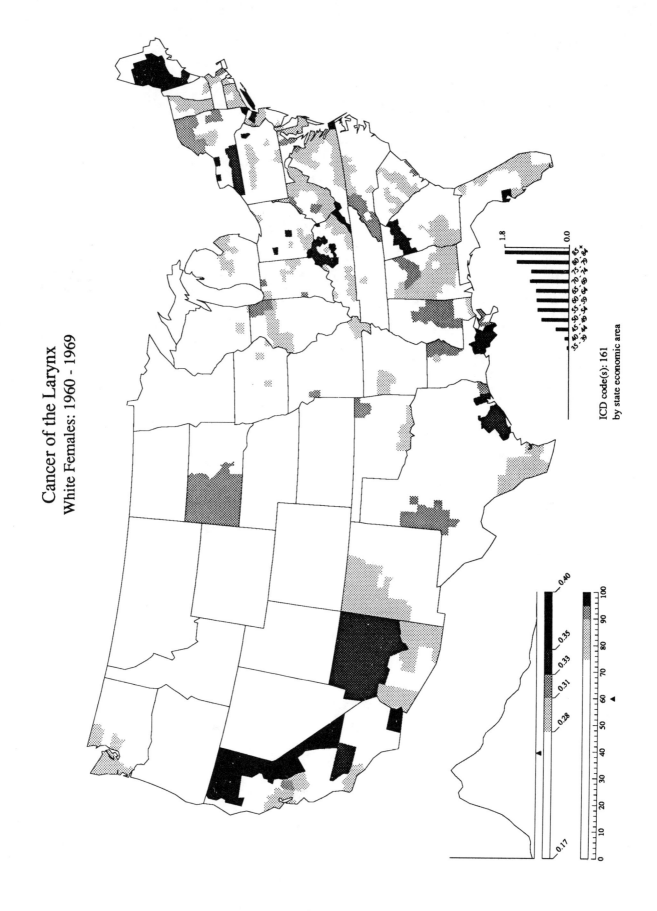

Cancer of the Larynx
White Females: 1960 - 1969

ICD code(s): 161
by state economic area

147

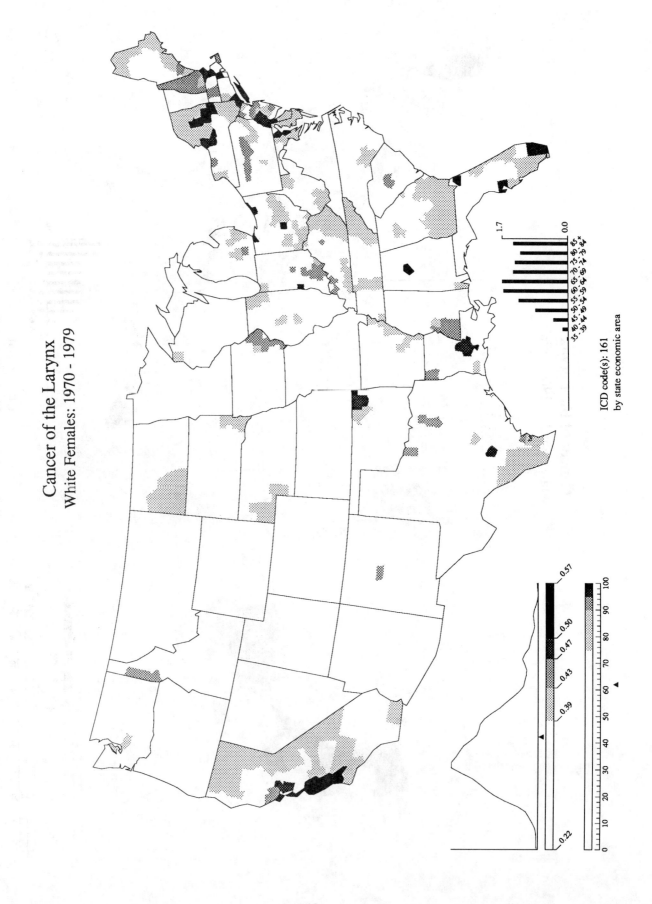

Cancer of the Larynx
White Females: 1970 - 1979

ICD code(s): 161
by state economic area

Cancer of the Larynx
White Females: Relative Change

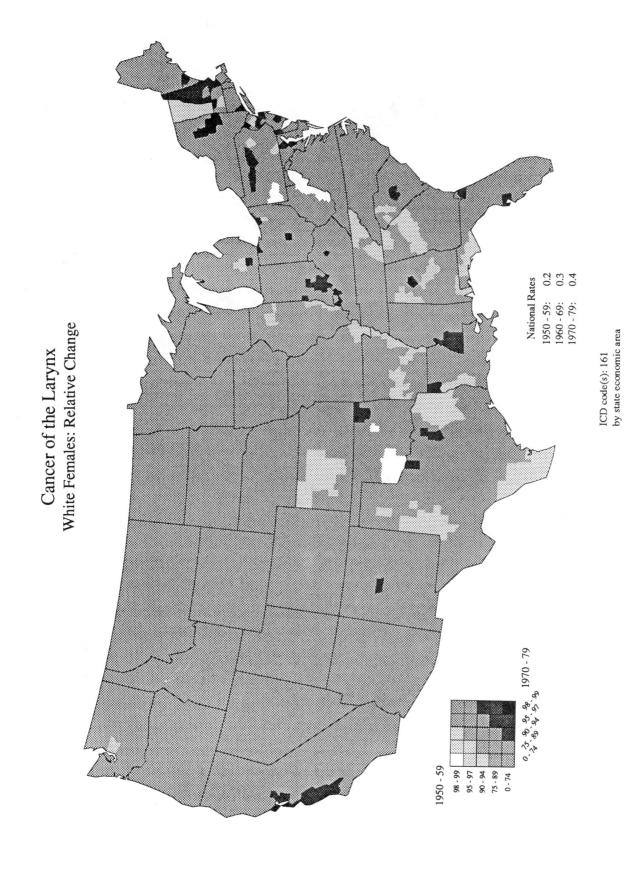

National Rates

1950 - 59: 0.2
1960 - 69: 0.3
1970 - 79: 0.4

ICD code(s): 161
by state economic area

1950 - 59

98 - 99
95 - 97
90 - 94
75 - 89
0 - 74

0 - 75 - 90 - 95 - 98 - 99
74   89   94   97   99
1970 - 79

149

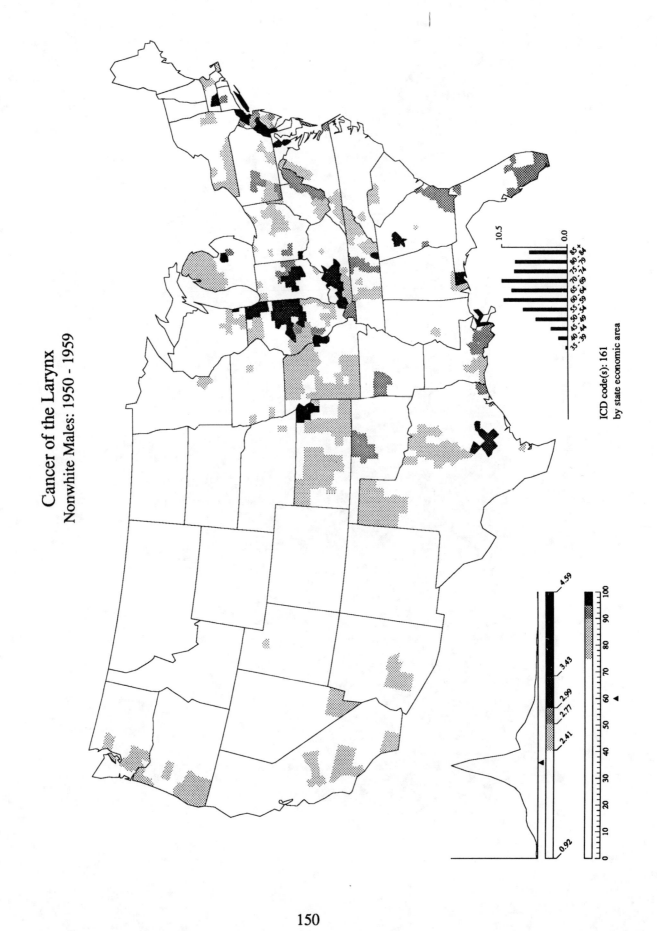

Cancer of the Larynx
Nonwhite Males: 1950 - 1959

ICD code(s): 161
by state economic area

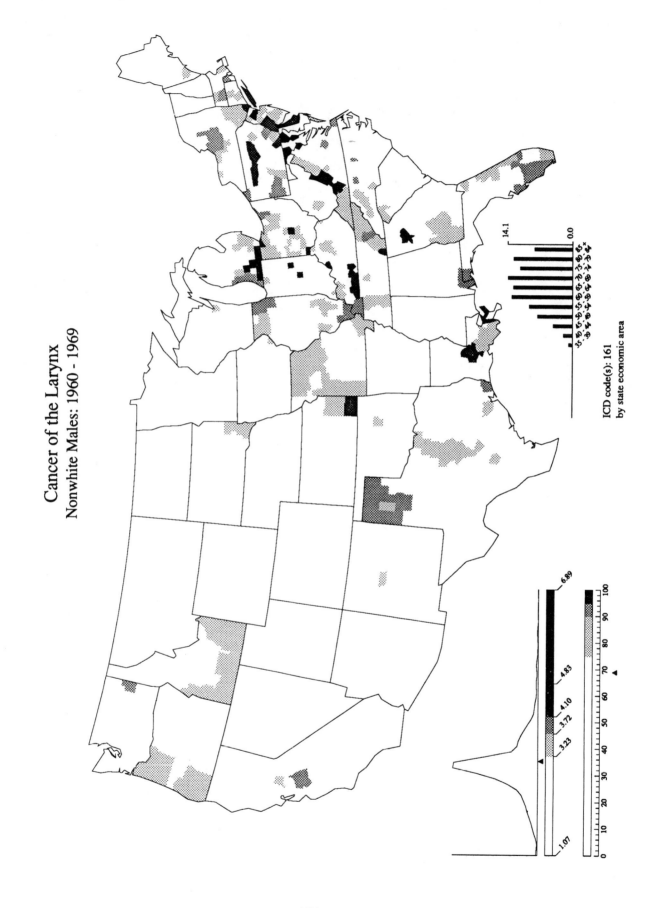

Cancer of the Larynx
Nonwhite Males: 1960 - 1969

ICD code(s): 161
by state economic area

151

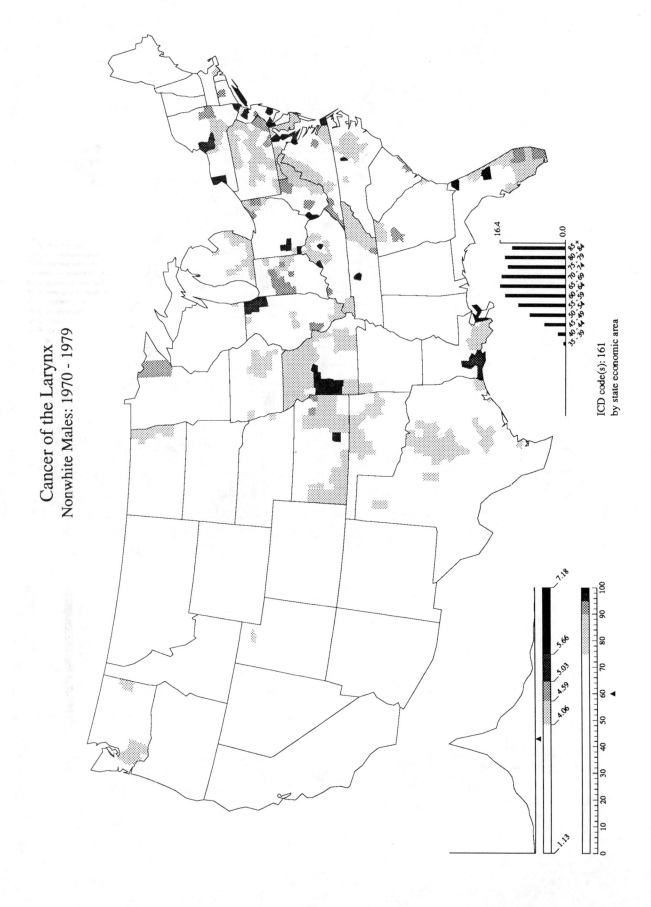

Cancer of the Larynx
Nonwhite Males: 1970 - 1979

ICD code(s): 161
by state economic area

Cancer of the Larynx
Nonwhite Males: Relative Change

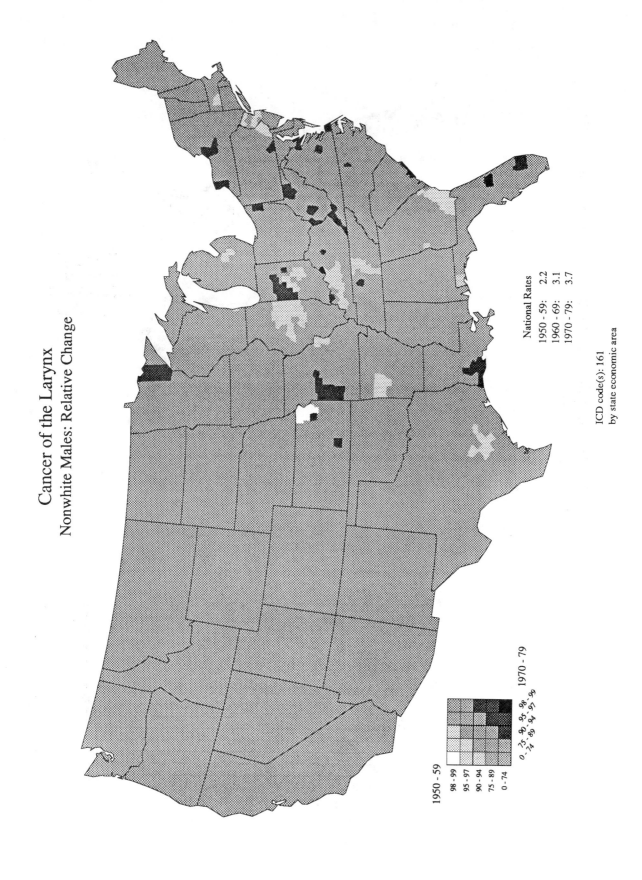

National Rates

1950 - 59:   2.2
1960 - 69:   3.1
1970 - 79:   3.7

ICD code(s): 161
by state economic area

1950 - 59

98 - 99
95 - 97
90 - 94
75 - 89
0 - 74

1970 - 79

0 - 75 - 90 - 95 - 98 - 99
  74 89 94 97

Cancer of the Trachea, Bronchus and Lung including Pleura and Other Respiratory Sites
White Males: 1950 - 1959

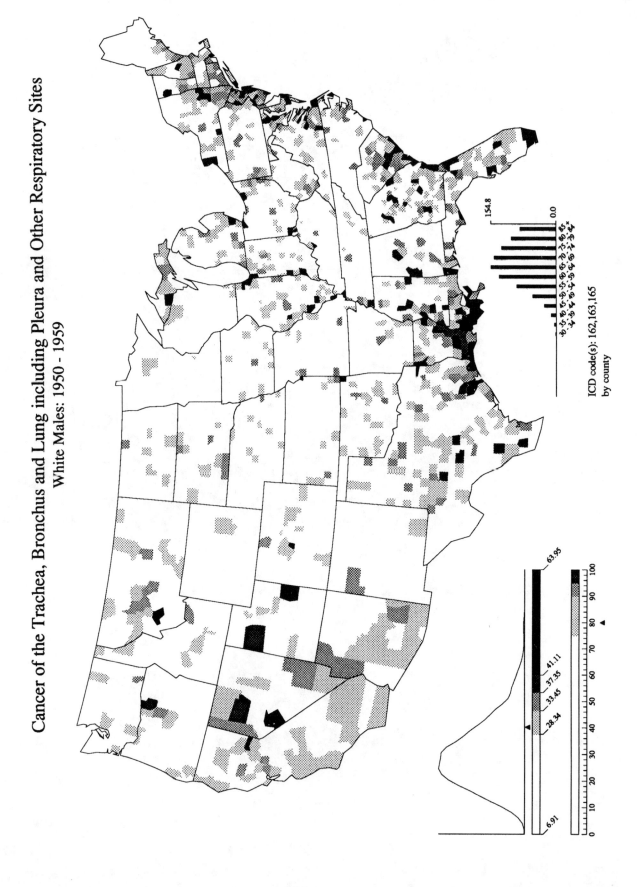

ICD code(s): 162,163,165
by county

Cancer of the Trachea, Bronchus and Lung including Pleura and Other Respiratory Sites
White Males: 1960 - 1969

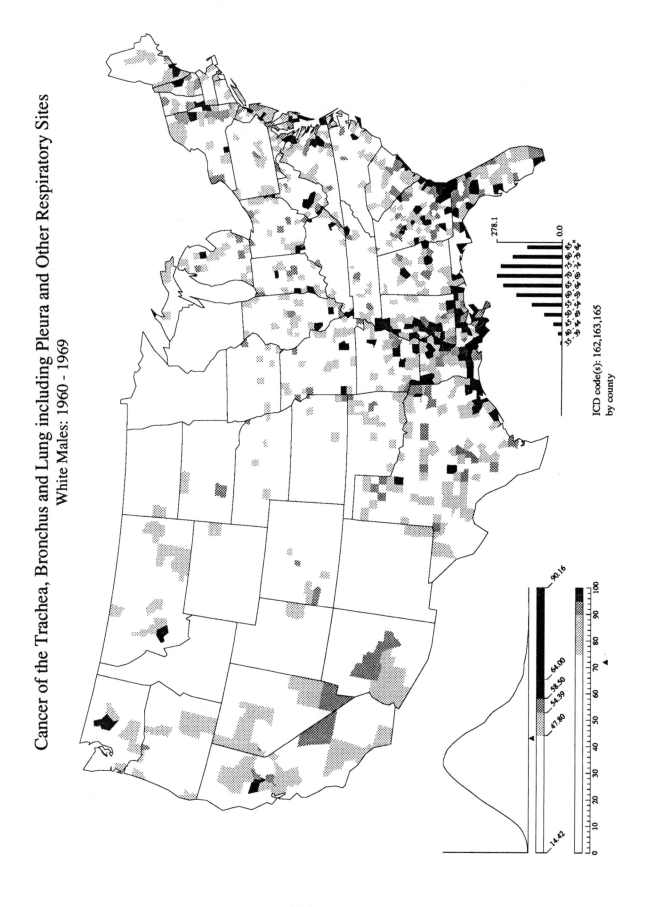

Cancer of the Trachea, Bronchus and Lung including Pleura and Other Respiratory Sites
White Males: 1970 - 1979

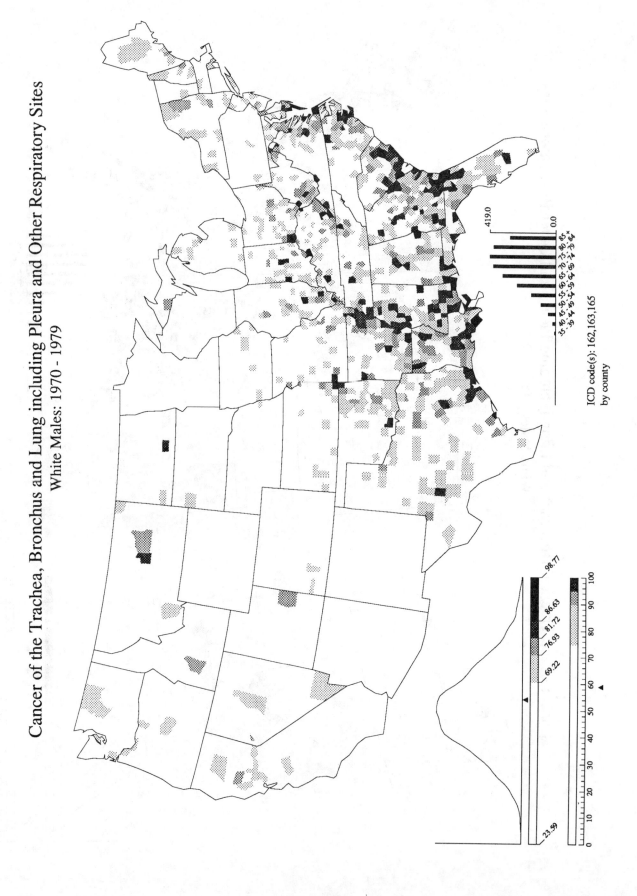

ICD code(s): 162,163,165
by county

156

Cancer of the Trachea, Bronchus and Lung including Pleura and Other Respiratory Sites
White Males: Relative Change

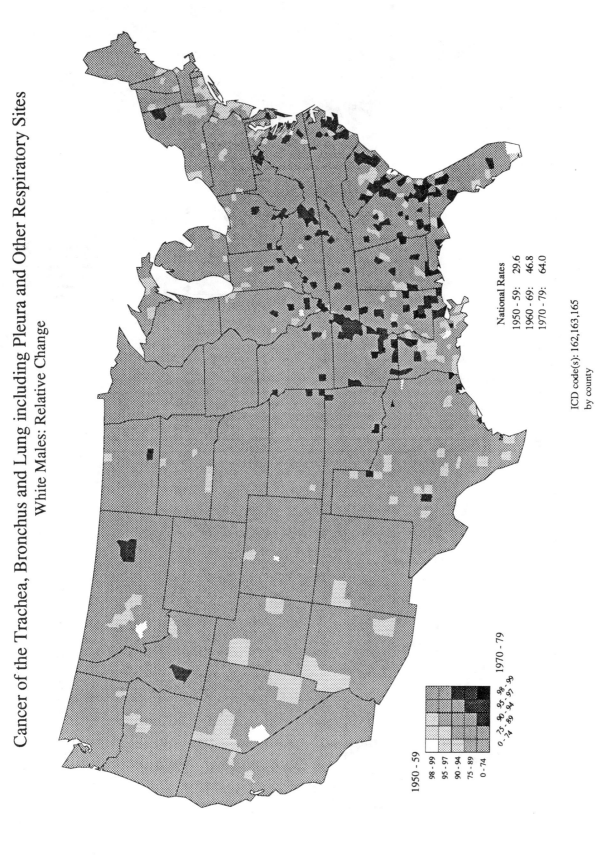

National Rates

1950 - 59:   29.6
1960 - 69:   46.8
1970 - 79:   64.0

ICD code(s): 162,163,165
by county

1950 - 59

98 - 99
95 - 97
90 - 94
75 - 89
0 - 74

1970 - 79

0 - 74 75 - 89 90 - 94 95 - 97 98 - 99

157

Cancer of the Trachea, Bronchus and Lung including Pleura and Other Respiratory Sites
White Females: 1950 - 1959

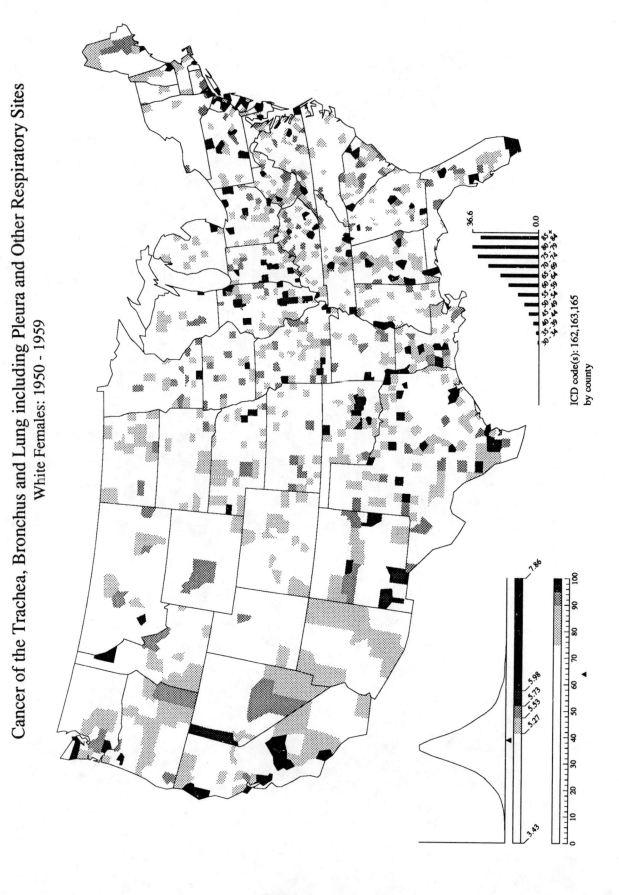

ICD code(s): 162,163,165
by county

Cancer of the Trachea, Bronchus and Lung including Pleura and Other Respiratory Sites
White Females: 1960 - 1969

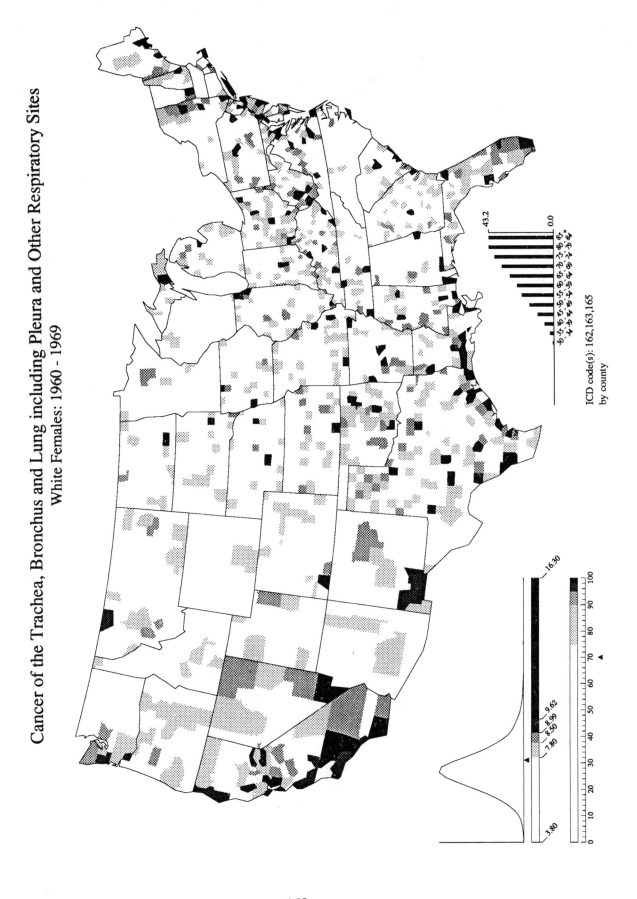

ICD code(s): 162,163,165
by county

Cancer of the Trachea, Bronchus and Lung including Pleura and Other Respiratory Sites
White Females: 1970 - 1979

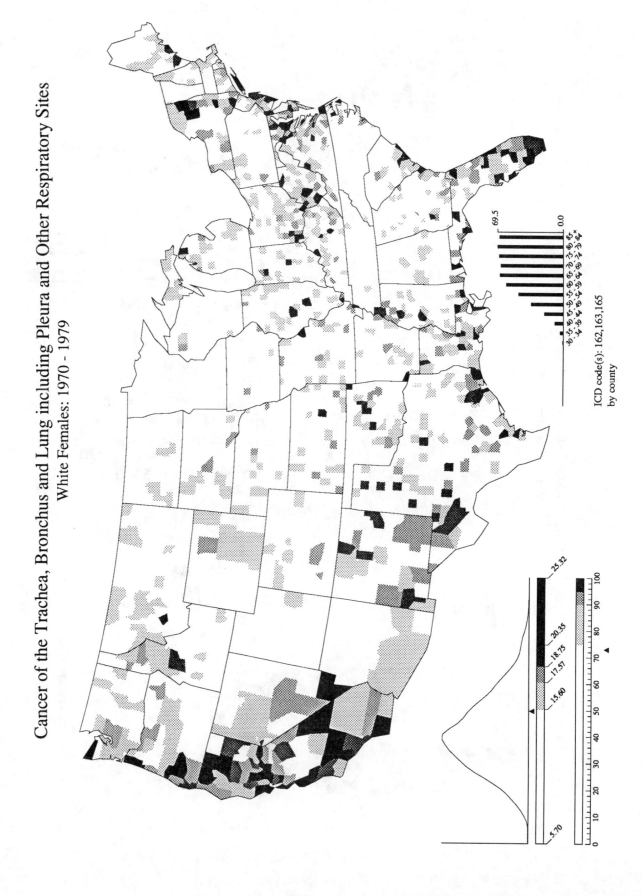

ICD code(s): 162,163,165
by county

Cancer of the Trachea, Bronchus and Lung including Pleura and Other Respiratory Sites
White Females: Relative Change

National Rates

1950 - 59:	5.1
1960 - 69:	7.6
1970 - 79:	15.3

ICD code(s): 162,163,165
by county

1950 - 59

98 - 99
95 - 97
90 - 94
75 - 89
0 - 74

1970 - 79

0 - 74 75 - 89 90 - 94 95 - 97 98 - 99

161

Cancer of the Trachea, Bronchus and Lung including Pleura and Other Respiratory Sites
Nonwhite Males: 1950 - 1959

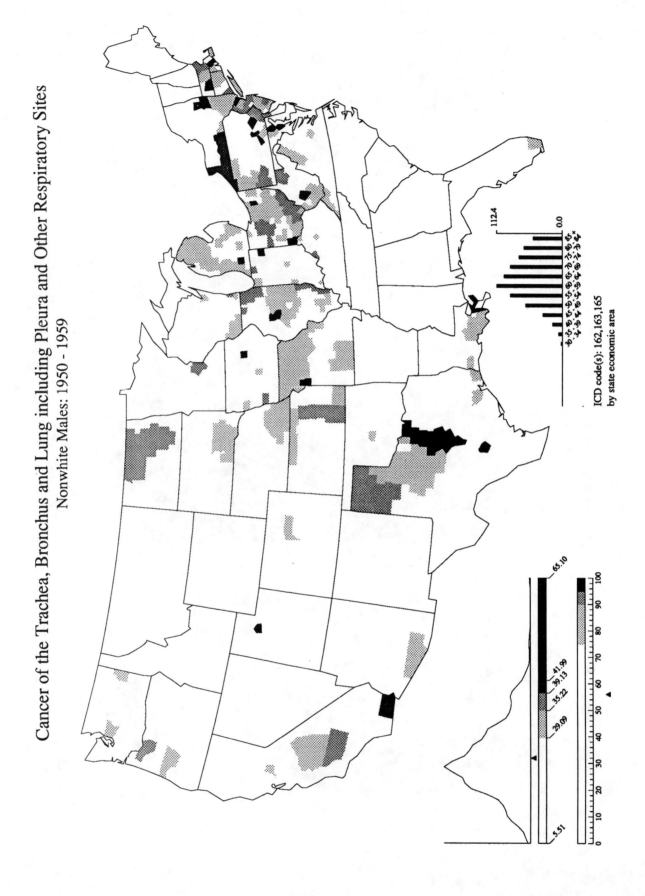

ICD code(s): 162,163,165
by state economic area

Cancer of the Trachea, Bronchus and Lung including Pleura and Other Respiratory Sites
Nonwhite Males: 1960 - 1969

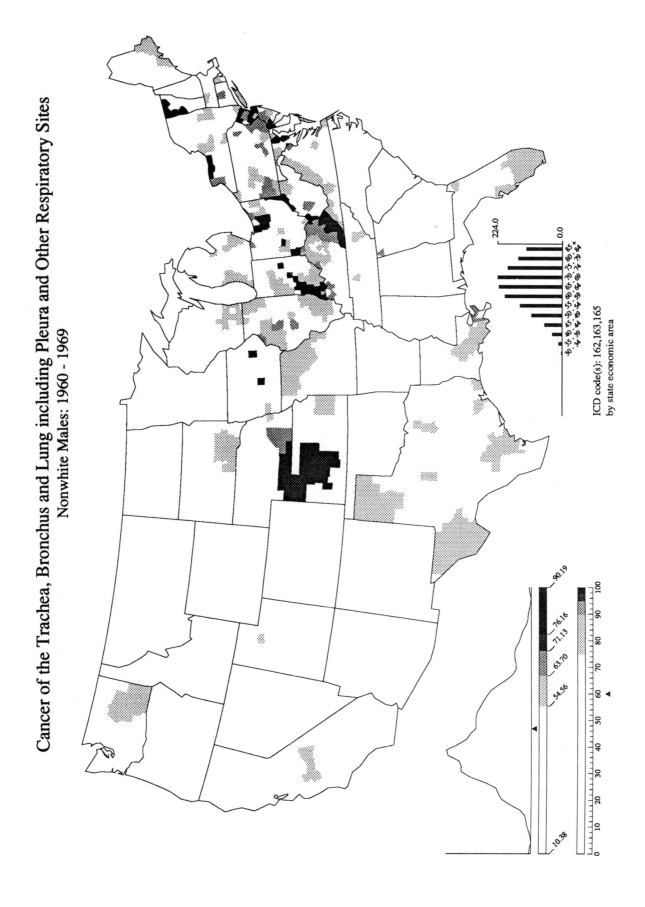

ICD code(s): 162,163,165
by state economic area

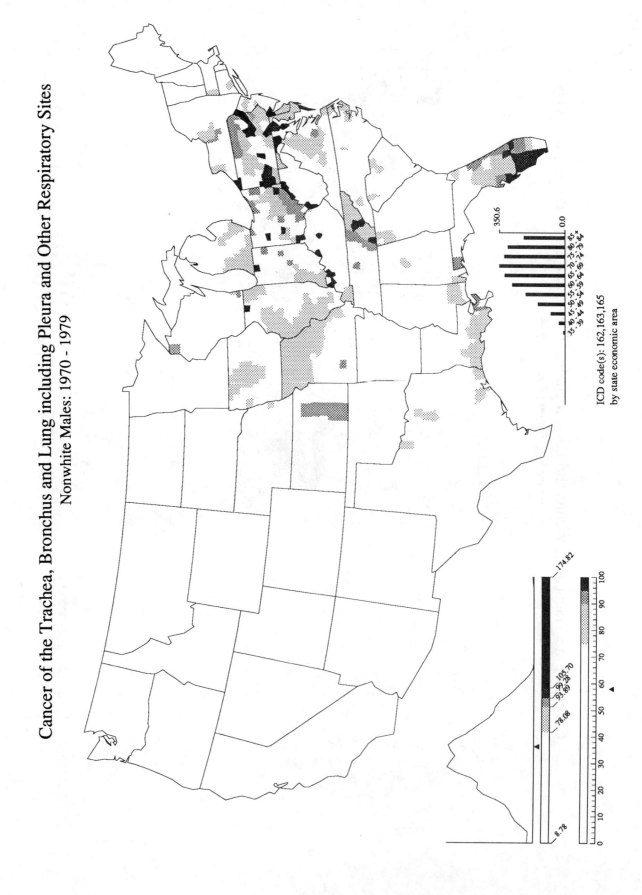

Cancer of the Trachea, Bronchus and Lung including Pleura and Other Respiratory Sites
Nonwhite Males: 1970 - 1979

ICD code(s): 162,163,165
by state economic area

Cancer of the Trachea, Bronchus and Lung including Pleura and Other Respiratory Sites
Nonwhite Males: Relative Change

National Rates

1950 - 59:	24.1
1960 - 69:	47.4
1970 - 79:	68.6

ICD code(s): 162,163,165
by state economic area

1950 - 59

1970 - 79

98 - 99
95 - 97
90 - 94
75 - 89
0 - 74

0 - 74   75 - 89   90 - 94   95 - 97   98 - 99

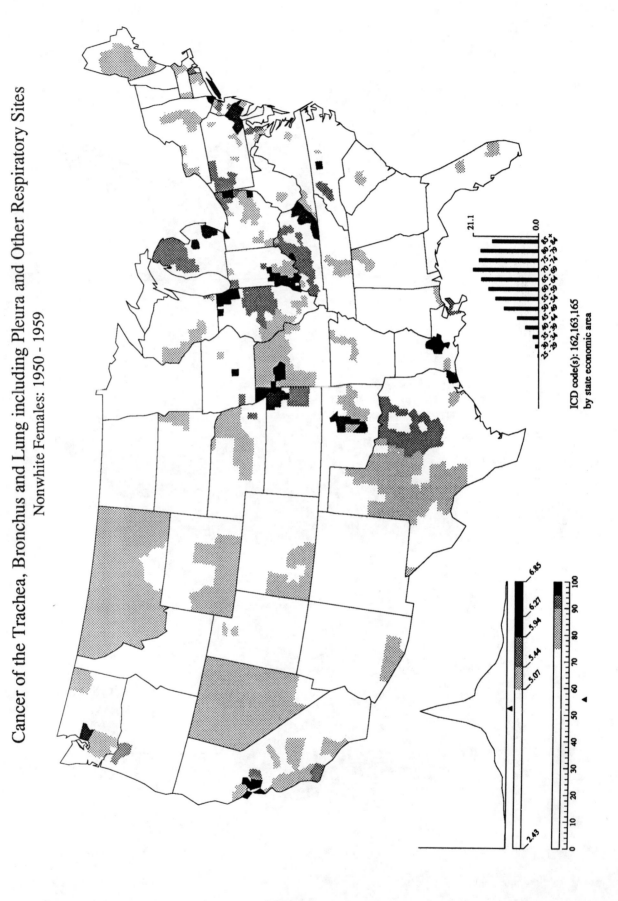

Cancer of the Trachea, Bronchus and Lung including Pleura and Other Respiratory Sites
Nonwhite Females: 1950 - 1959

ICD code(s): 162,163,165
by state economic area

Cancer of the Trachea, Bronchus and Lung including Pleura and Other Respiratory Sites
Nonwhite Females: 1960 - 1969

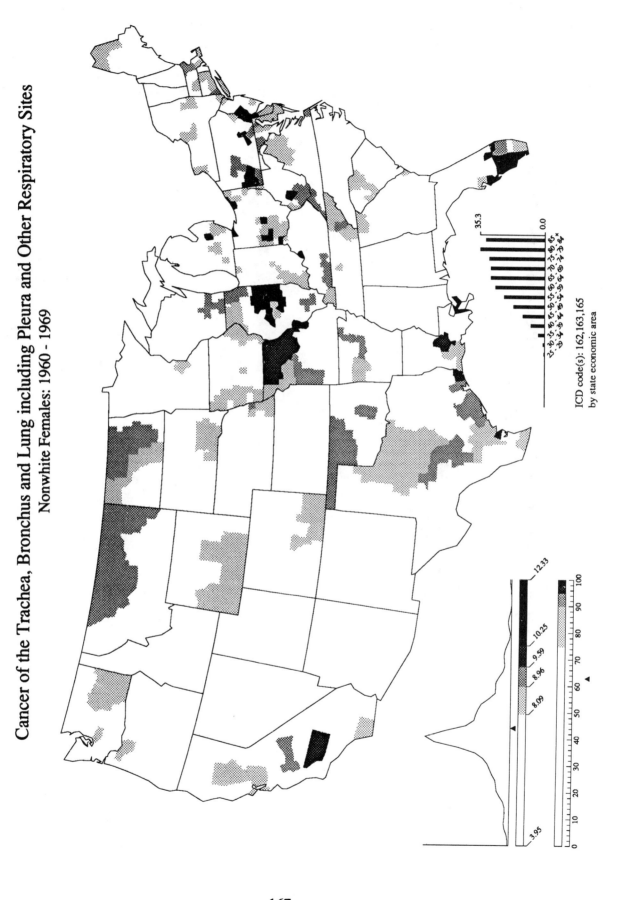

ICD code(s): 162,163,165
by state economic area

Cancer of the Trachea, Bronchus and Lung including Pleura and Other Respiratory Sites
Nonwhite Females: 1970 - 1979

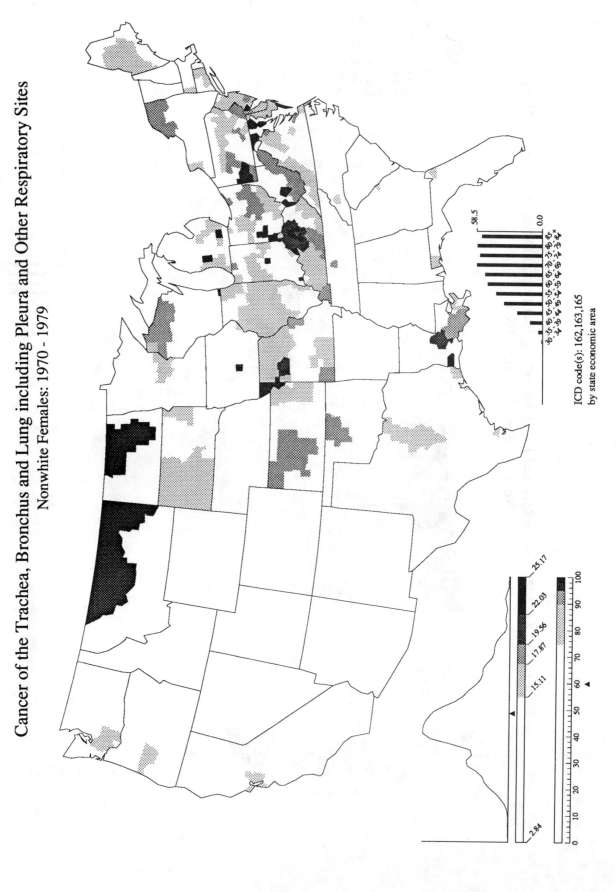

ICD code(s): 162,163,165
by state economic area

168

Cancer of the Trachea, Bronchus and Lung including Pleura and Other Respiratory Sites
Nonwhite Females: Relative Change

National Rates

1950 - 59:	4.7
1960 - 69:	7.5
1970 - 79:	13.5

ICD code(s): 162,163,165
by state economic area

1950 - 59

98 - 99
95 - 97
90 - 94
75 - 89
0 - 74

0 - 75 - 90 - 95 - 98 - 99
74   89   94   97   99

1970 - 79

Connective and Soft Tissue Cancer
White Males: 1950 - 1959

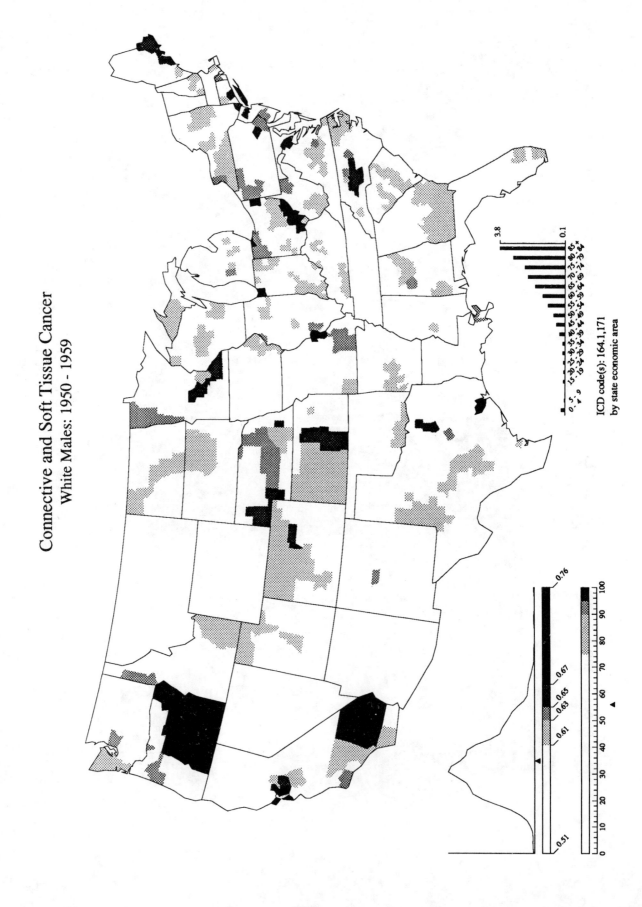

ICD code(s): 164.1,171
by state economic area

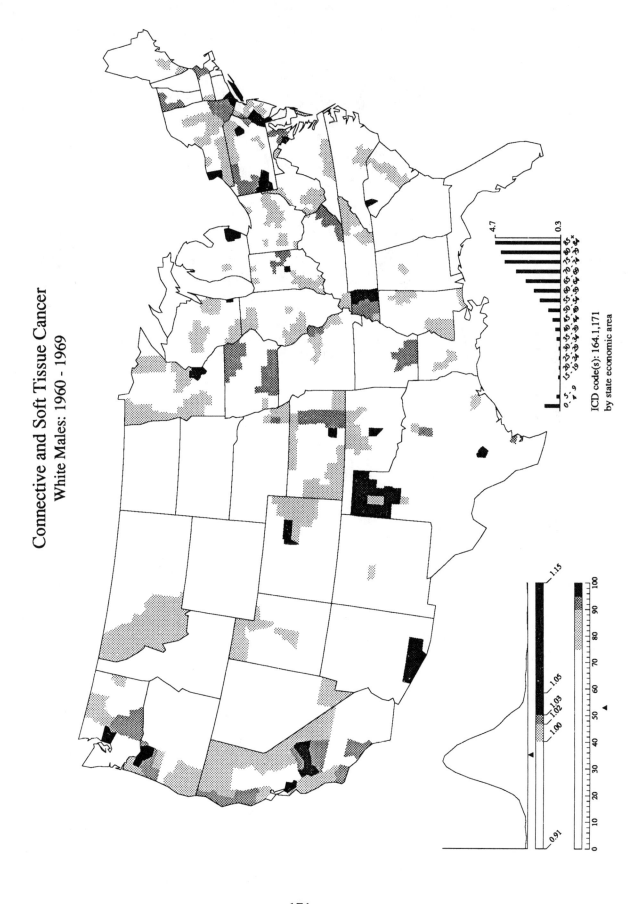

Connective and Soft Tissue Cancer
White Males: 1960 - 1969

ICD code(s): 164.1,171
by state economic area

Connective and Soft Tissue Cancer
White Males: 1970 - 1979

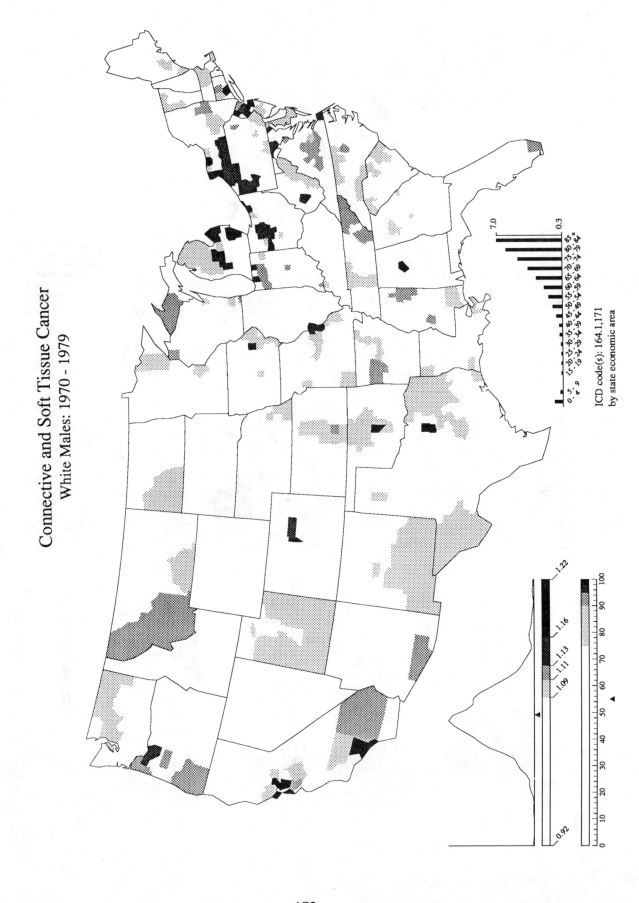

ICD code(s): 164.1,171
by state economic area

172

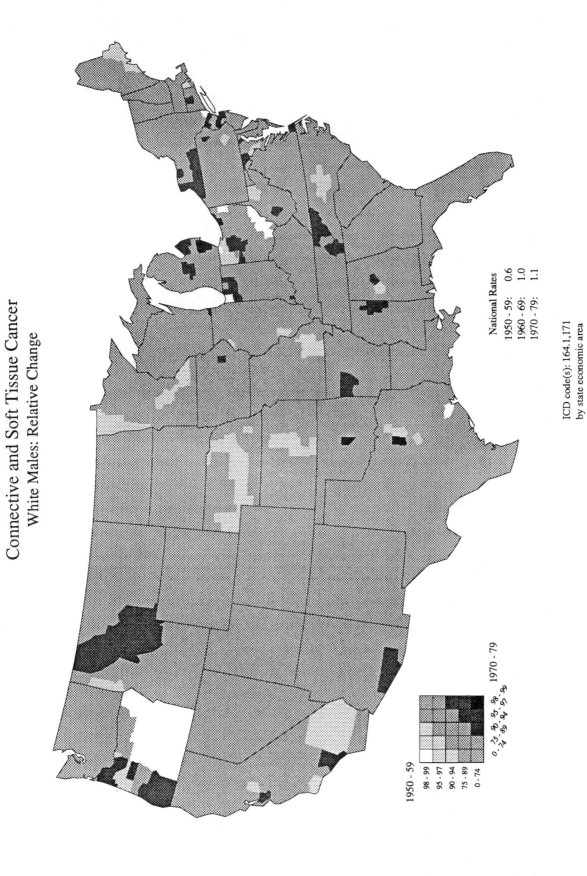

Connective and Soft Tissue Cancer
White Males: Relative Change

National Rates

1950 - 59:	0.6
1960 - 69:	1.0
1970 - 79:	1.1

ICD code(s): 164.1,171
by state economic area

1950 - 59

98 - 99
95 - 97
90 - 94
75 - 89
0 - 74

1970 - 79

98 - 99
95 - 97
90 - 94
75 - 89
0 - 74

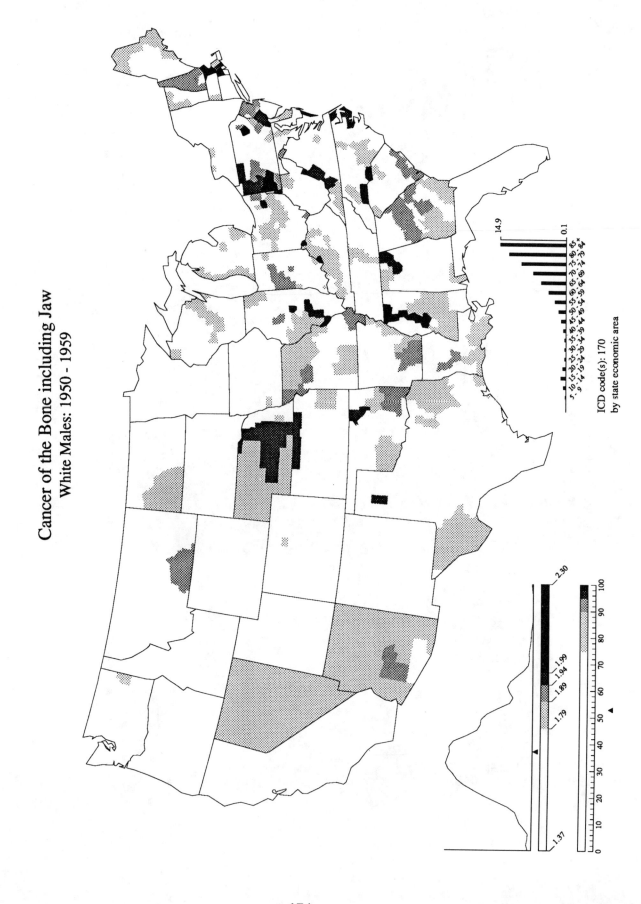

Cancer of the Bone including Jaw
White Males: 1950 - 1959

ICD code(s): 170
by state economic area

174

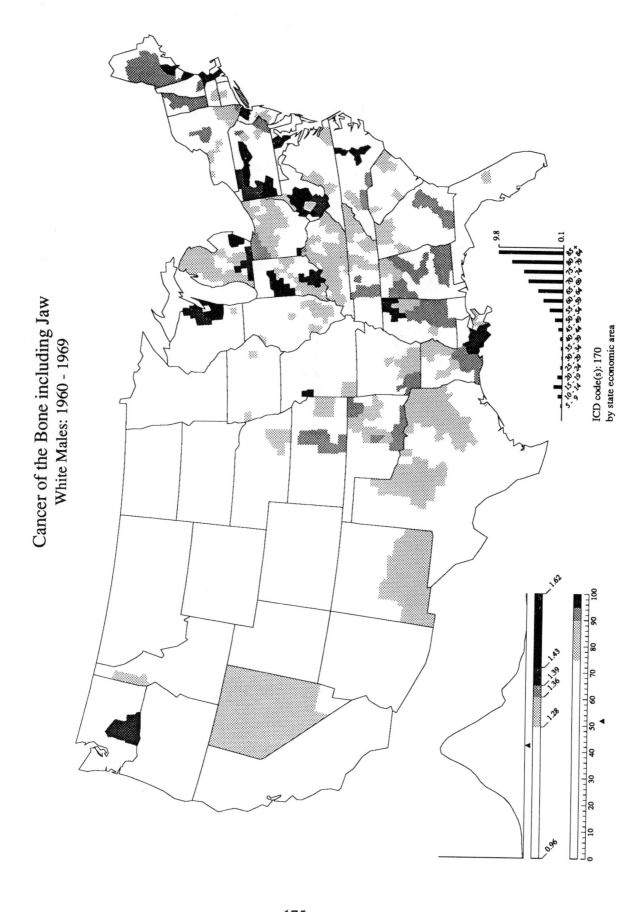

Cancer of the Bone including Jaw
White Males: 1960 - 1969

ICD code(s): 170
by state economic area

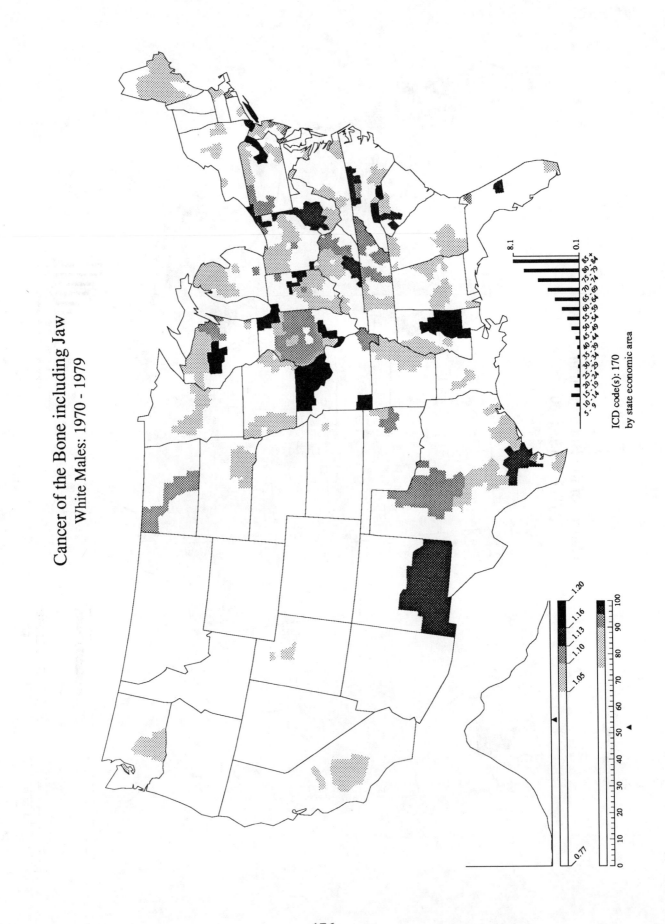

Cancer of the Bone including Jaw
White Males: 1970 - 1979

ICD code(s): 170
by state economic area

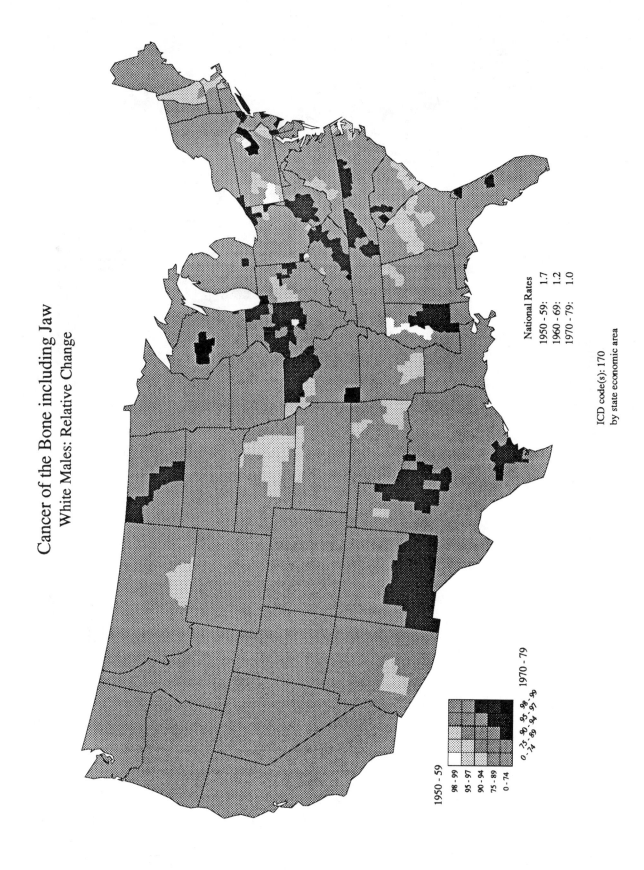

Cancer of the Bone including Jaw
White Males: Relative Change

National Rates

1950 - 59:   1.7
1960 - 69:   1.2
1970 - 79:   1.0

ICD code(s): 170
by state economic area

1950 - 59

98 - 99
95 - 97
90 - 94
75 - 89
0 - 74

1970 - 79

98 - 99
95 - 97
90 - 94
75 - 89
0 - 74

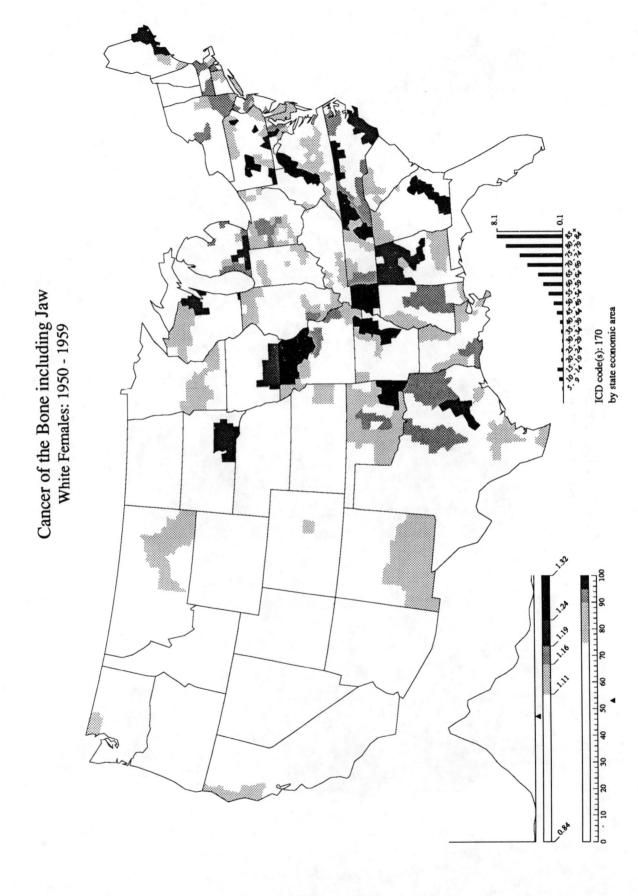

Cancer of the Bone including Jaw
White Females: 1950 - 1959

ICD code(s): 170
by state economic area

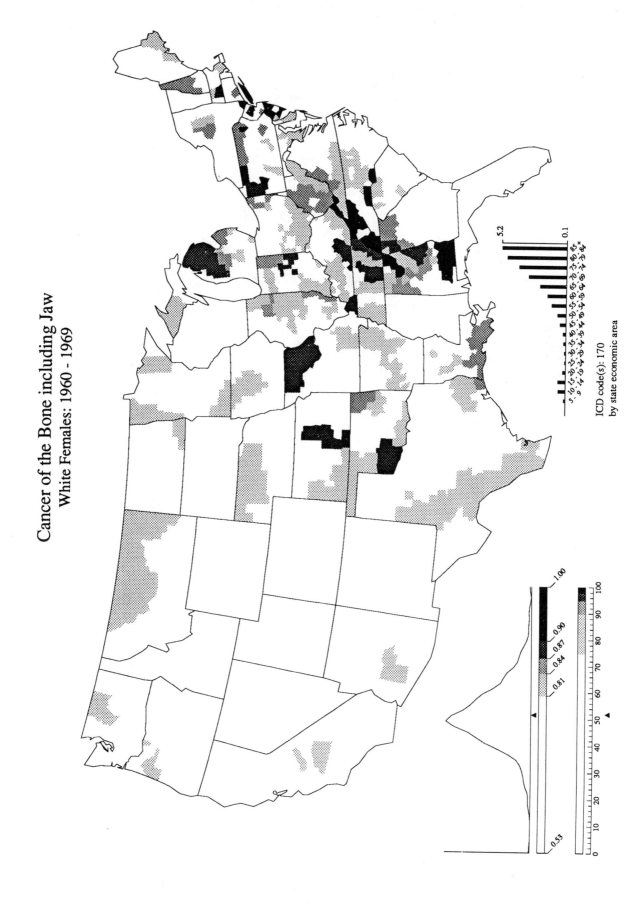

Cancer of the Bone including Jaw
White Females: 1960 - 1969

ICD code(s): 170
by state economic area

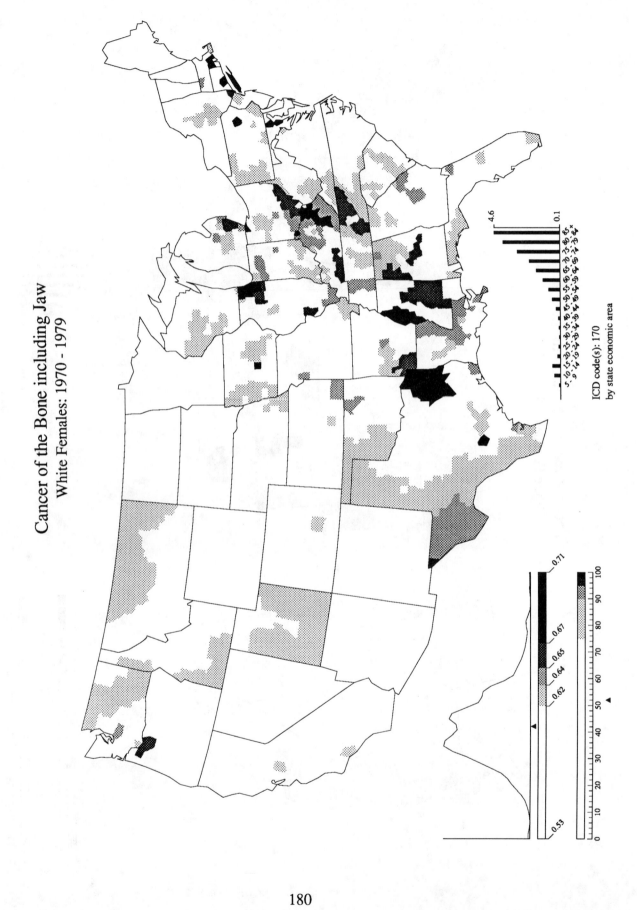

Cancer of the Bone including Jaw
White Females: 1970 - 1979

ICD code(s): 170
by state economic area

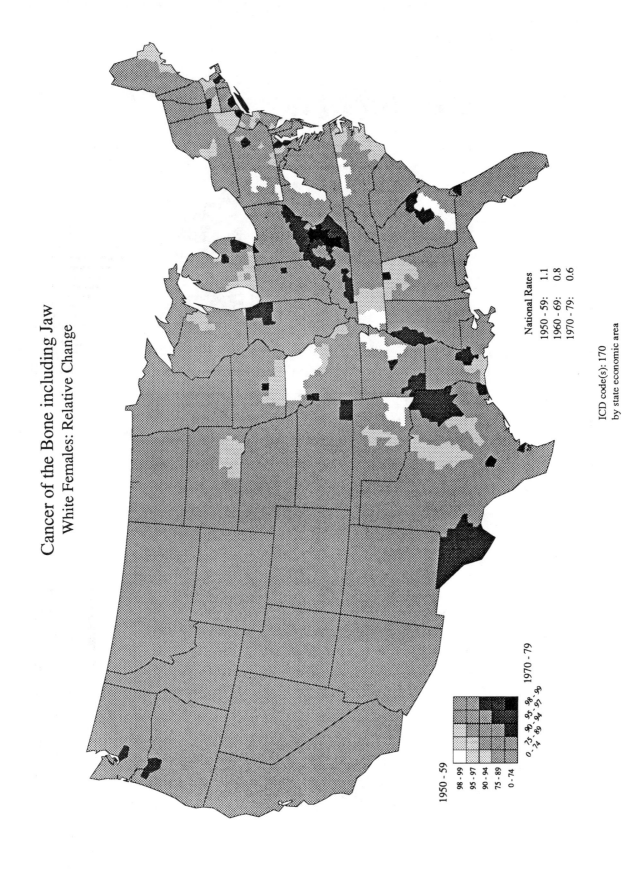

Cancer of the Bone including Jaw
White Females: Relative Change

National Rates

1950 - 59: 1.1
1960 - 69: 0.8
1970 - 79: 0.6

ICD code(s): 170
by state economic area

1950 - 59

98 - 99
95 - 97
90 - 94
75 - 89
0 - 74

1970 - 79

0 - 74
75 - 89
90 - 94
95 - 97
98 - 99

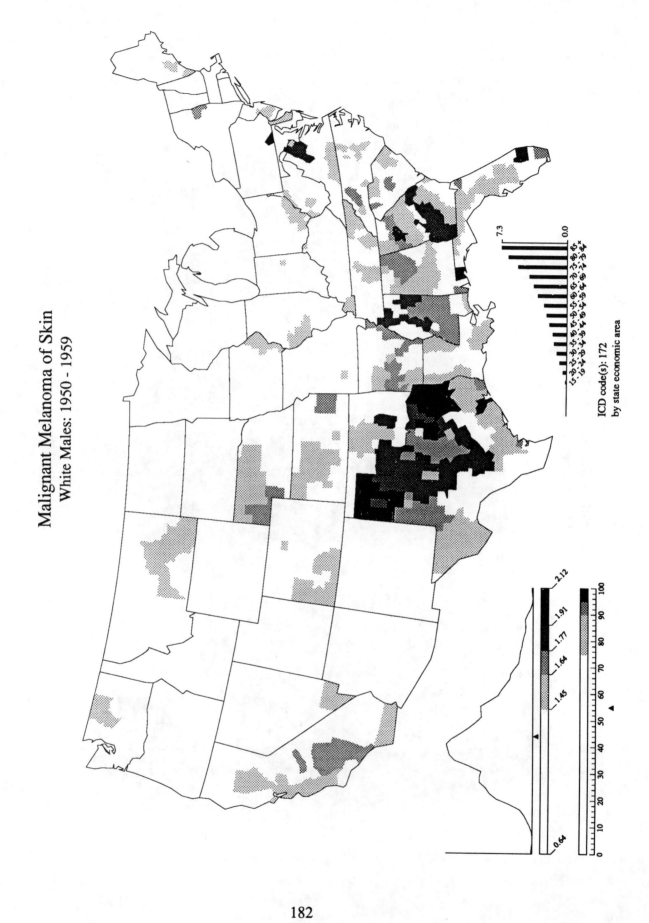

Malignant Melanoma of Skin
White Males: 1950 - 1959

ICD code(s): 172
by state economic area

182

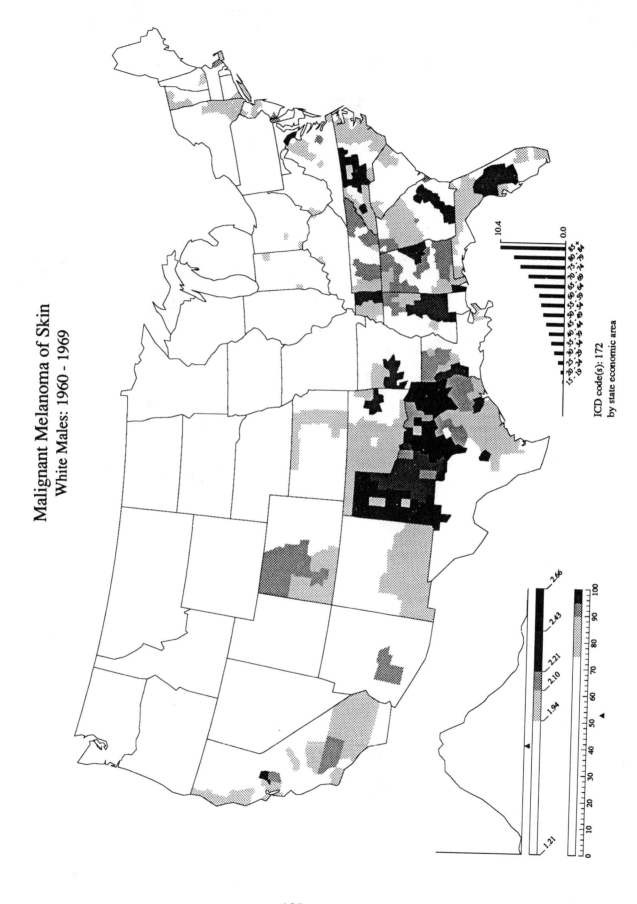

Malignant Melanoma of Skin
White Males: 1960 - 1969

ICD code(s): 172
by state economic area

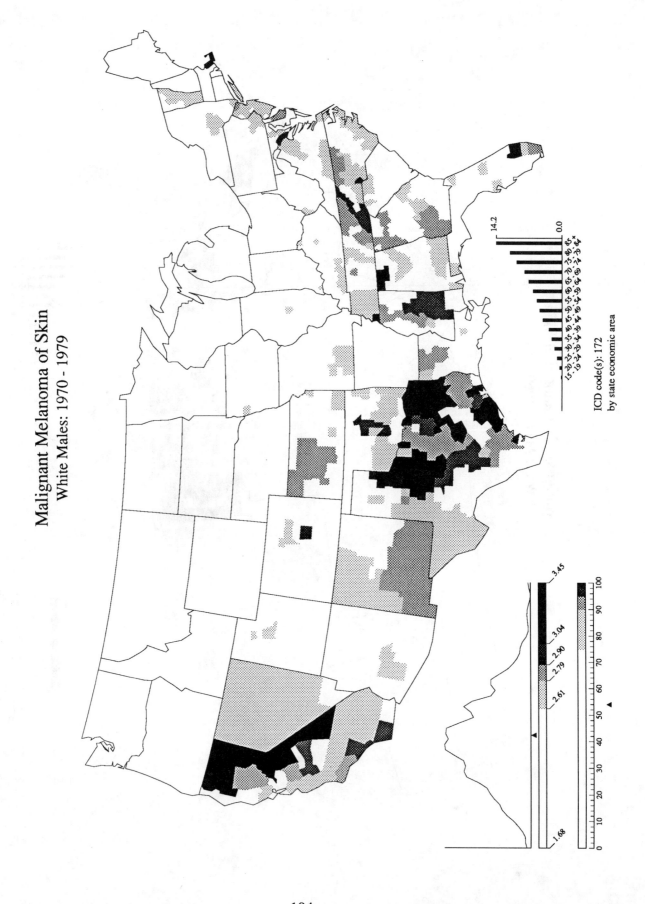

Malignant Melanoma of Skin
White Males: 1970 - 1979

ICD code(s): 172
by state economic area

Malignant Melanoma of Skin
White Males: Relative Change

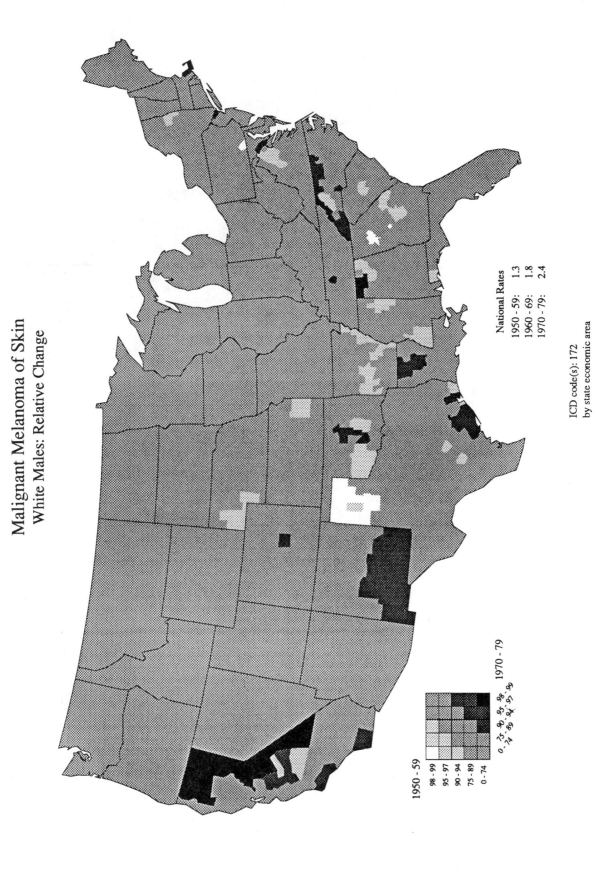

National Rates

1950 - 59:	1.3
1960 - 69:	1.8
1970 - 79:	2.4

ICD code(s): 172
by state economic area

1950 - 59
98 - 99
95 - 97
90 - 94
75 - 89
0 - 74

1970 - 79
0 - 74 89 94 97 99
75 - 90 95 98 98

185

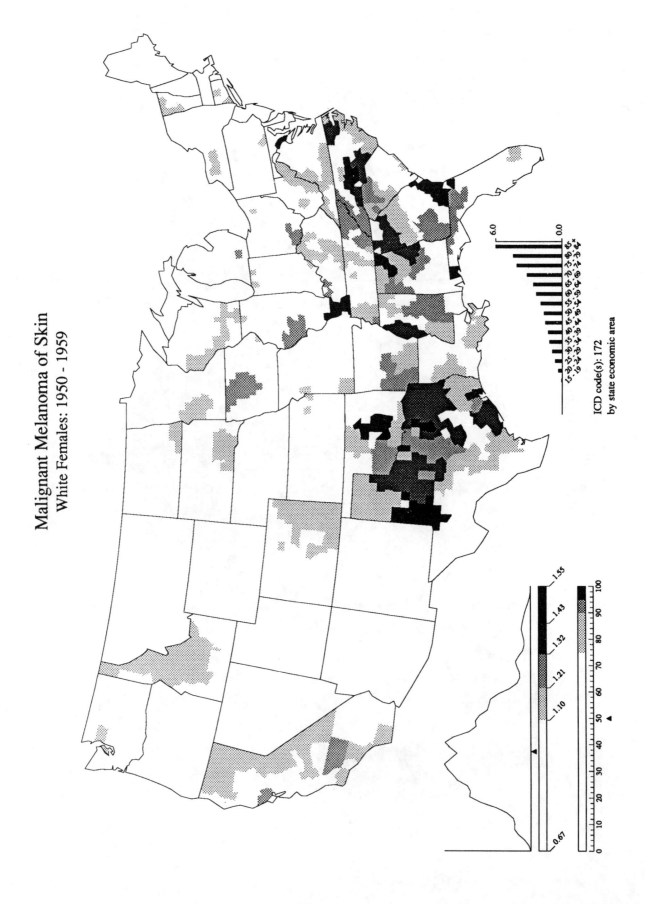

Malignant Melanoma of Skin
White Females: 1950 - 1959

ICD code(s): 172
by state economic area

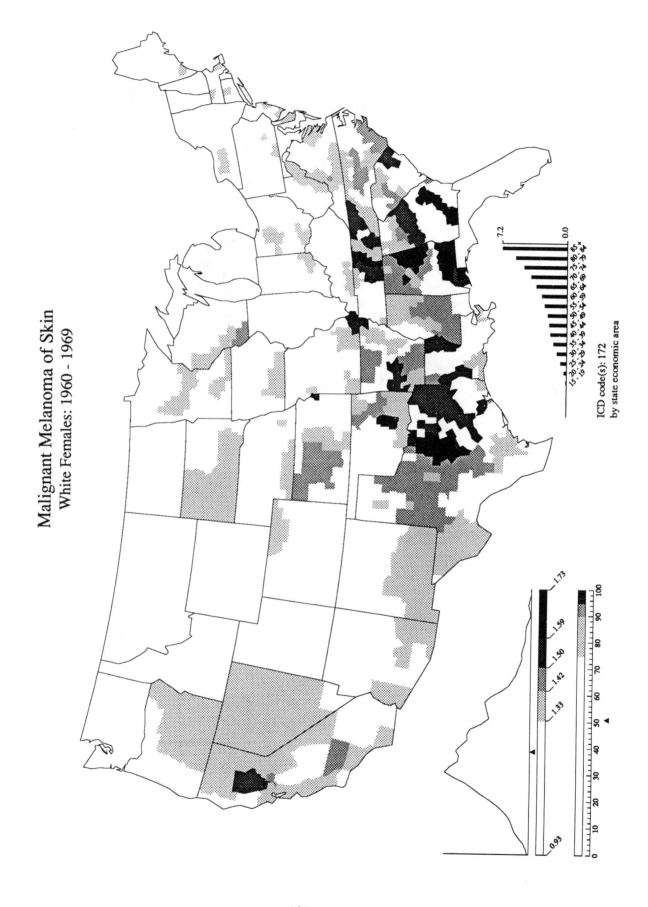

Malignant Melanoma of Skin
White Females: 1960 - 1969

ICD code(s): 172
by state economic area

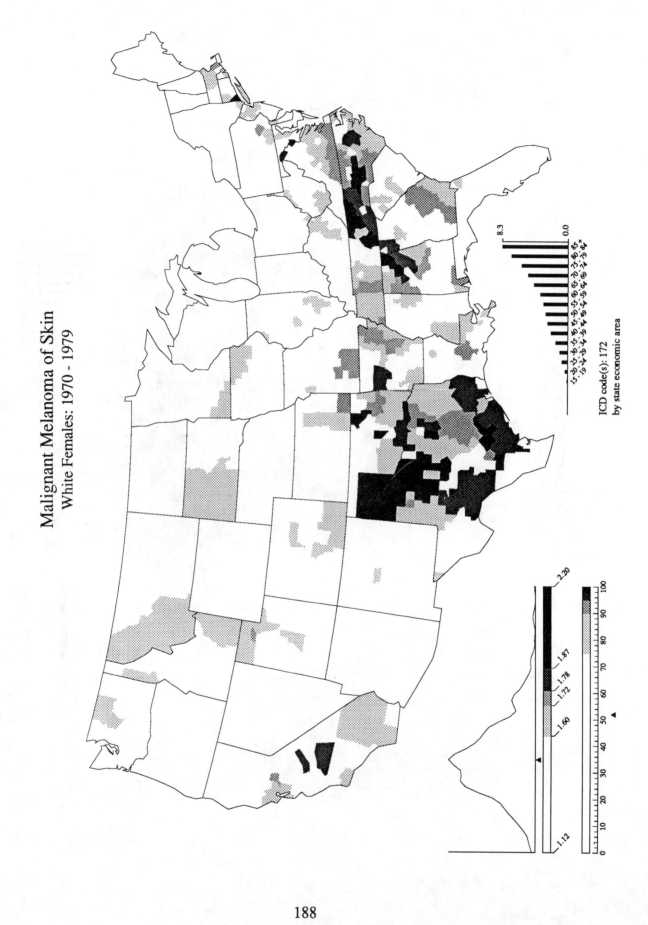

Malignant Melanoma of Skin
White Females: 1970 - 1979

ICD code(s): 172
by state economic area

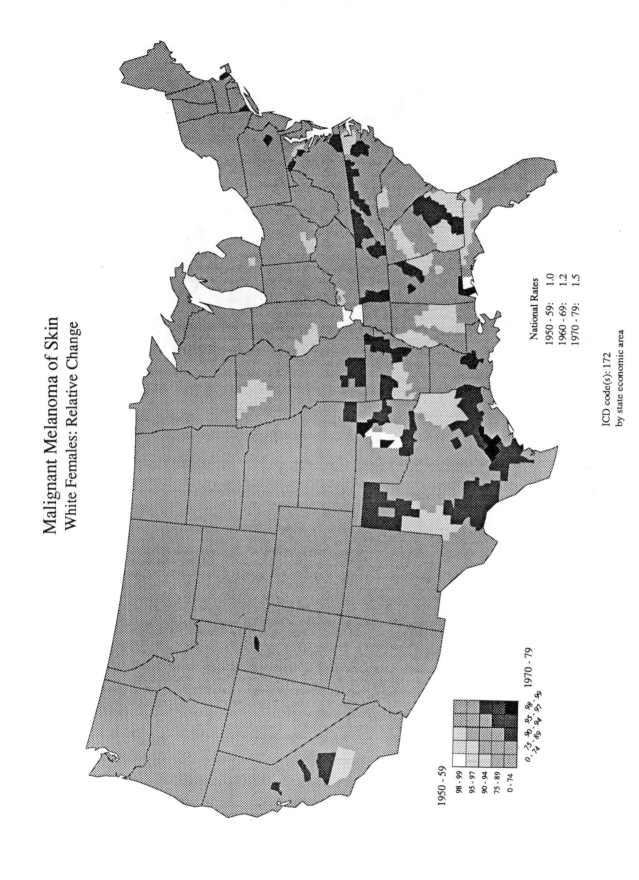

Malignant Melanoma of Skin
White Females: Relative Change

National Rates

1950 - 59: 1.0
1960 - 69: 1.2
1970 - 79: 1.5

ICD code(s): 172
by state economic area

1950 - 59

98 - 99
95 - 97
90 - 94
75 - 89
0 - 74

0 - 74 75 - 89 90 - 94 95 - 97 98 - 99
1970 - 79

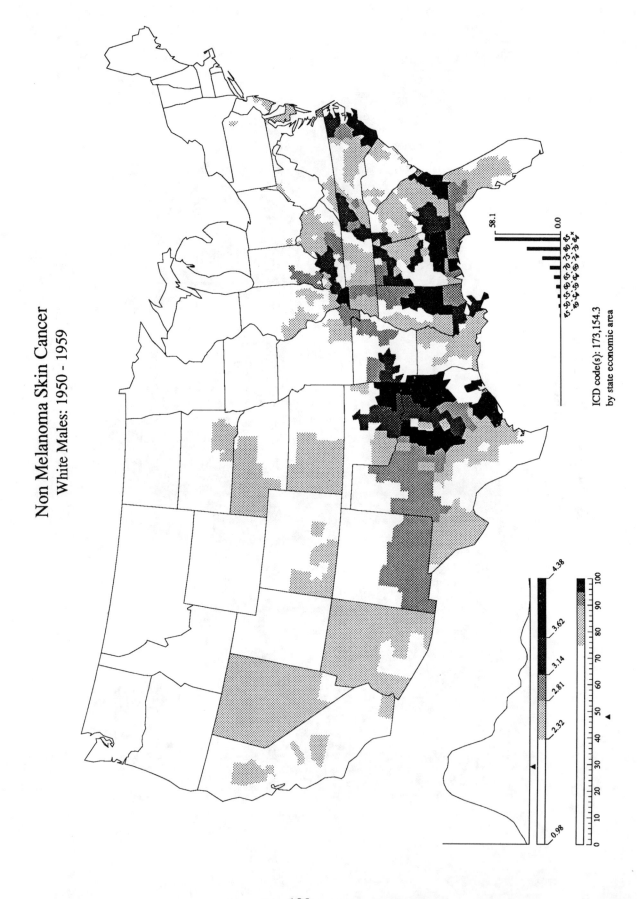

Non Melanoma Skin Cancer
White Males: 1950 - 1959

ICD code(s): 173,154.3
by state economic area

190

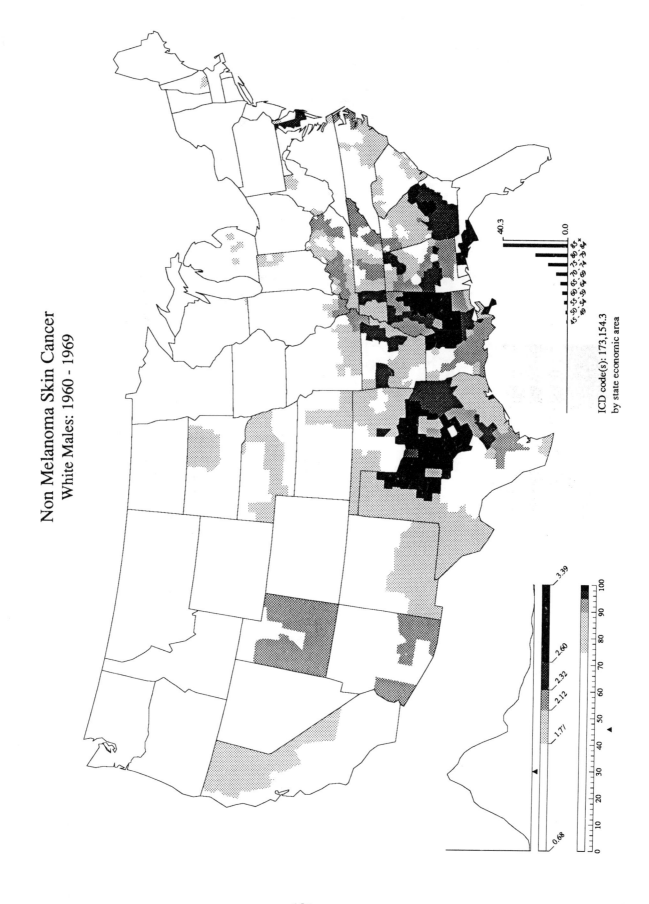

Non Melanoma Skin Cancer
White Males: 1960 - 1969

ICD code(s): 173,154.3
by state economic area

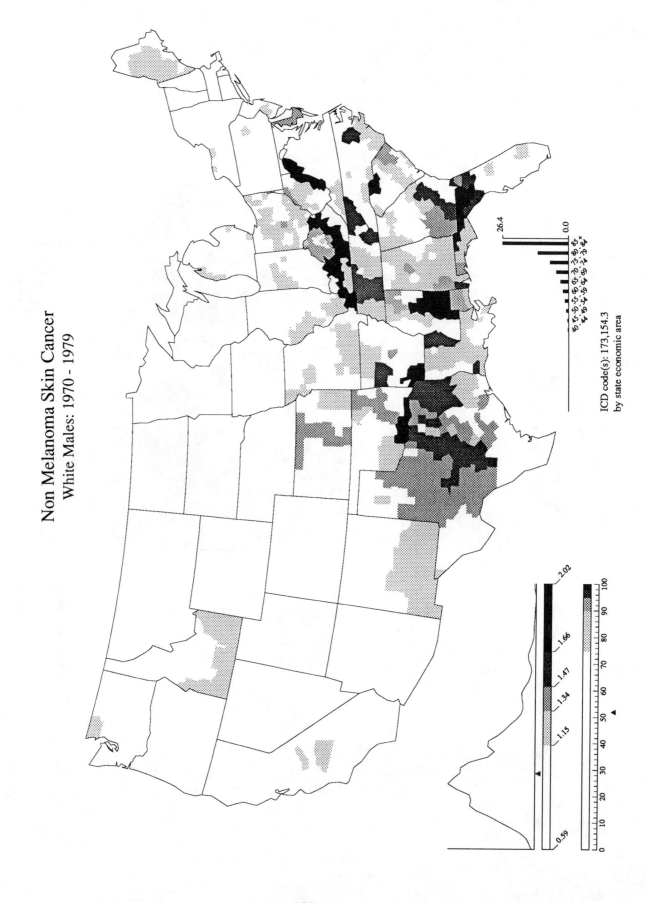

Non Melanoma Skin Cancer
White Males: 1970 - 1979

ICD code(s): 173,154.3
by state economic area

Non Melanoma Skin Cancer
White Males: Relative Change

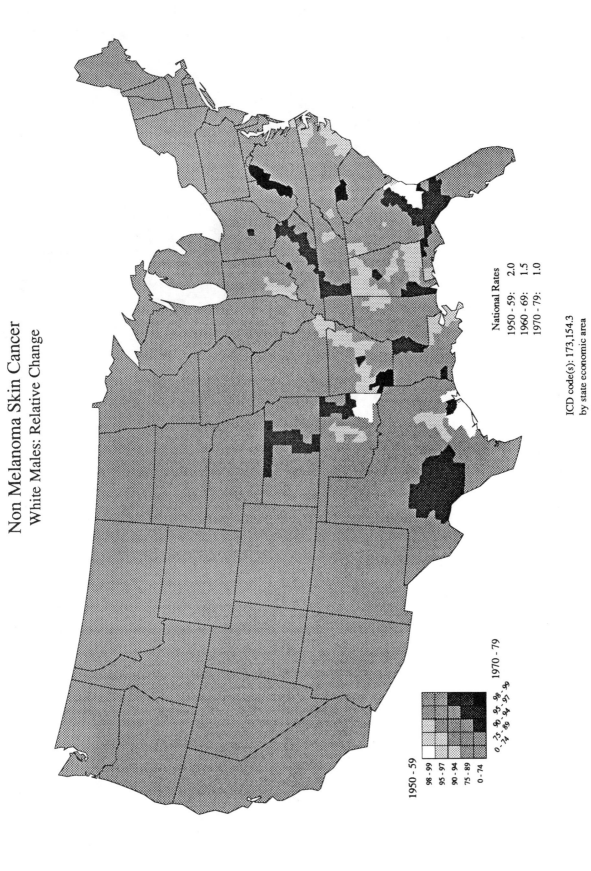

National Rates

1950 - 59:	2.0
1960 - 69:	1.5
1970 - 79:	1.0

ICD code(s): 173,154.3
by state economic area

1950 - 59

98 - 99
95 - 97
90 - 94
75 - 89
0 - 74

1970 - 79

0 - 74 75 - 89 90 - 94 95 - 97 98 - 99

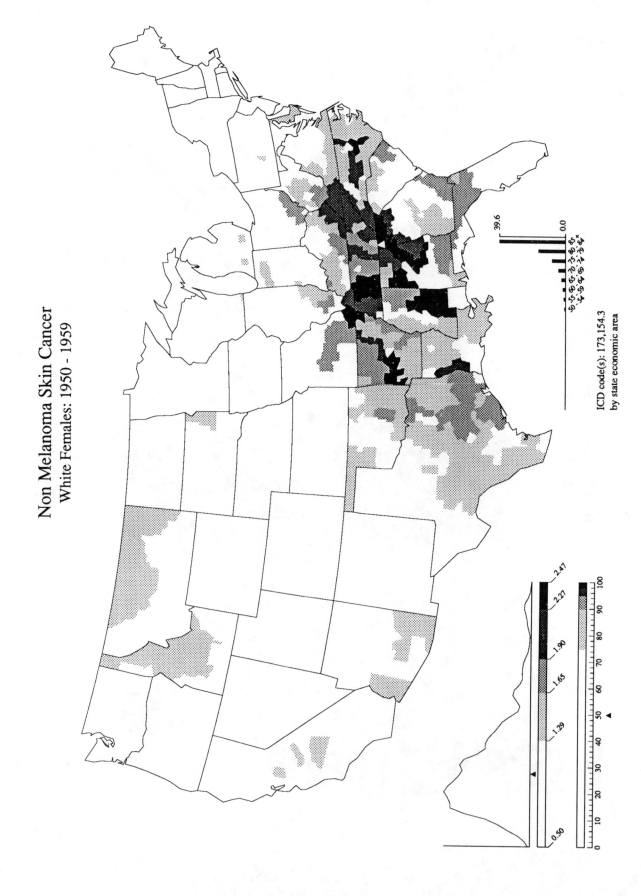

Non Melanoma Skin Cancer
White Females: 1950 - 1959

ICD code(s): 173,154.3
by state economic area

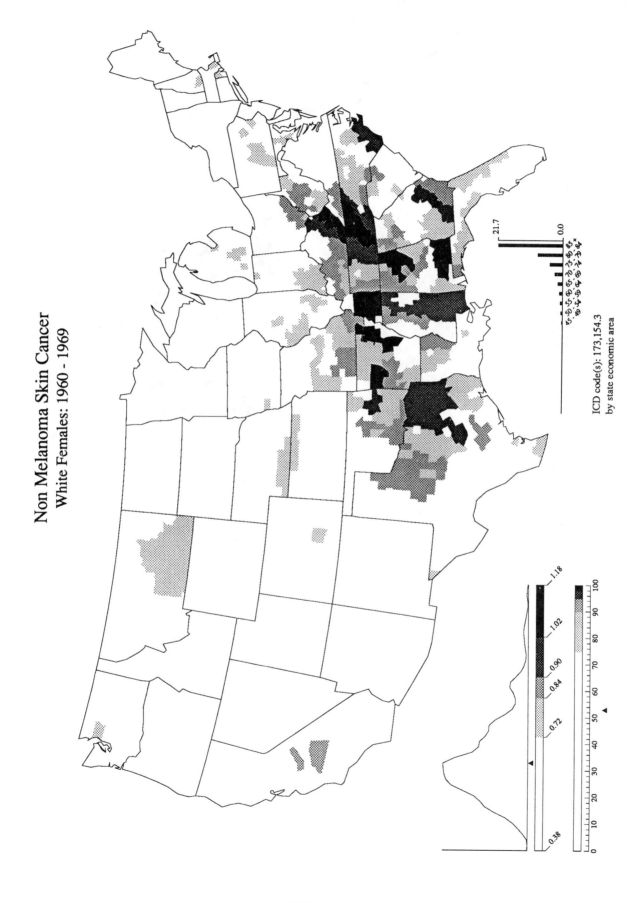

Non Melanoma Skin Cancer
White Females: 1960 - 1969

ICD code(s): 173,154.3
by state economic area

195

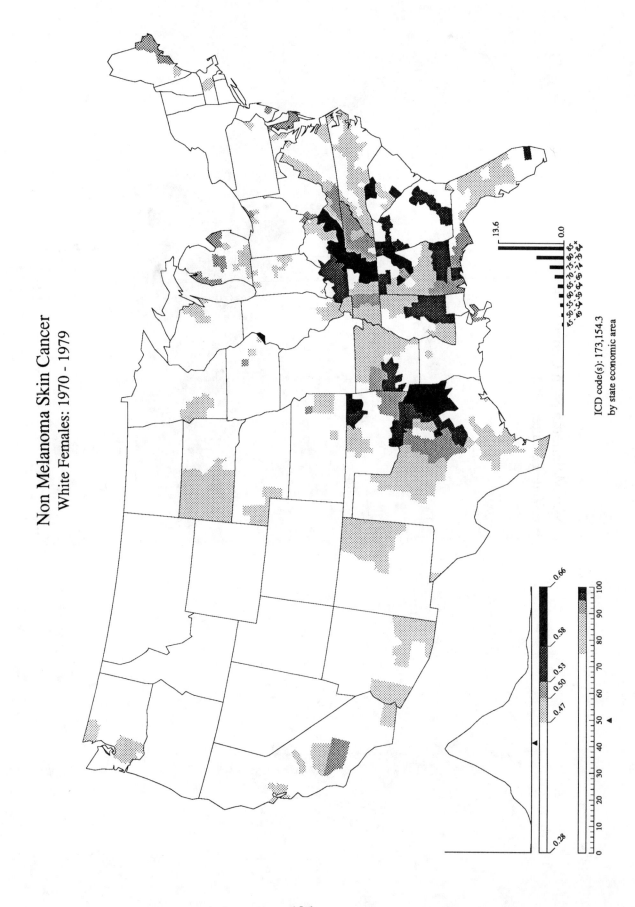

Non Melanoma Skin Cancer
White Females: 1970 - 1979

ICD code(s): 173,154.3
by state economic area

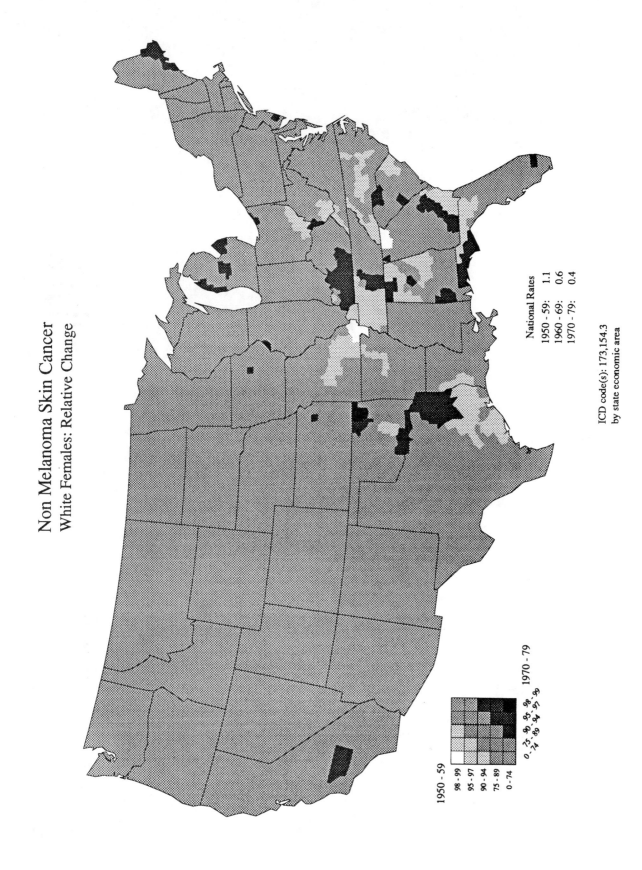

Non Melanoma Skin Cancer
White Females: Relative Change

National Rates

1950 - 59:	1.1
1960 - 69:	0.6
1970 - 79:	0.4

ICD code(s): 173,154.3
by state economic area

1950 - 59

98 - 99
95 - 97
90 - 94
75 - 89
0 - 74

0 - 75 90 95 98 99
74 89 94 97 99

1970 - 79

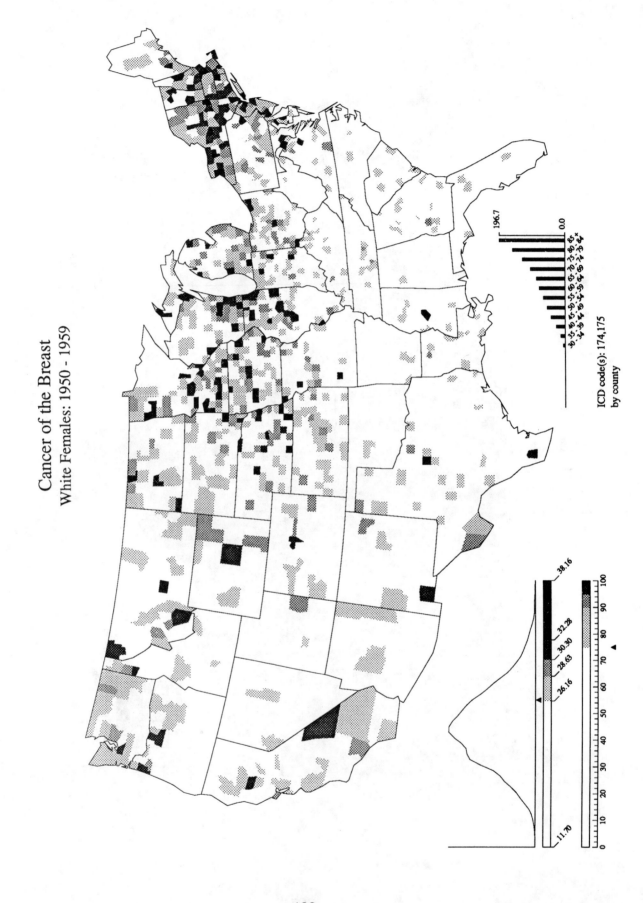

Cancer of the Breast
White Females: 1950 - 1959

ICD code(s): 174,175
by county

198

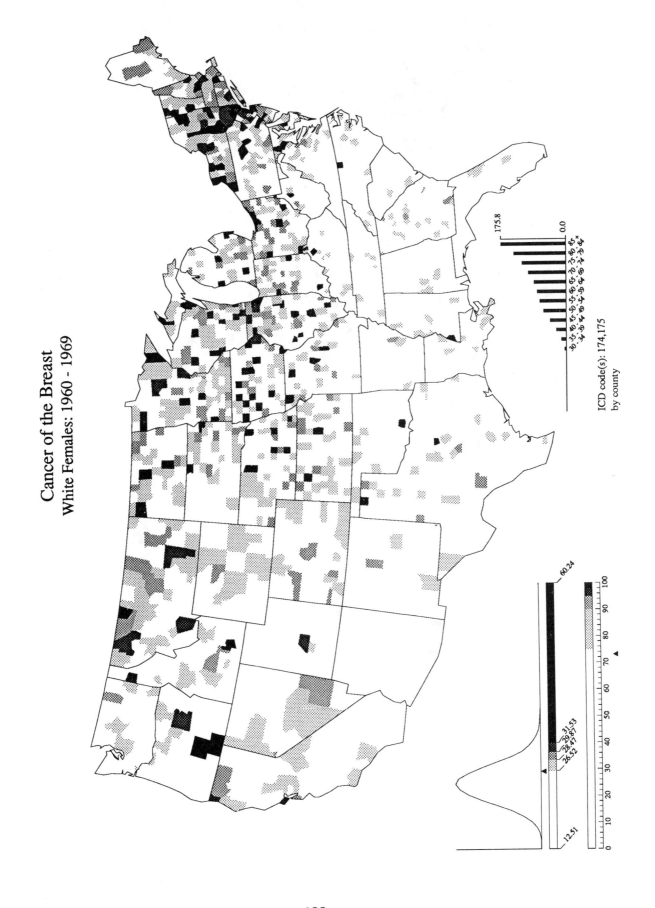

Cancer of the Breast
White Females: 1960 - 1969

ICD code(s): 174,175
by county

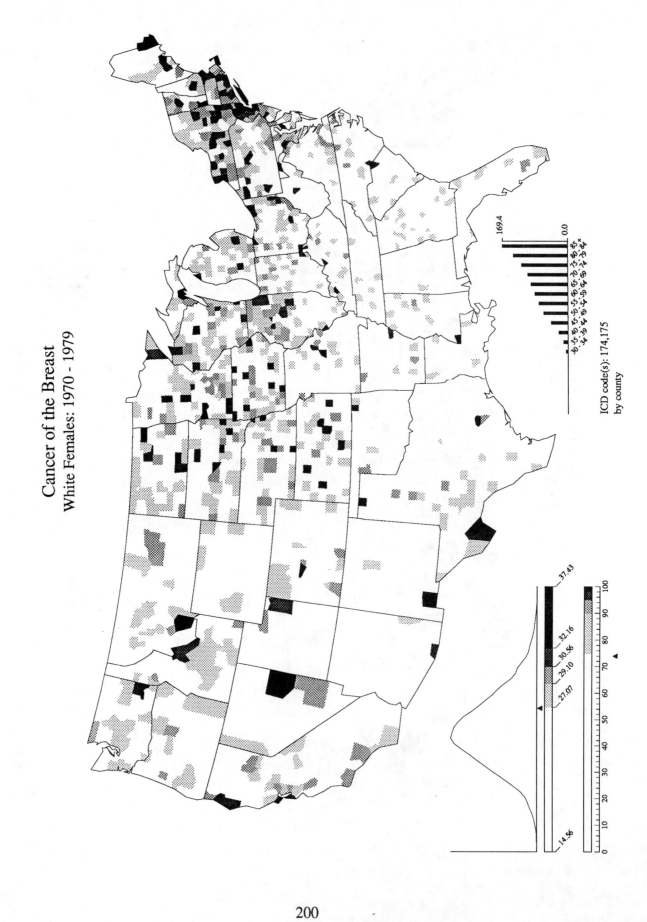

Cancer of the Breast
White Females: 1970 - 1979

ICD code(s): 174,175
by county

Cancer of the Breast
White Females: Relative Change

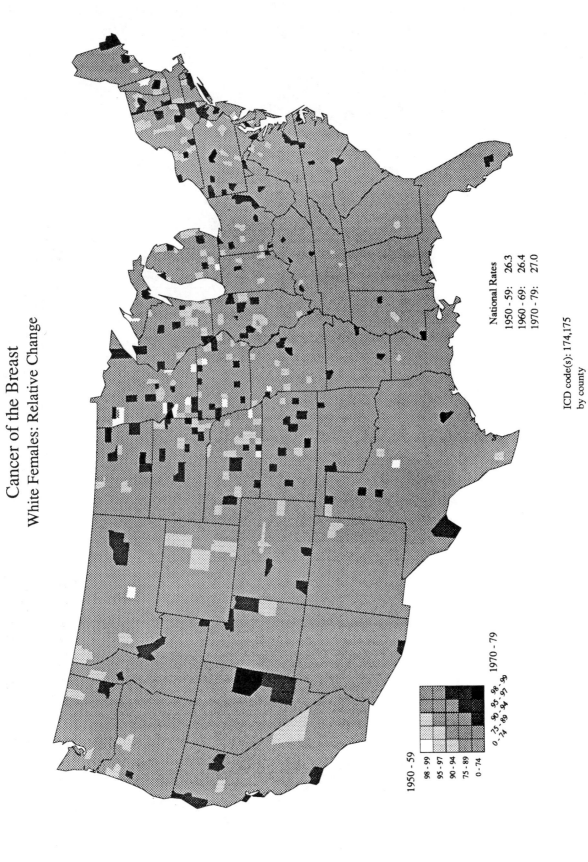

National Rates

1950 - 59:	26.3
1960 - 69:	26.4
1970 - 79:	27.0

ICD code(s): 174,175
by county

1950 - 59
98 - 99
95 - 97
90 - 94
75 - 89
0 - 74

1970 - 79

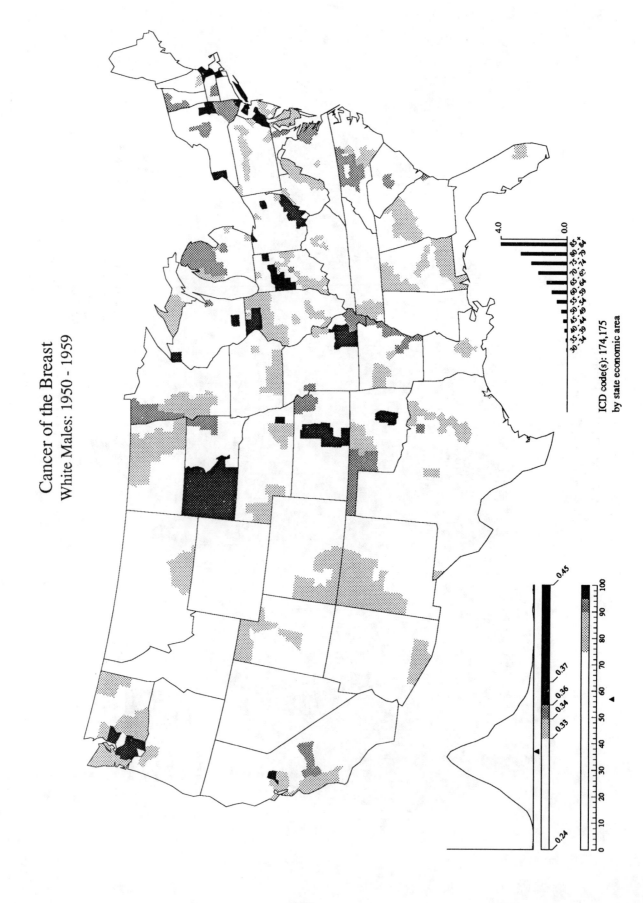

Cancer of the Breast
White Males: 1950 - 1959

ICD code(s): 174,175
by state economic area

202

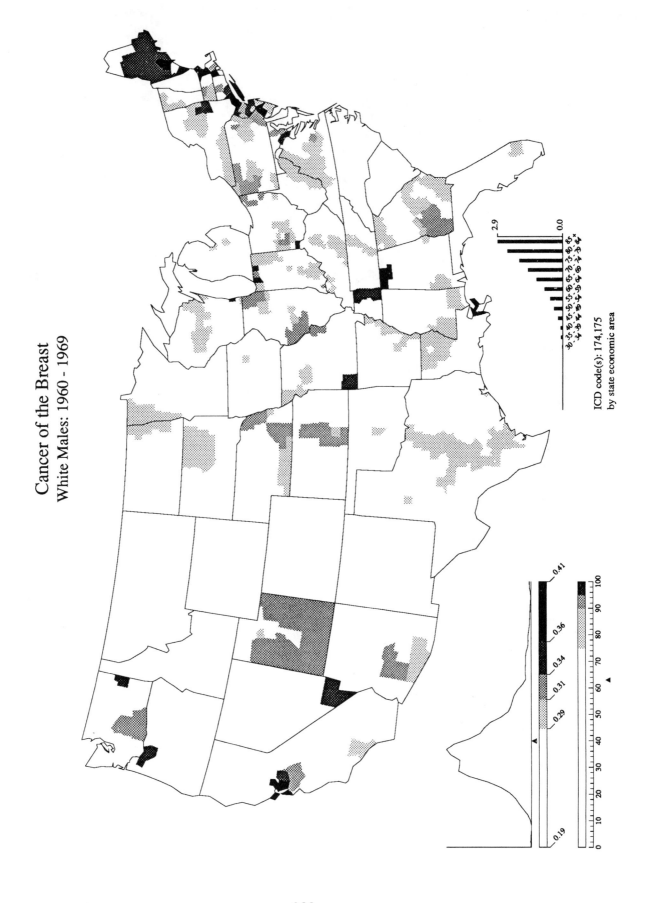

Cancer of the Breast
White Males: 1960 - 1969

ICD code(s): 174,175
by state economic area

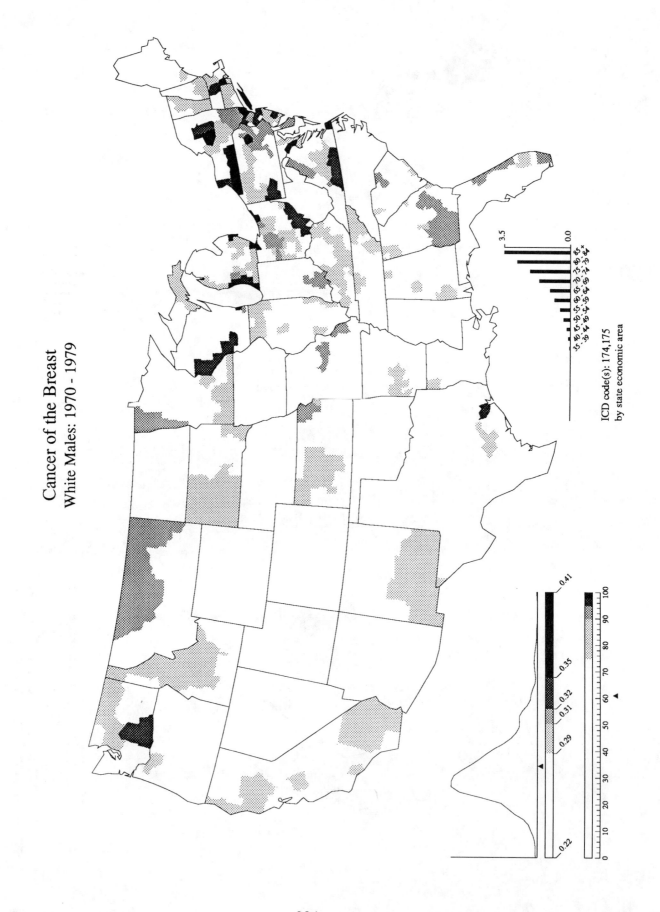

Cancer of the Breast
White Males: 1970 - 1979

ICD code(s): 174,175
by state economic area

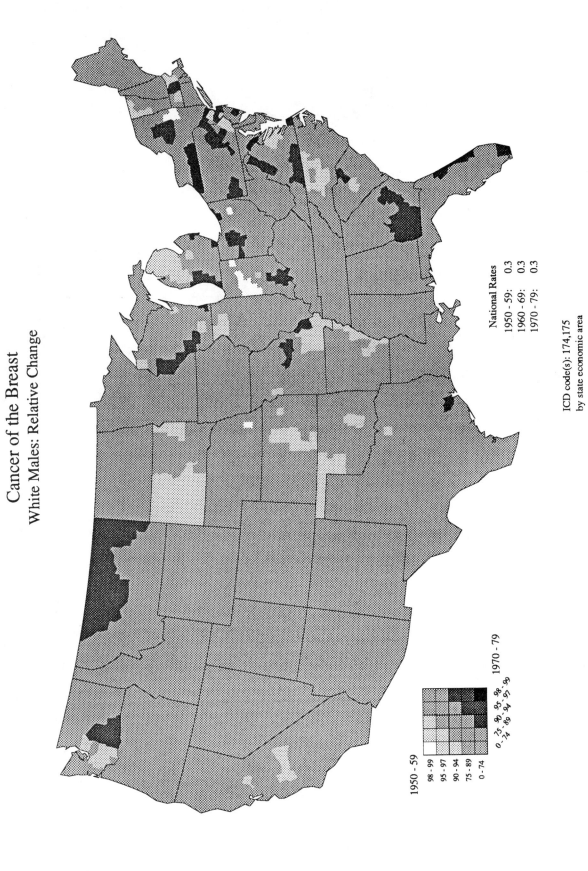

Cancer of the Breast
White Males: Relative Change

National Rates

1950 - 59:	0.3
1960 - 69:	0.3
1970 - 79:	0.3

ICD code(s): 174,175
by state economic area

1950 - 59

1970 - 79

98 - 99
95 - 97
90 - 94
75 - 89
0 - 74

98 - 99
95 - 97
90 - 94
75 - 89
0 - 74

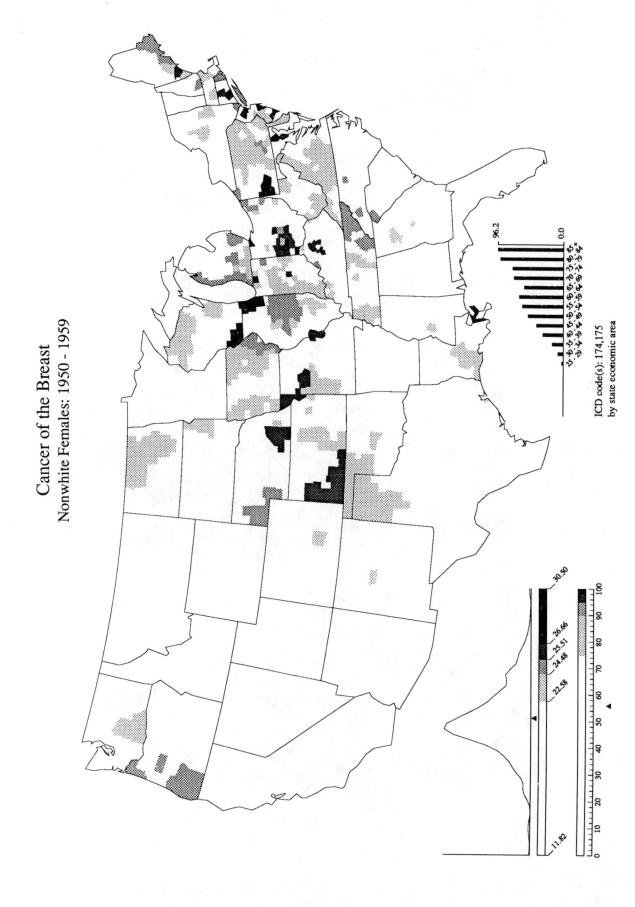

Cancer of the Breast
Nonwhite Females: 1950 - 1959

ICD code(s): 174,175
by state economic area

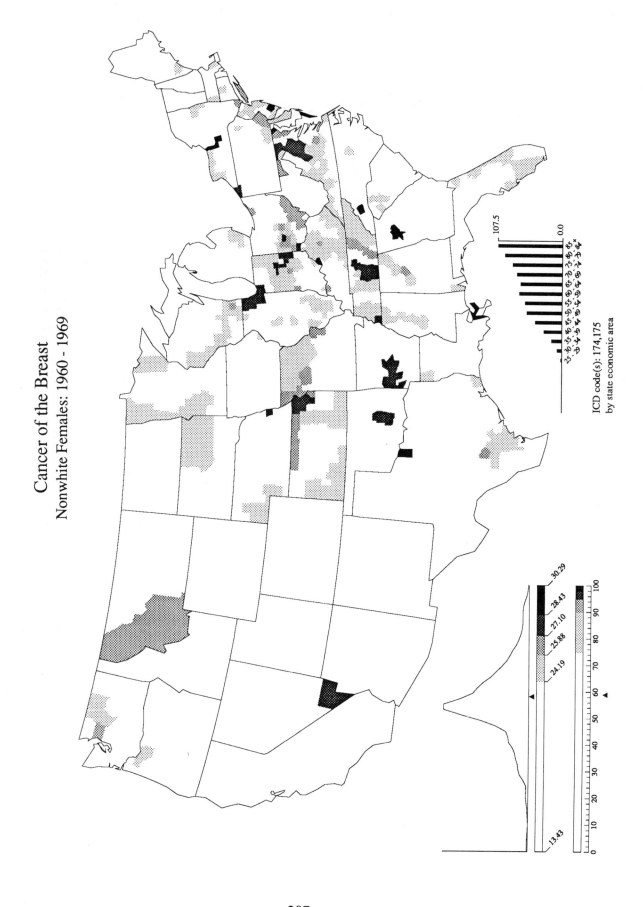

Cancer of the Breast
Nonwhite Females: 1960 - 1969

ICD code(s): 174,175
by state economic area

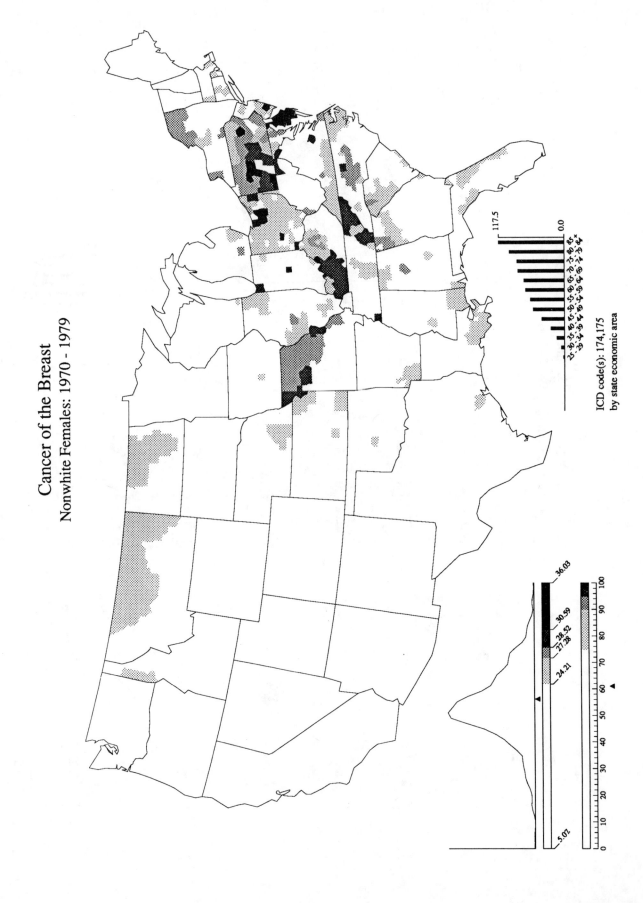

Cancer of the Breast
Nonwhite Females: 1970 - 1979

ICD code(s): 174,175
by state economic area

208

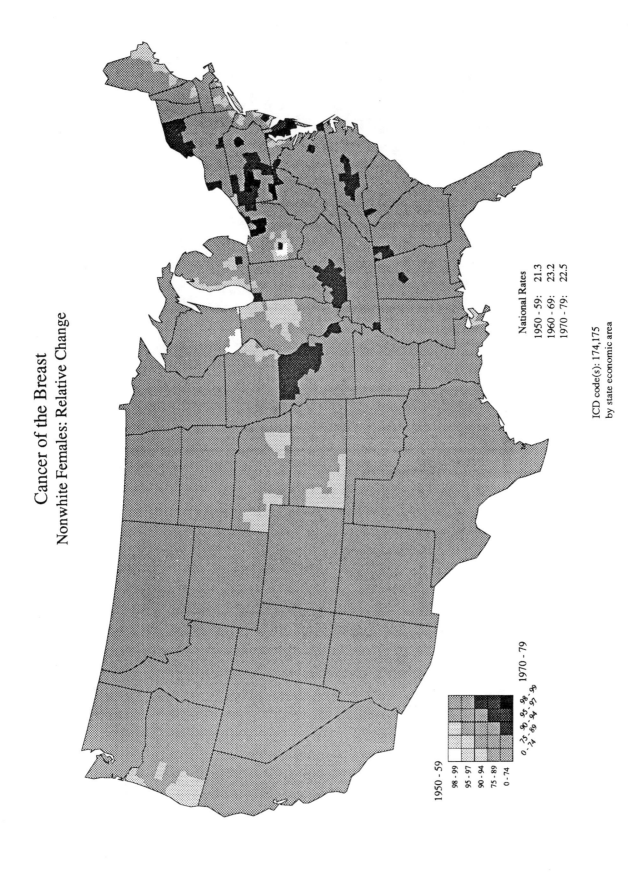

Cancer of the Breast
Nonwhite Females: Relative Change

National Rates

1950 - 59:	21.3
1960 - 69:	23.2
1970 - 79:	22.5

ICD code(s): 174,175
by state economic area

1950 - 59

98 - 99
95 - 97
90 - 94
75 - 89
0 - 74

0 - 74
75 - 89
90 - 94
95 - 97
98 - 99

1970 - 79

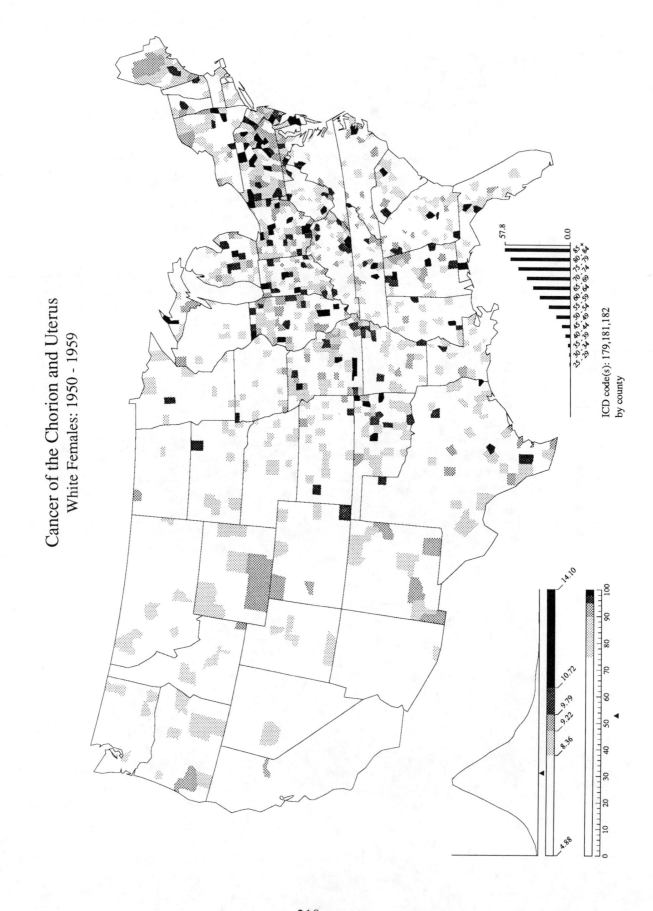

Cancer of the Chorion and Uterus
White Females: 1950 - 1959

ICD code(s): 179,181,182
by county

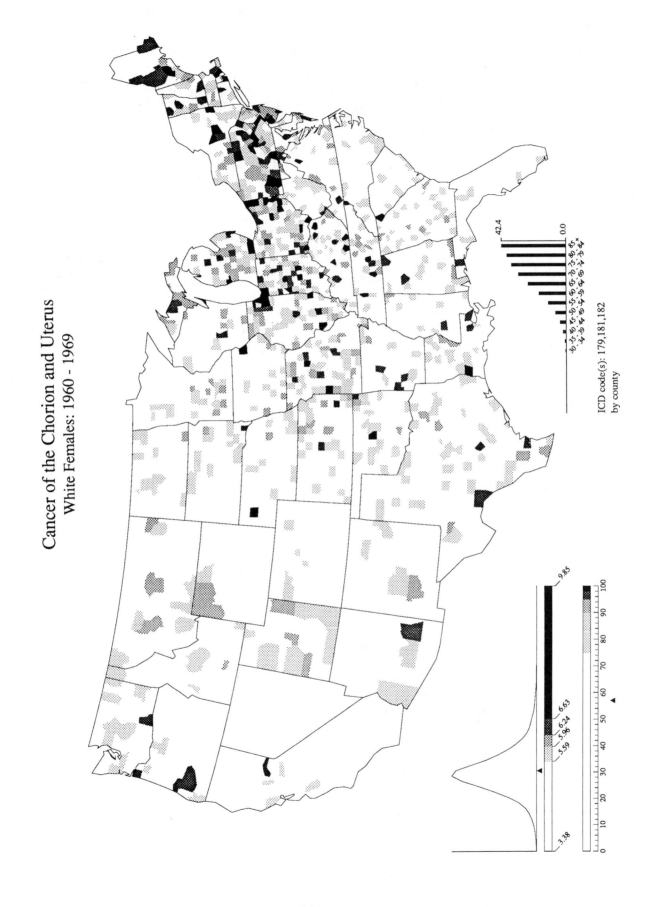

Cancer of the Chorion and Uterus
White Females: 1960 - 1969

ICD code(s): 179,181,182
by county

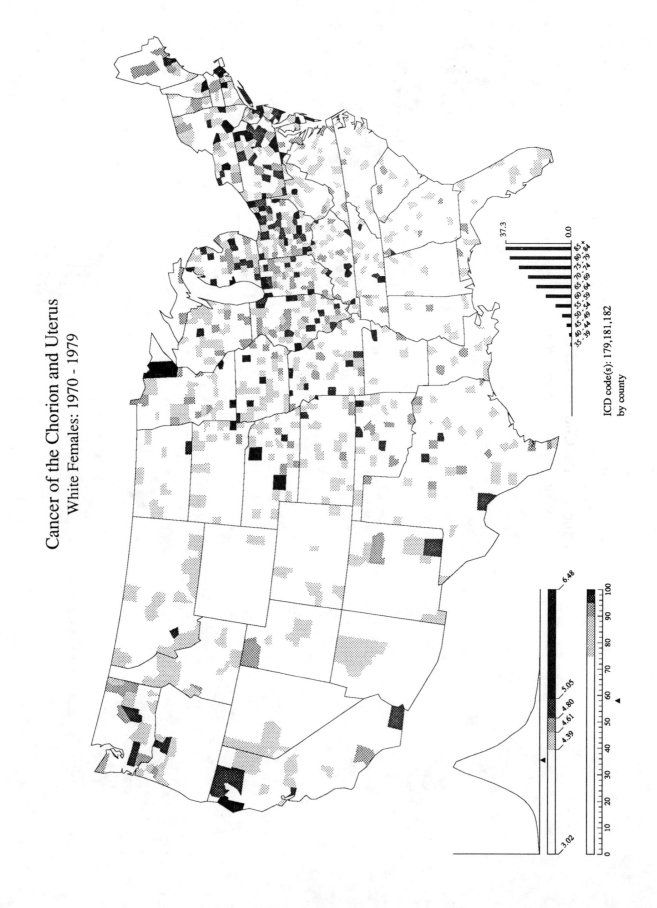

Cancer of the Chorion and Uterus
White Females: 1970 - 1979

ICD code(s): 179,181,182
by county

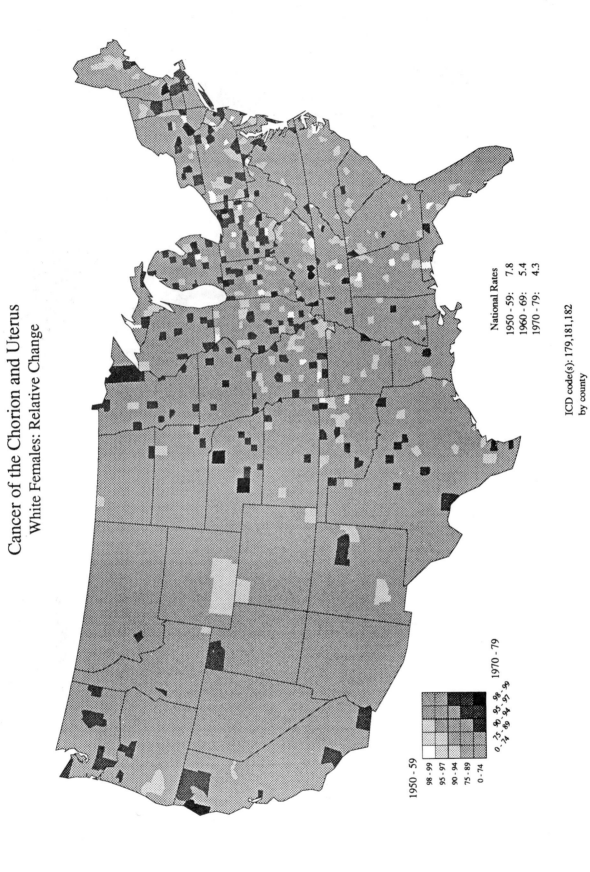

Cancer of the Chorion and Uterus
White Females: Relative Change

National Rates

1950 - 59: 7.8
1960 - 69: 5.4
1970 - 79: 4.3

ICD code(s): 179,181,182
by county

1950 - 59

98 - 99
95 - 97
90 - 94
75 - 89
0 - 74

1970 - 79

98 - 99
95 - 97
90 - 94
75 - 89
0 - 74

213

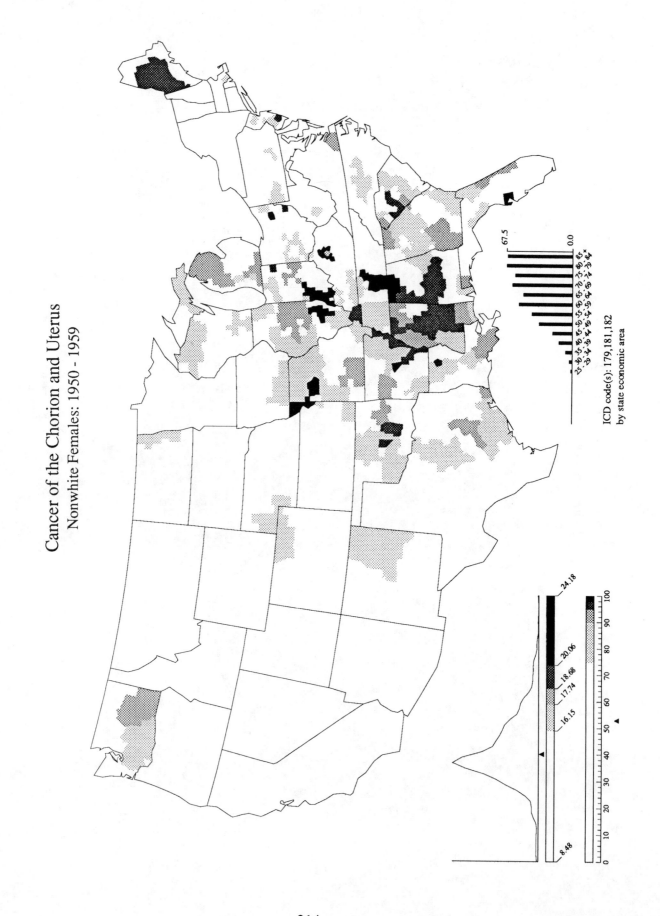

Cancer of the Chorion and Uterus
Nonwhite Females: 1950 - 1959

ICD code(s): 179,181,182
by state economic area

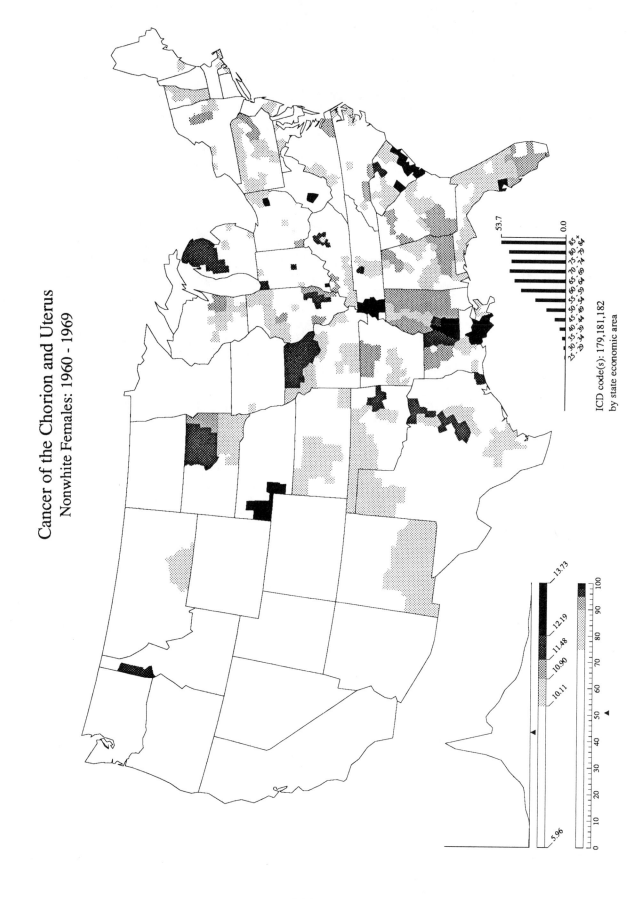

Cancer of the Chorion and Uterus
Nonwhite Females: 1960 - 1969

ICD code(s): 179,181,182
by state economic area

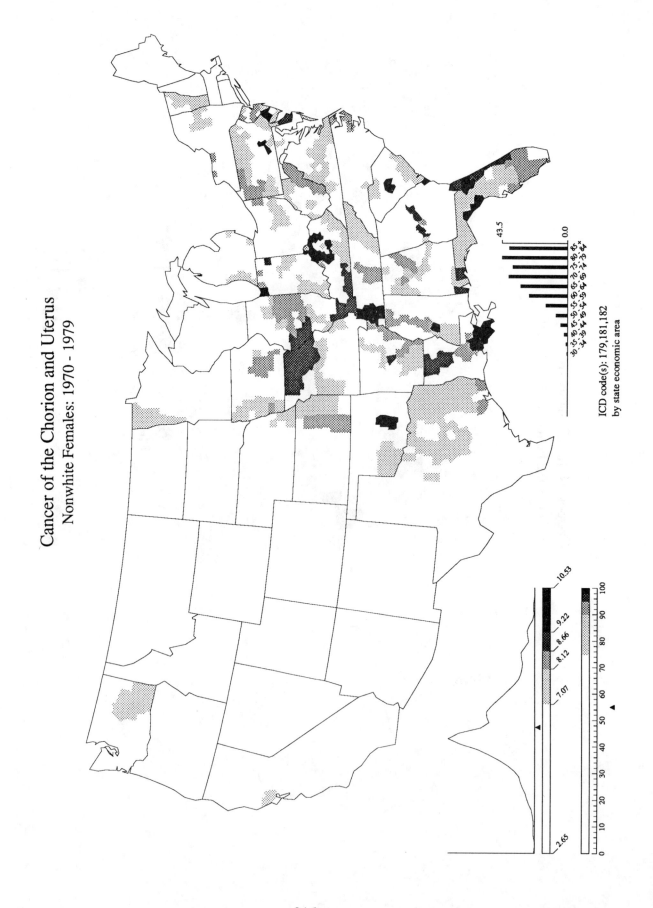

Cancer of the Chorion and Uterus
Nonwhite Females: 1970 - 1979

ICD code(s): 179,181,182
by state economic area

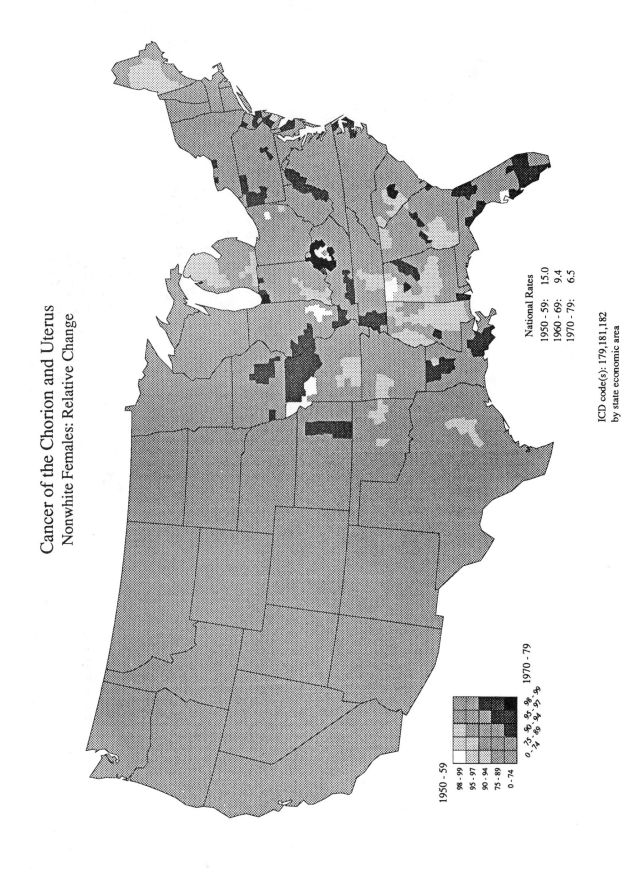

Cancer of the Chorion and Uterus
Nonwhite Females: Relative Change

National Rates

1950 - 59:	15.0
1960 - 69:	9.4
1970 - 79:	6.5

ICD code(s): 179,181,182
by state economic area

1950 - 59

98 - 99
95 - 97
90 - 94
75 - 89
0 - 74

0 - .73 .90 .95 .98 .99
.74 .89 .94 .97 .98

1970 - 79

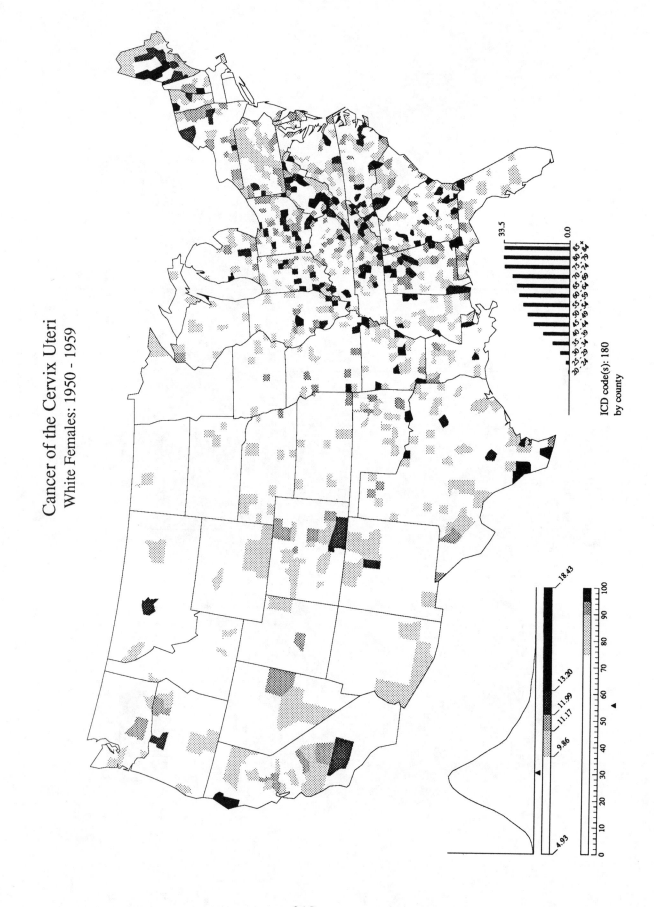

Cancer of the Cervix Uteri
White Females: 1950 - 1959

ICD code(s): 180
by county

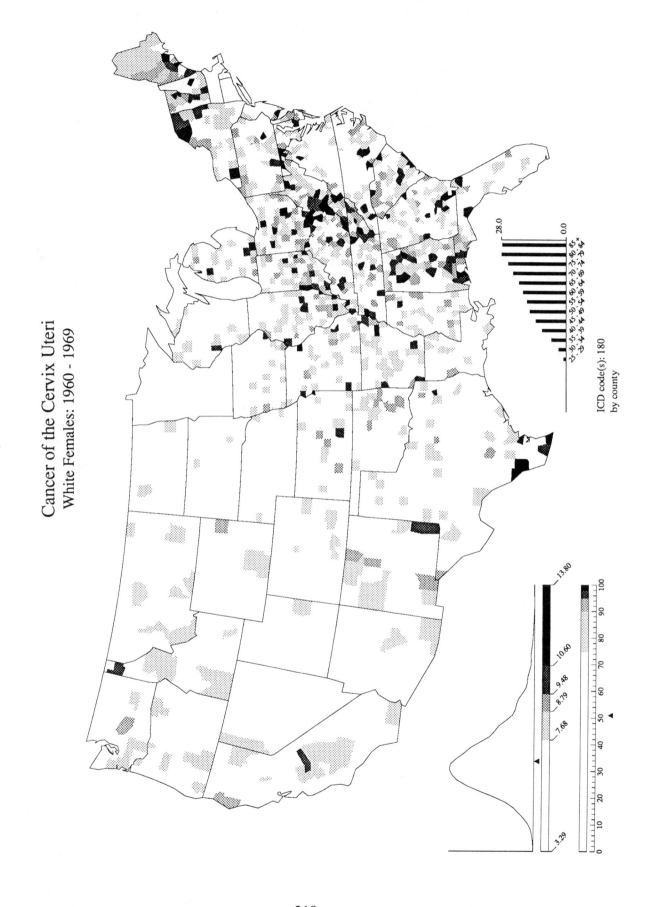

Cancer of the Cervix Uteri
White Females: 1960 - 1969

ICD code(s): 180
by county

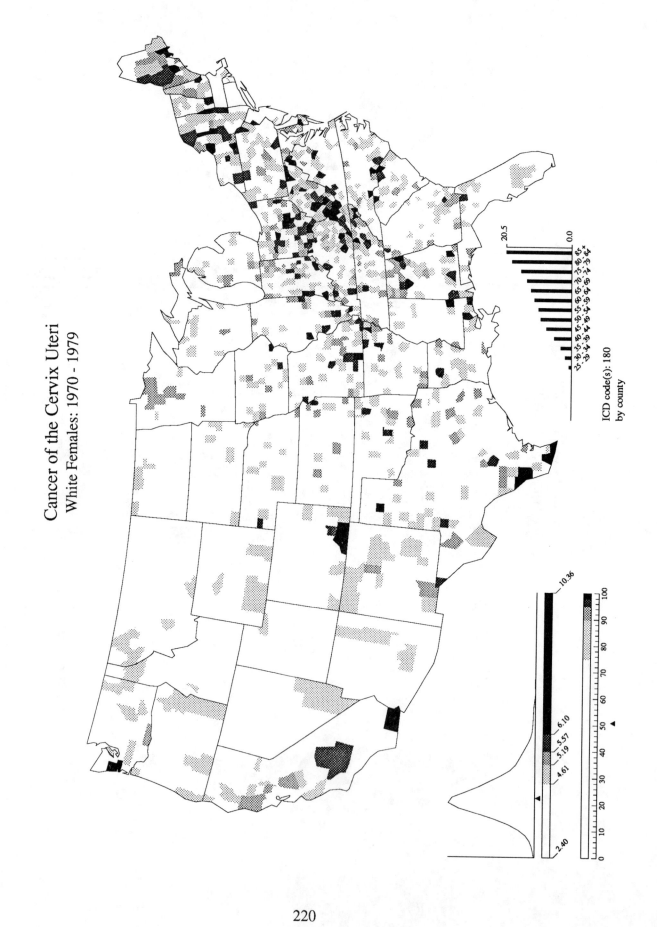

Cancer of the Cervix Uteri
White Females: 1970 - 1979

ICD code(s): 180
by county

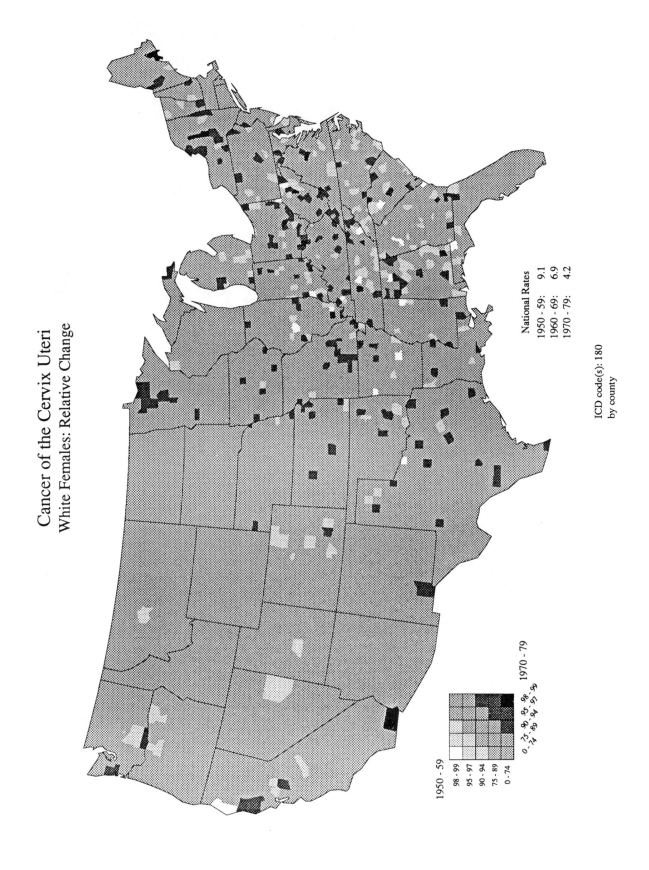

Cancer of the Cervix Uteri
White Females: Relative Change

National Rates

1950 - 59:   9.1
1960 - 69:   6.9
1970 - 79:   4.2

ICD code(s): 180
by county

1950 - 59
98 - 99
95 - 97
90 - 94
75 - 89
0 - 74

1970 - 79
98 - 99
95 - 97
90 - 94
75 - 89
0 - 74

221

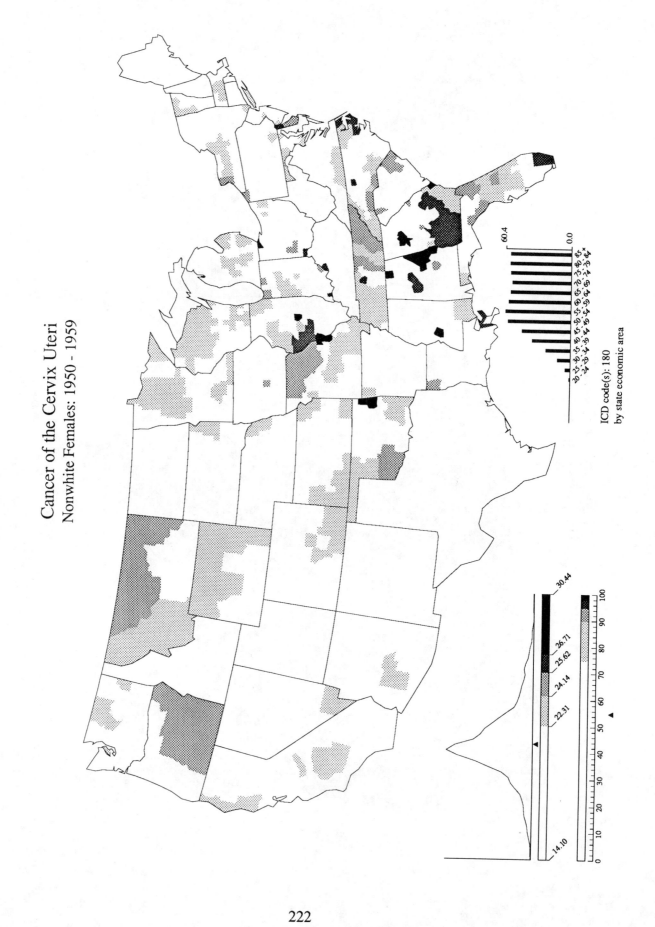

Cancer of the Cervix Uteri
Nonwhite Females: 1950 - 1959

ICD code(s): 180
by state economic area

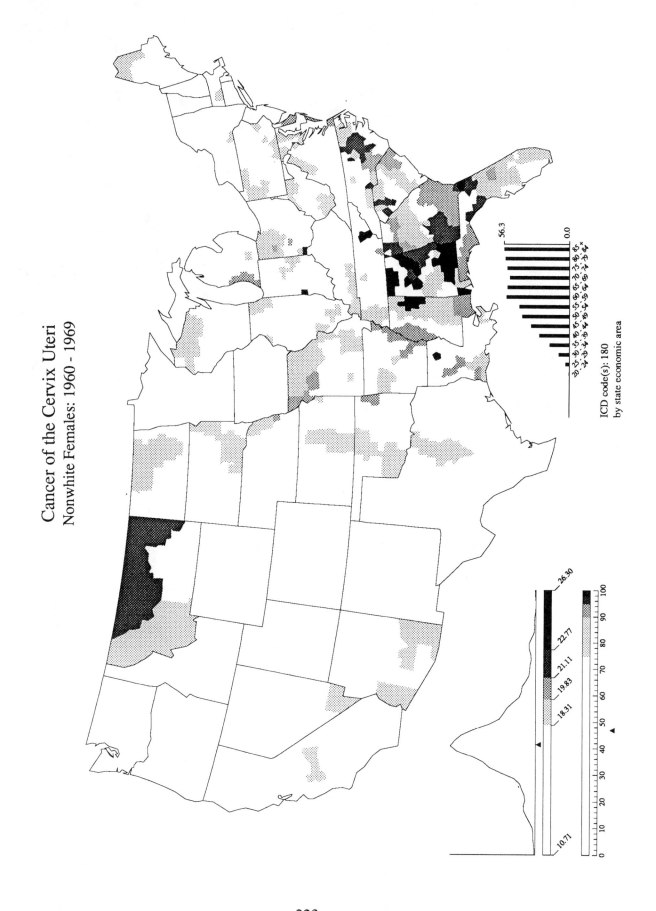

Cancer of the Cervix Uteri
Nonwhite Females: 1960 - 1969

ICD code(s): 180
by state economic area

223

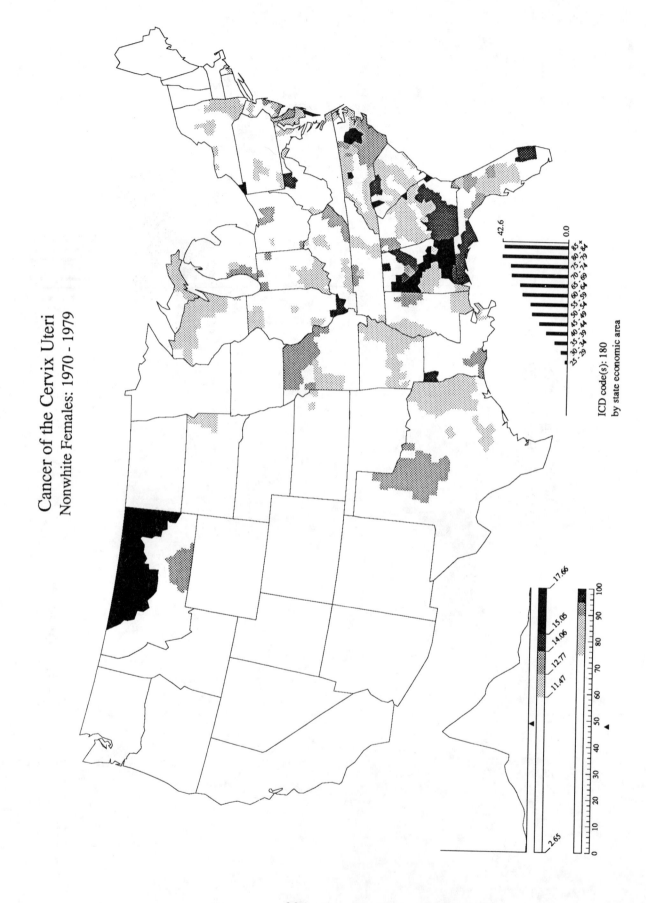

Cancer of the Cervix Uteri
Nonwhite Females: 1970 - 1979

ICD code(s): 180
by state economic area

Cancer of the Cervix Uteri
Nonwhite Females: Relative Change

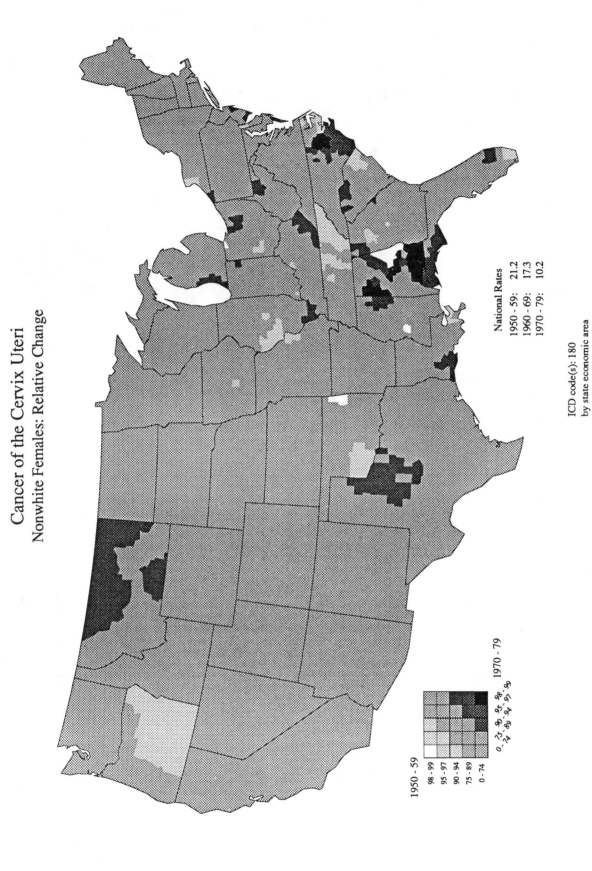

National Rates
1950 - 59: 21.2
1960 - 69: 17.3
1970 - 79: 10.2

ICD code(s): 180
by state economic area

1950 - 59
98 - 99
95 - 97
90 - 94
75 - 89
0 - 74

1970 - 79
0 - 74   75 - 89   90 - 94   95 - 97   98 - 99

225

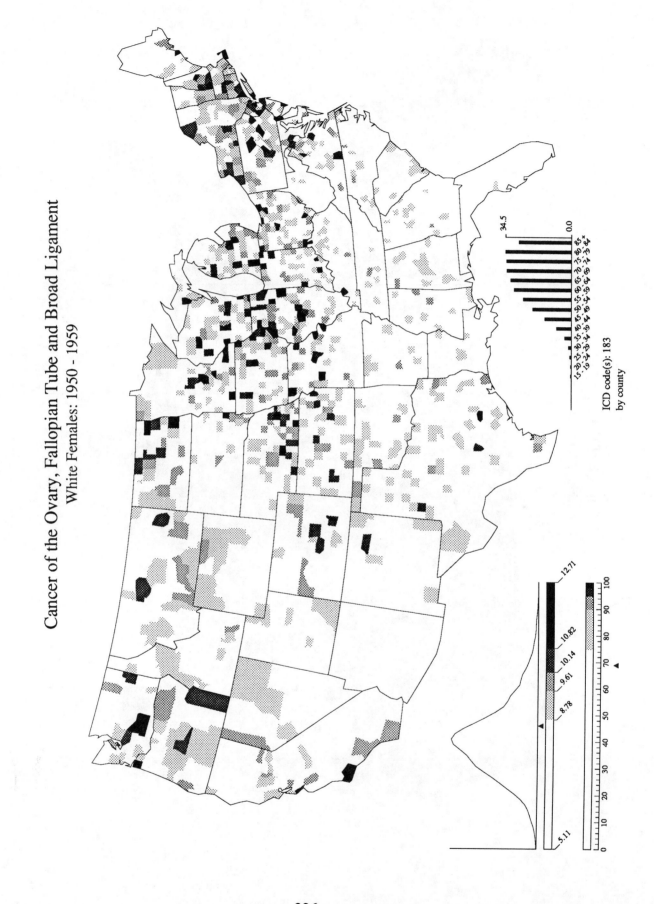

Cancer of the Ovary, Fallopian Tube and Broad Ligament
White Females: 1950 - 1959

ICD code(s): 183
by county

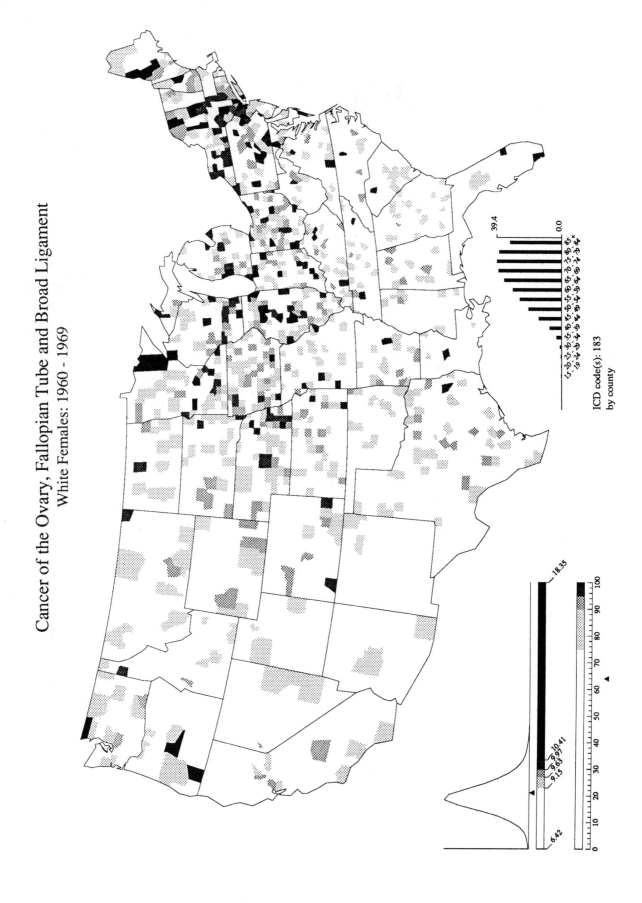

Cancer of the Ovary, Fallopian Tube and Broad Ligament
White Females: 1960 - 1969

ICD code(s): 183
by county

227

Cancer of the Ovary, Fallopian Tube and Broad Ligament
White Females: 1970 - 1979

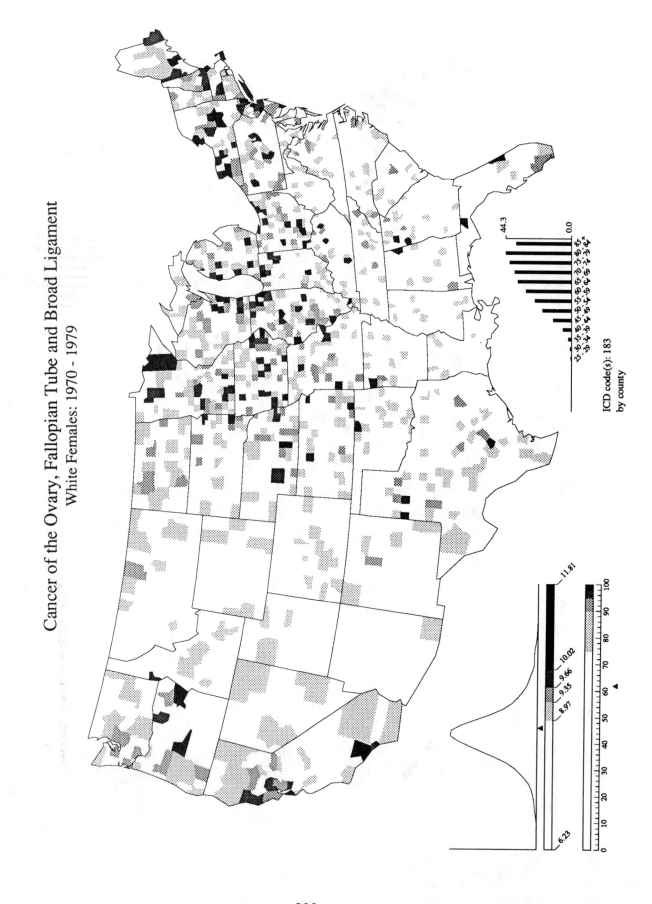

ICD code(s): 183
by county

Cancer of the Ovary, Fallopian Tube and Broad Ligament
White Females: Relative Change

National Rates

1950 - 59:   8.6
1960 - 69:   8.9
1970 - 79:   8.8

ICD code(s): 183
by county

1950 - 59

98 - 99
95 - 97
90 - 94
75 - 89
0 - 74

1970 - 79
0 - 73 75 - 89 90 - 94 95 - 97 98 - 99

Cancer of the Ovary, Fallopian Tube and Broad Ligament
Nonwhite Females: 1950 - 1959

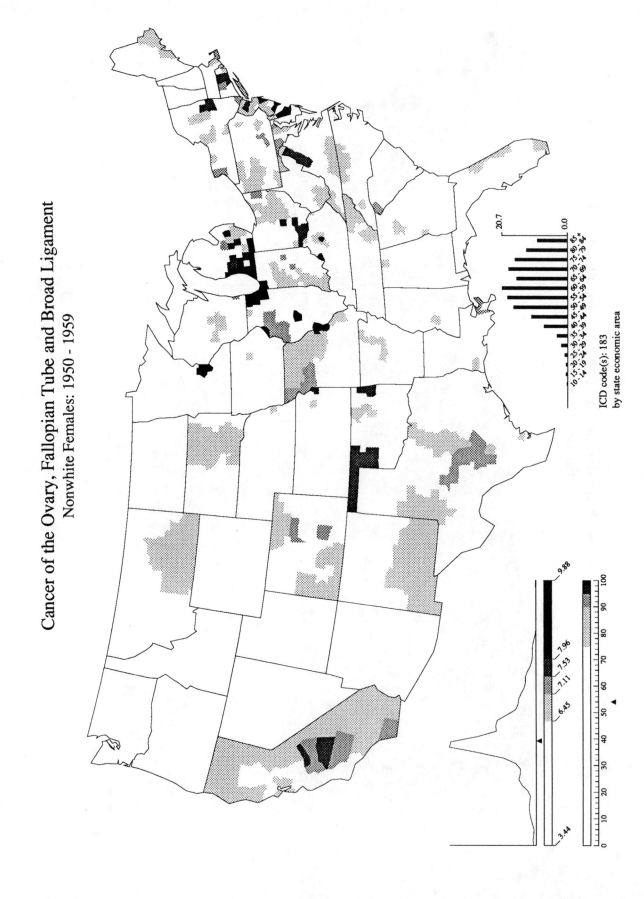

ICD code(s): 183
by state economic area

230

Cancer of the Ovary, Fallopian Tube and Broad Ligament
Nonwhite Females: 1960 - 1969

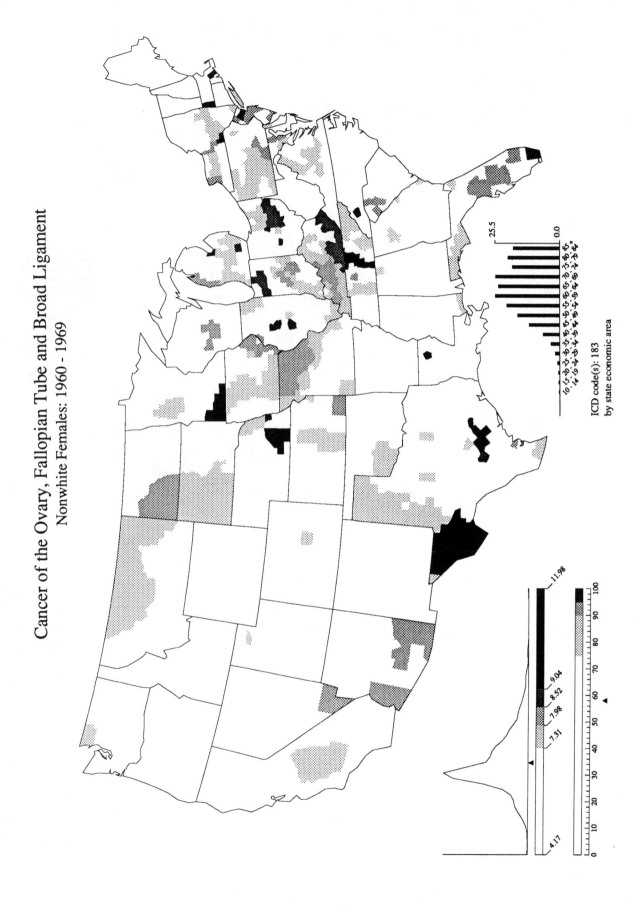

ICD code(s): 183
by state economic area

Cancer of the Ovary, Fallopian Tube and Broad Ligament
Nonwhite Females: 1970 - 1979

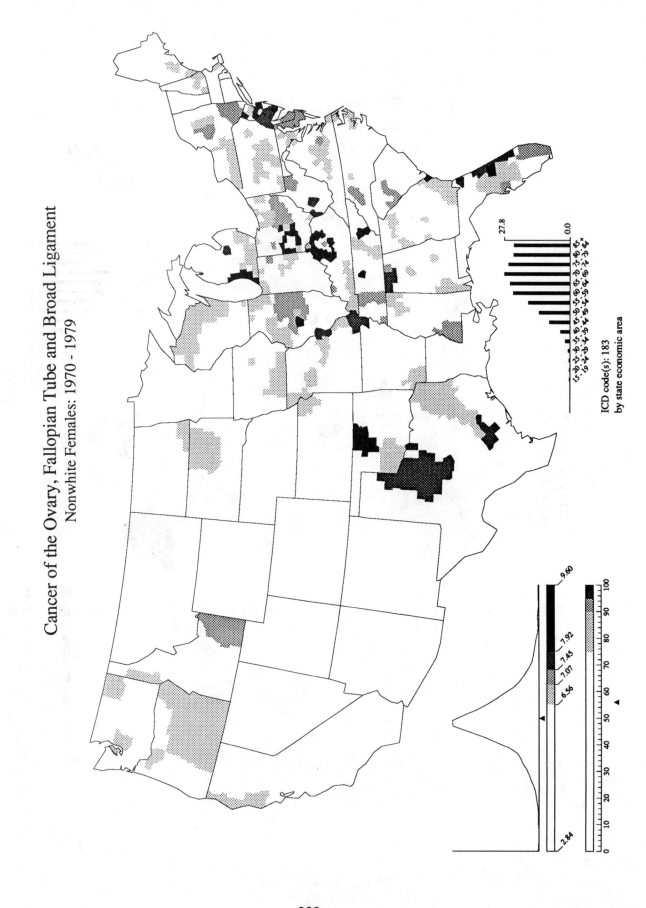

ICD code(s): 183
by state economic area

Cancer of the Ovary, Fallopian Tube and Broad Ligament
Nonwhite Females: Relative Change

National Rates

1950 - 59:	5.9
1960 - 69:	6.9
1970 - 79:	6.3

ICD code(s): 183
by state economic area

233

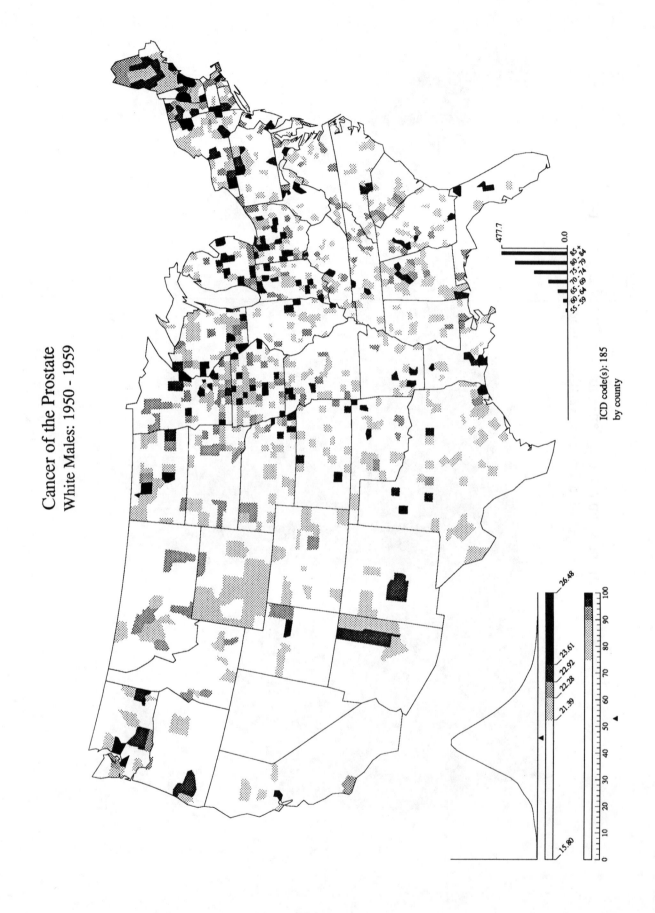

Cancer of the Prostate
White Males: 1950 - 1959

ICD code(s): 185
by county

Cancer of the Prostate
White Males: 1960 - 1969

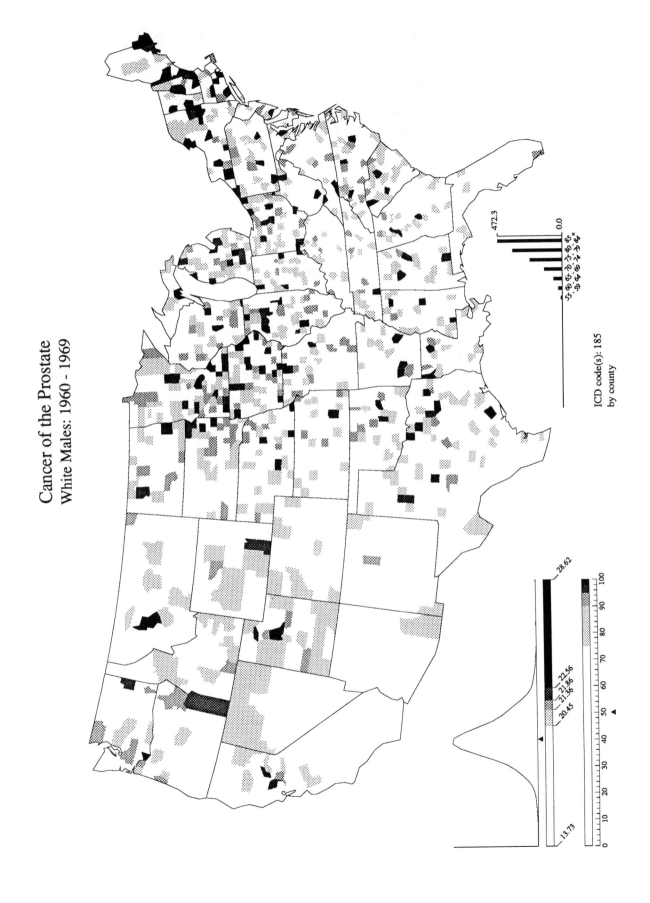

ICD code(s): 185
by county

Cancer of the Prostate
White Males: 1970 - 1979

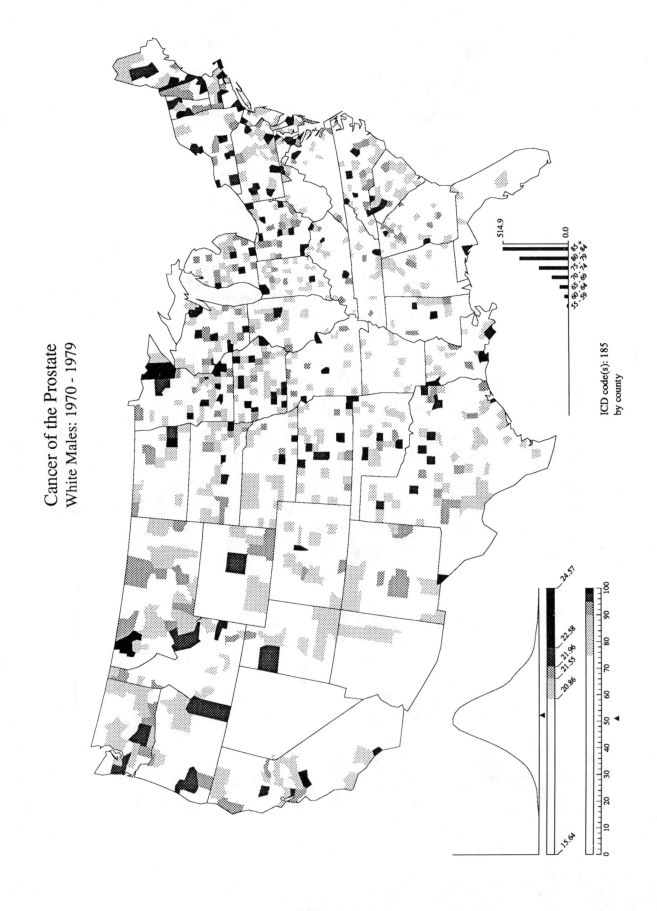

ICD code(s): 185
by county

Cancer of the Prostate
White Males: Relative Change

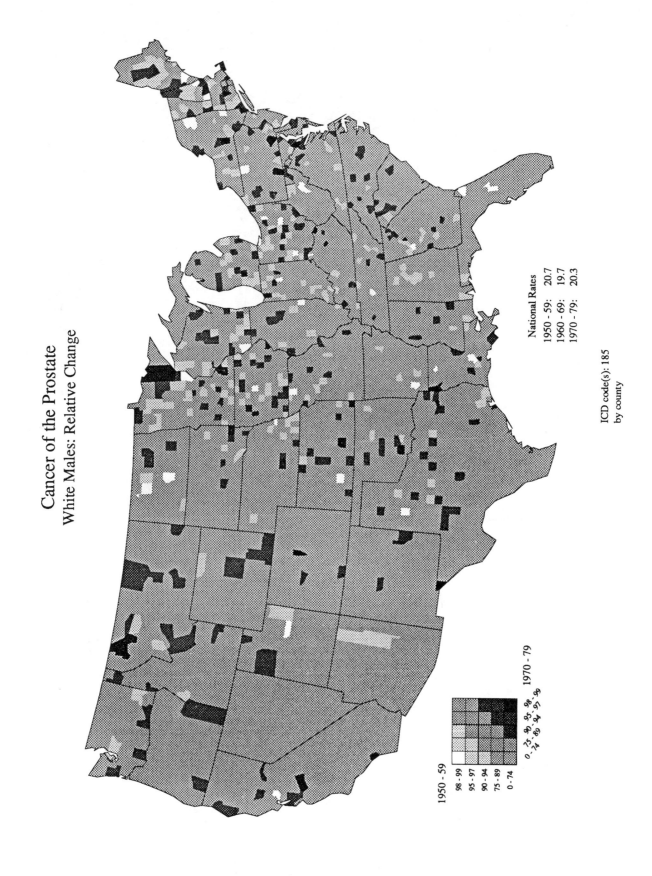

National Rates

1950 - 59:	20.7
1960 - 69:	19.7
1970 - 79:	20.3

ICD code(s): 185
by county

1950 - 59

98 - 99
95 - 97
90 - 94
75 - 89
0 - 74

0 - 74 75 - 89 90 - 94 95 - 97 98 - 99

1970 - 79

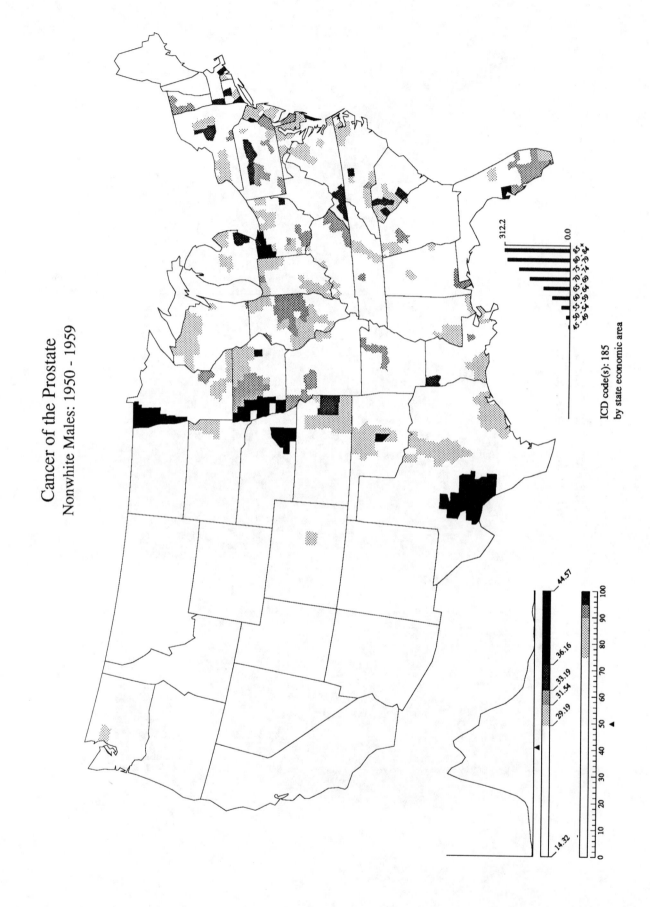

Cancer of the Prostate
Nonwhite Males: 1950 - 1959

ICD code(s): 185
by state economic area

238

Cancer of the Prostate
Nonwhite Males: 1960 - 1969

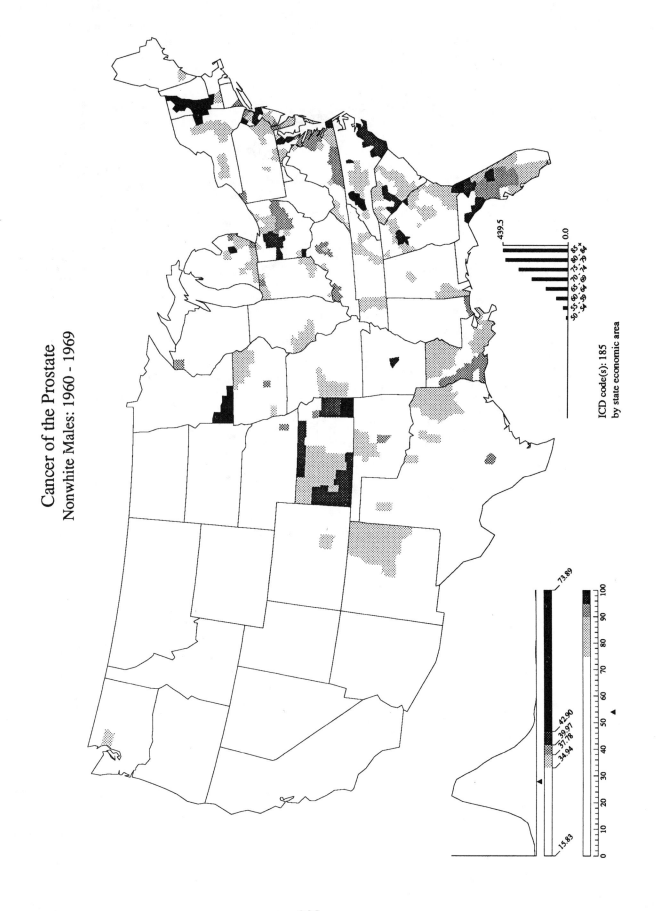

ICD code(s): 185
by state economic area

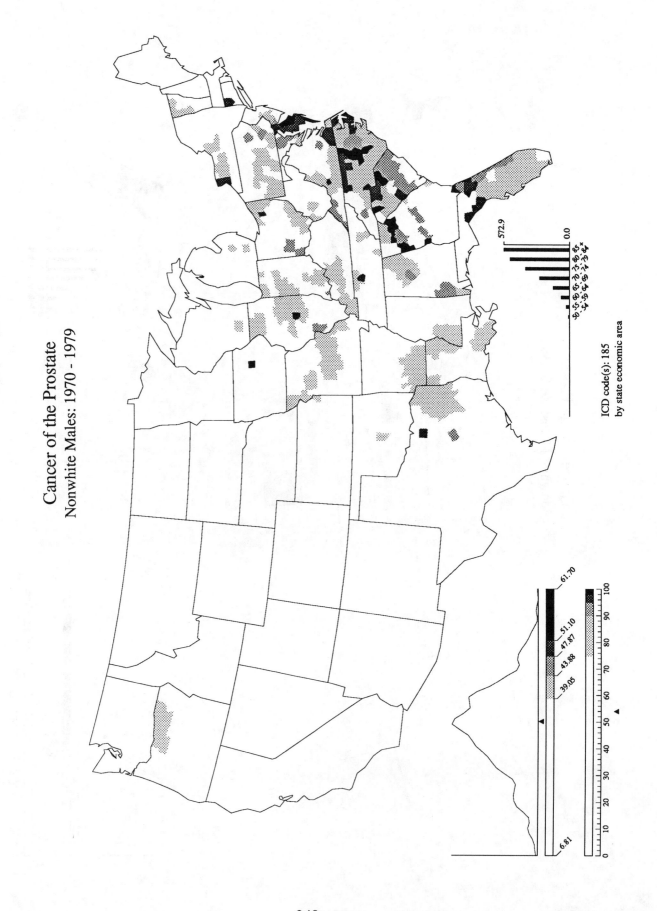

Cancer of the Prostate
Nonwhite Males: 1970 - 1979

ICD code(s): 185
by state economic area

Cancer of the Prostate
Nonwhite Males: Relative Change

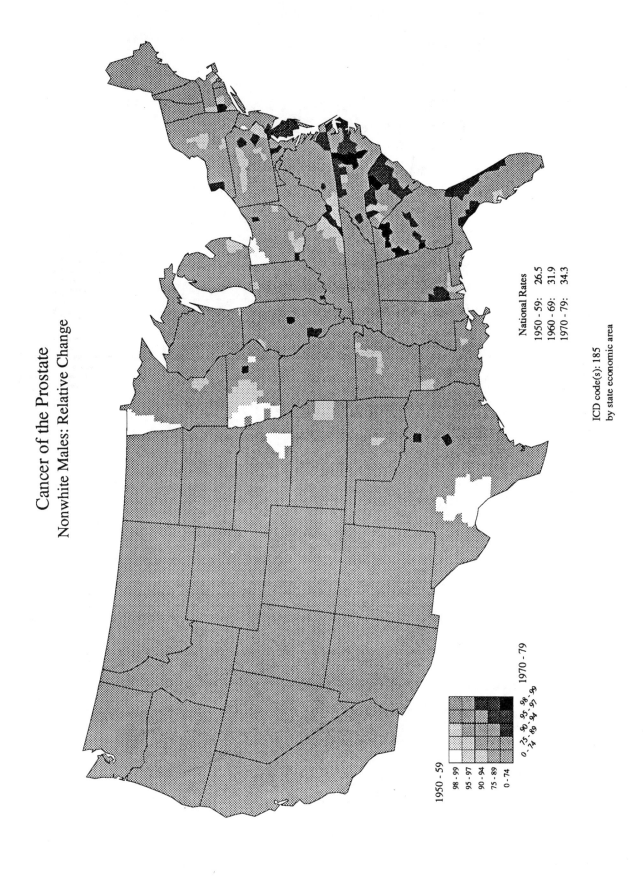

National Rates

1950 - 59: 26.5
1960 - 69: 31.9
1970 - 79: 34.3

ICD code(s): 185
by state economic area

1950 - 59

98 - 99
95 - 97
90 - 94
75 - 89
0 - 74

1970 - 79

98 - 99
95 - 97
90 - 94
75 - 89
0 - 74

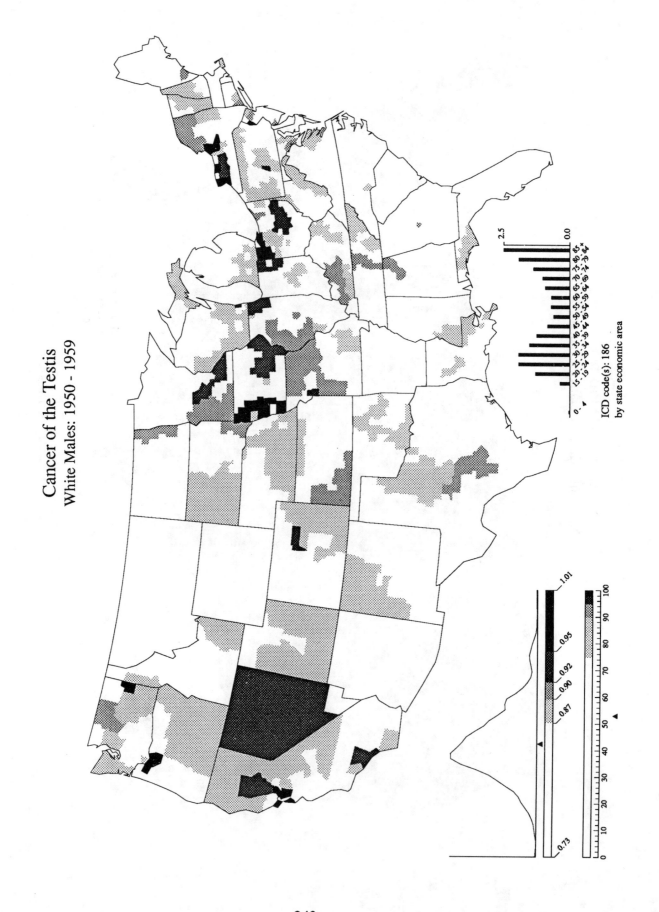

Cancer of the Testis
White Males: 1950 - 1959

ICD code(s): 186
by state economic area

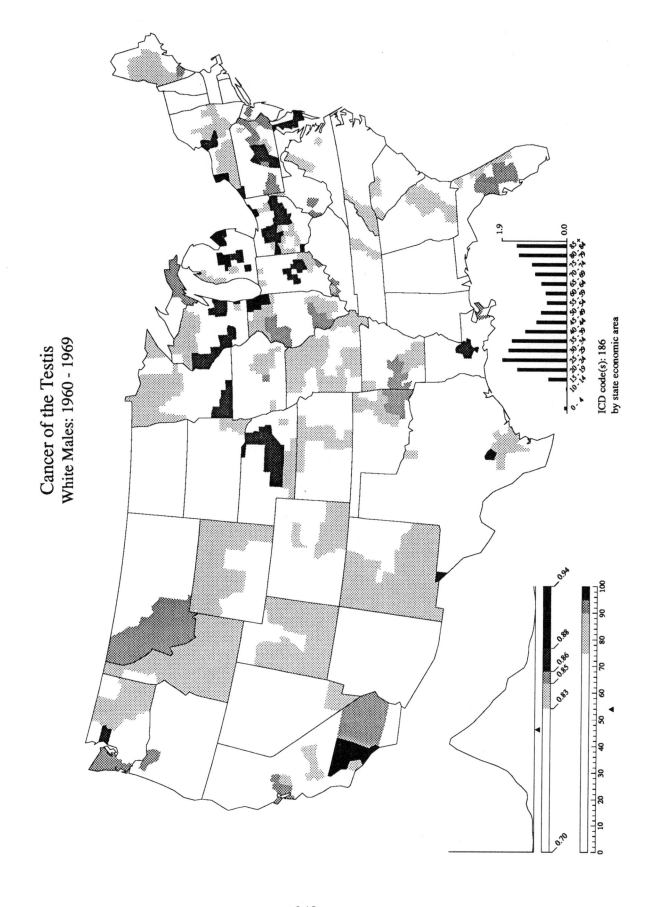

Cancer of the Testis
White Males: 1960 - 1969

ICD code(s): 186
by state economic area

243

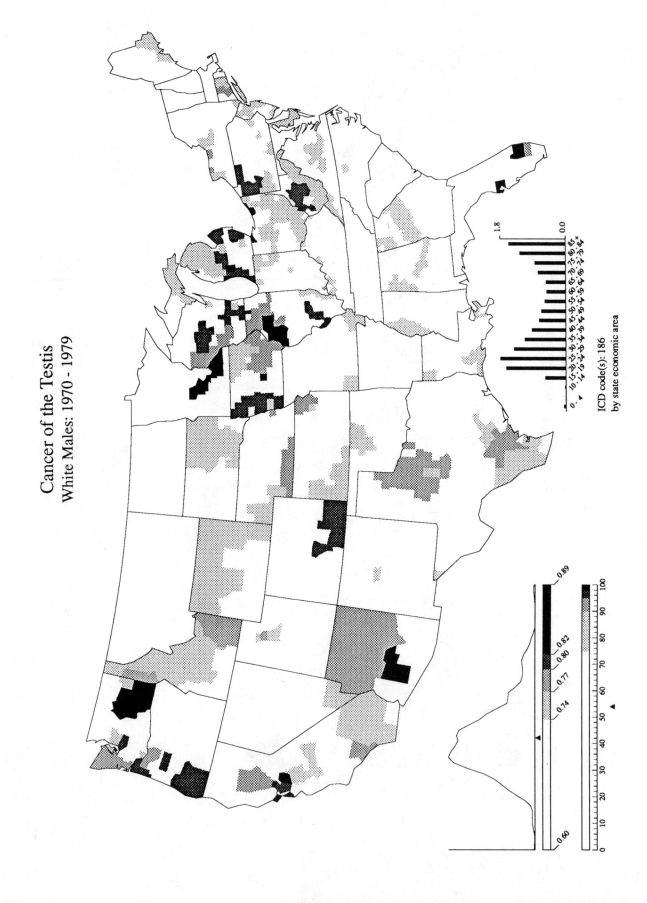

Cancer of the Testis
White Males: 1970 - 1979

ICD code(s): 186
by state economic area

244

Cancer of the Testis
White Males: Relative Change

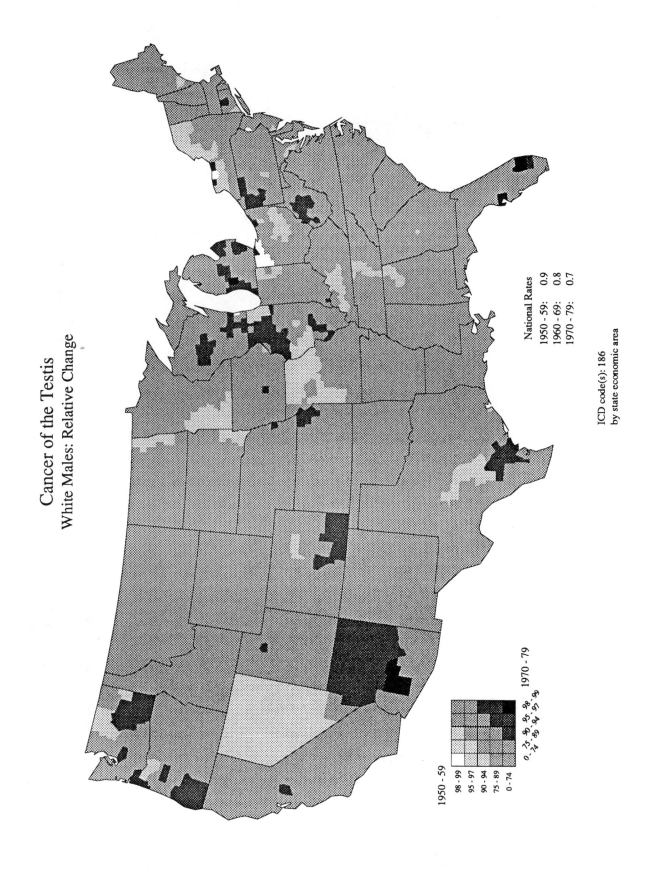

National Rates

1950 - 59:	0.9
1960 - 69:	0.8
1970 - 79:	0.7

ICD code(s): 186
by state economic area

Cancer of the Bladder and other Urinary Organs
White Males: 1950 - 1959

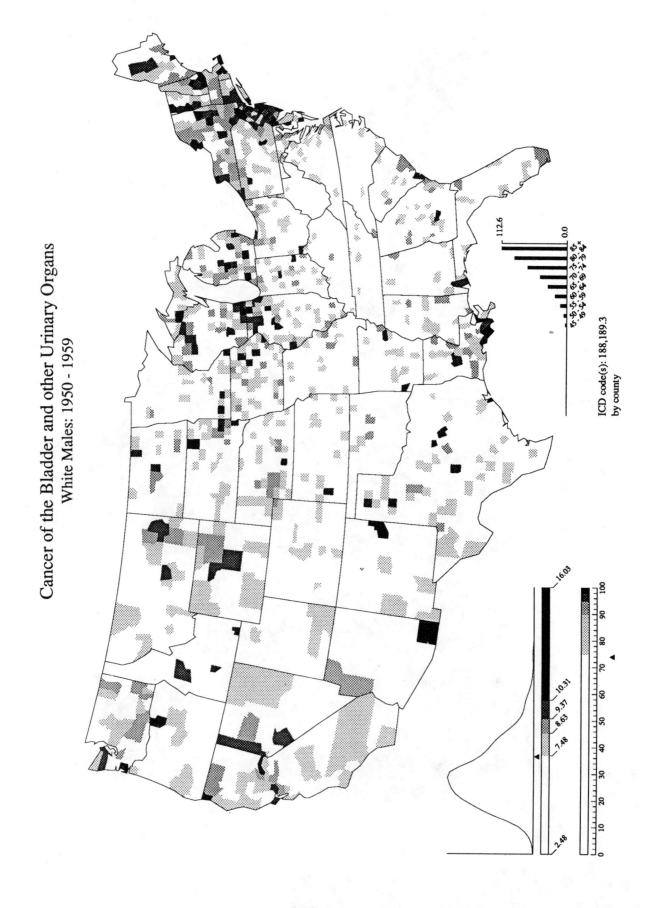

ICD code(s): 188,189.3
by county

Cancer of the Bladder and other Urinary Organs
White Males: 1960 - 1969

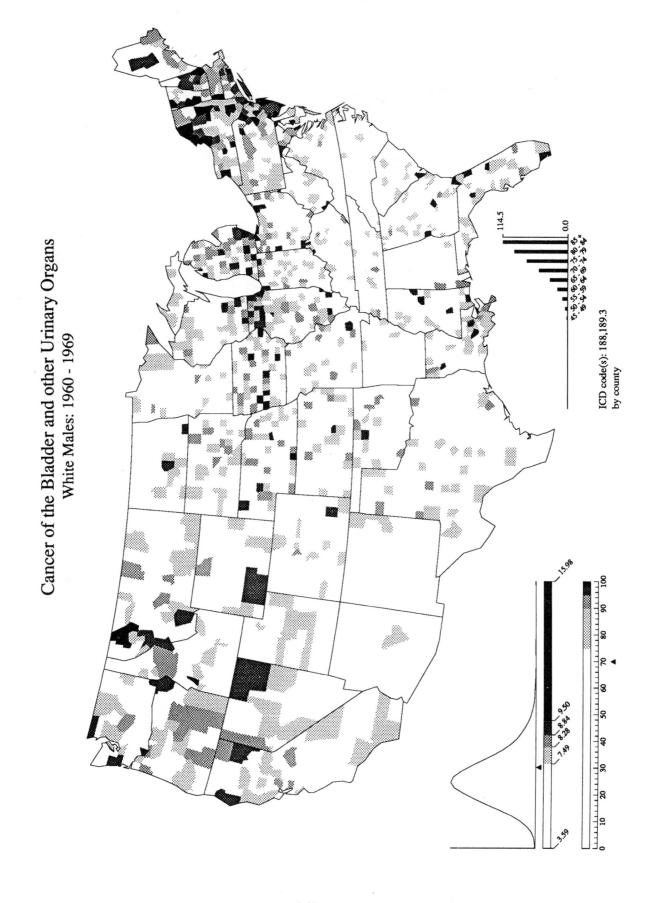

ICD code(s): 188,189.3
by county

Cancer of the Bladder and other Urinary Organs
White Males: 1970 - 1979

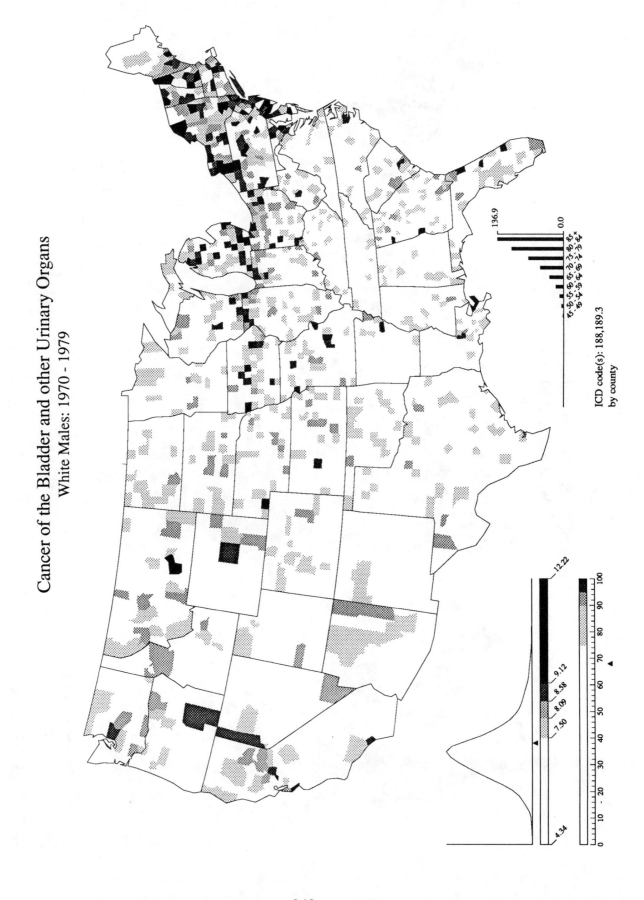

ICD code(s): 188,189.3
by county

248

Cancer of the Bladder and other Urinary Organs
White Males: Relative Change

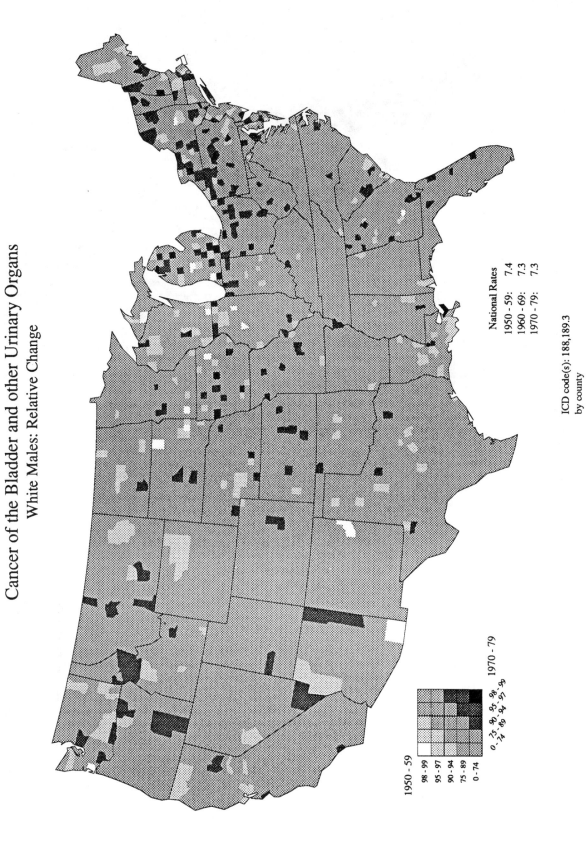

National Rates

1950 - 59:	7.4
1960 - 69:	7.3
1970 - 79:	7.3

ICD code(s): 188,189.3
by county

1950 - 59

| 98 - 99 |
| 95 - 97 |
| 90 - 94 |
| 75 - 89 |
| 0 - 74 |

0 - 74 75 - 89 90 - 94 95 - 97 98 - 99

1970 - 79

Cancer of the Bladder and other Urinary Organs
White Females: 1950 - 1959

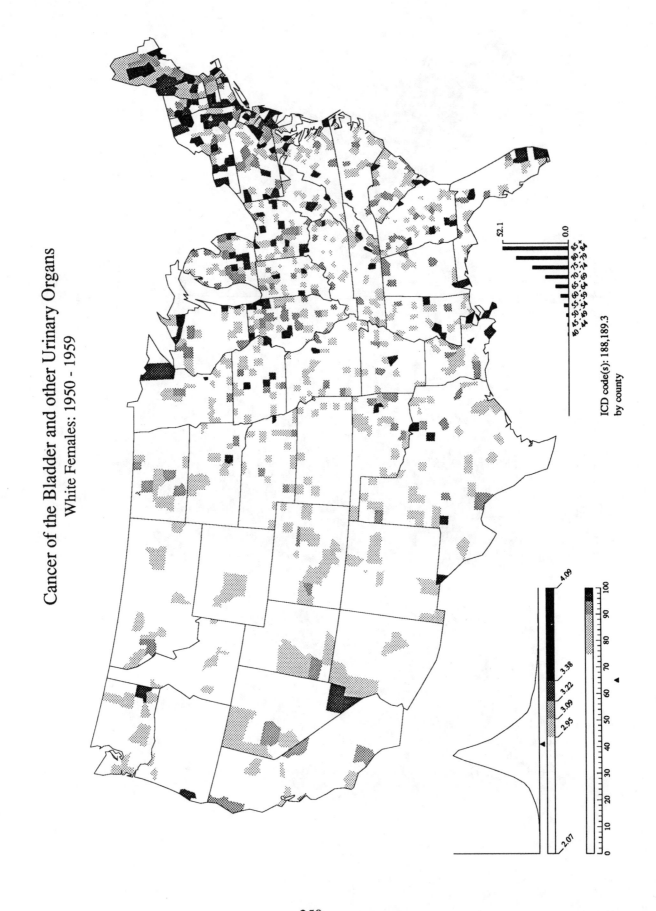

ICD code(s): 188,189.3
by county

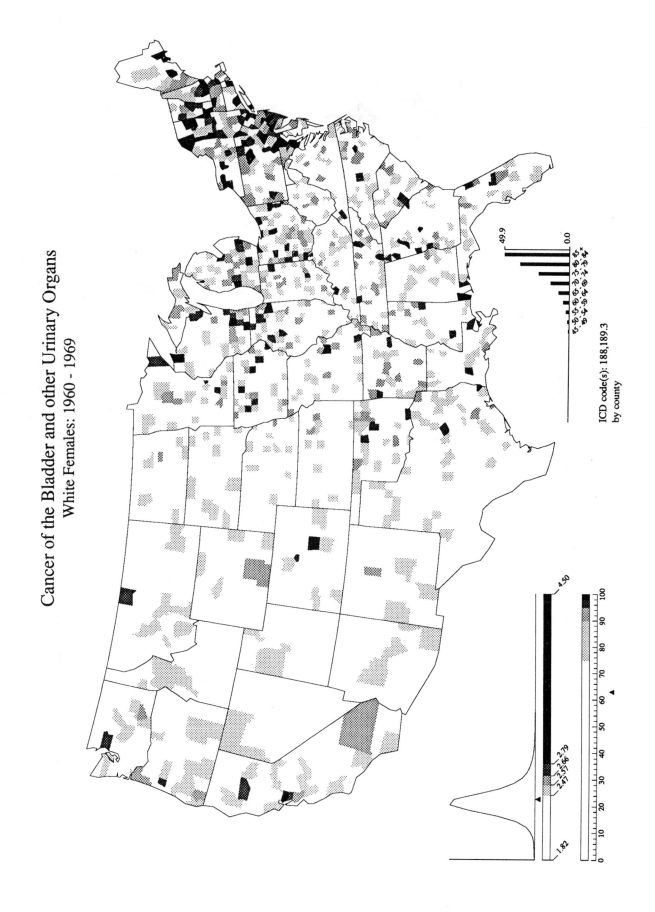

Cancer of the Bladder and other Urinary Organs
White Females: 1960 - 1969

ICD code(s): 188,189.3
by county

251

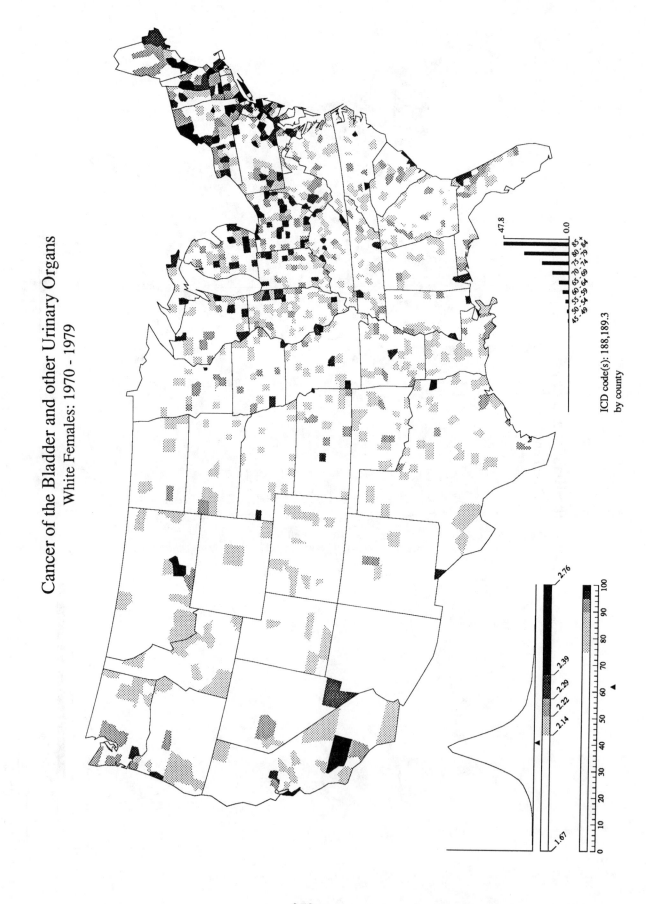

Cancer of the Bladder and other Urinary Organs
White Females: 1970 - 1979

ICD code(s): 188,189.3
by county

Cancer of the Bladder and other Urinary Organs
White Females: Relative Change

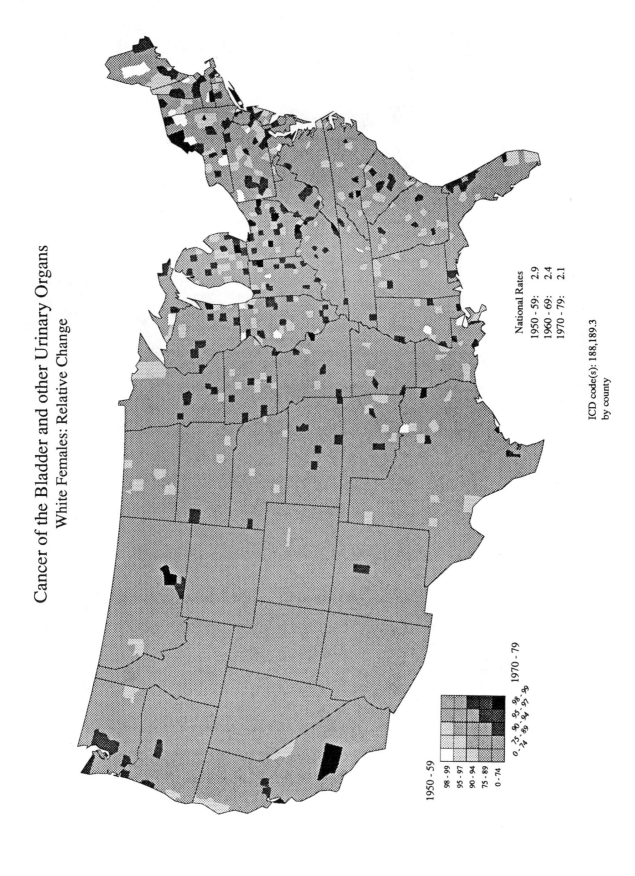

National Rates

1950 - 59:	2.9
1960 - 69:	2.4
1970 - 79:	2.1

ICD code(s): 188,189.3
by county

1950 - 59

1970 - 79

98 - 99
95 - 97
90 - 94
75 - 89
0 - 74

0 - 74   75 - 89   90 - 94   95 - 97   98 - 99

Cancer of the Bladder and other Urinary Organs
Nonwhite Males: 1950 - 1959

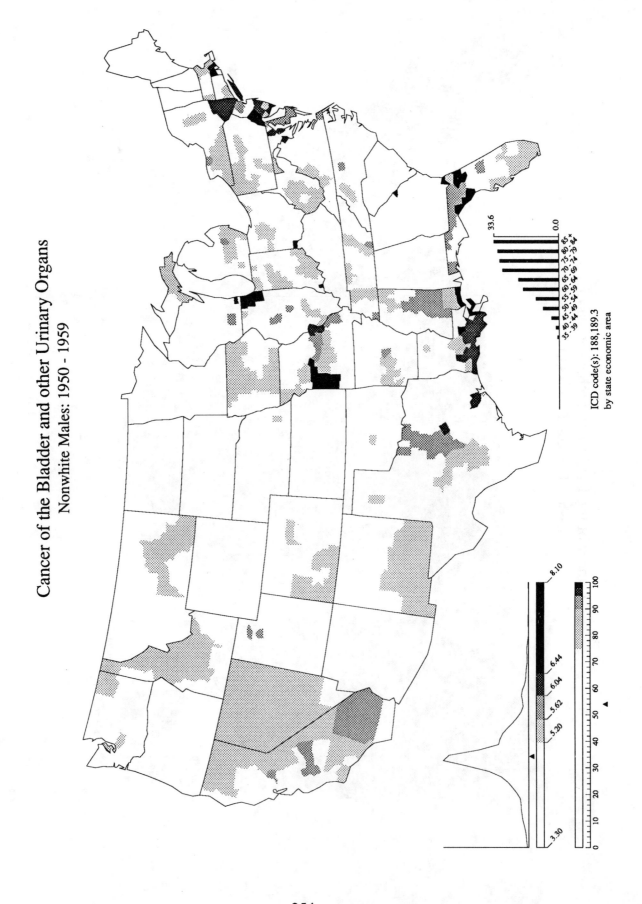

ICD code(s): 188,189.3
by state economic area

Cancer of the Bladder and other Urinary Organs
Nonwhite Males: 1960 - 1969

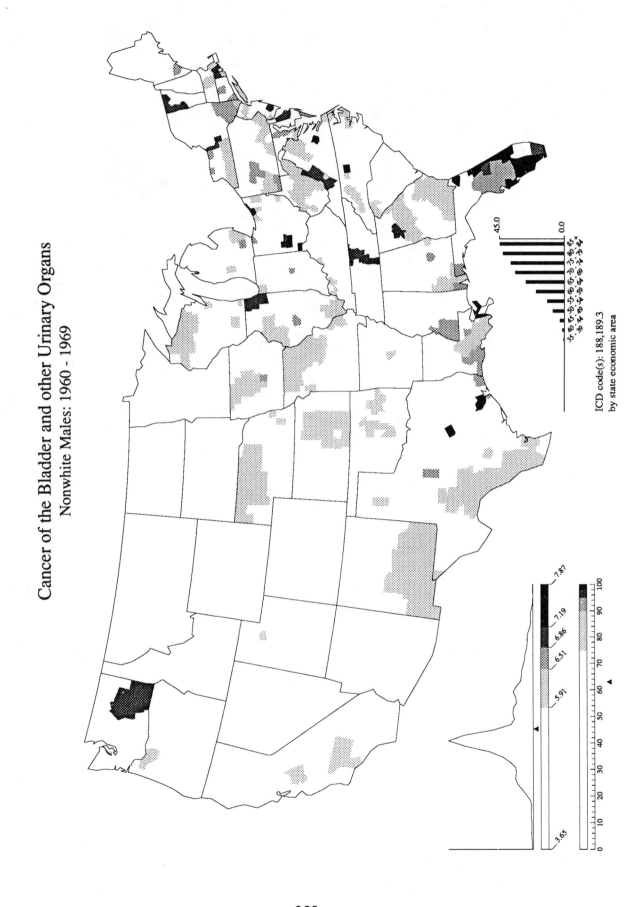

ICD code(s): 188,189.3
by state economic area

Cancer of the Bladder and other Urinary Organs
Nonwhite Males: 1970 - 1979

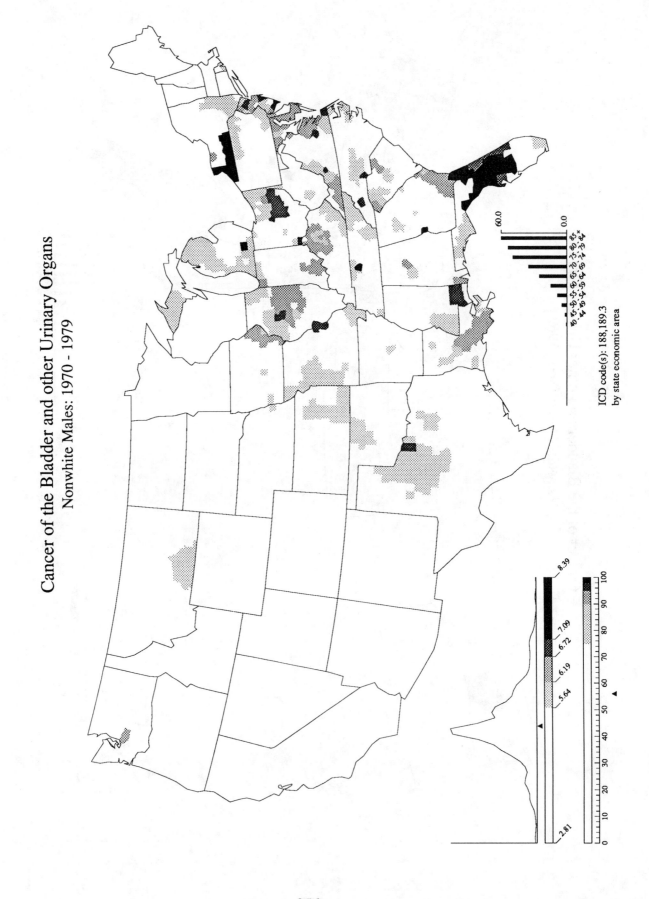

ICD code(s): 188,189.3
by state economic area

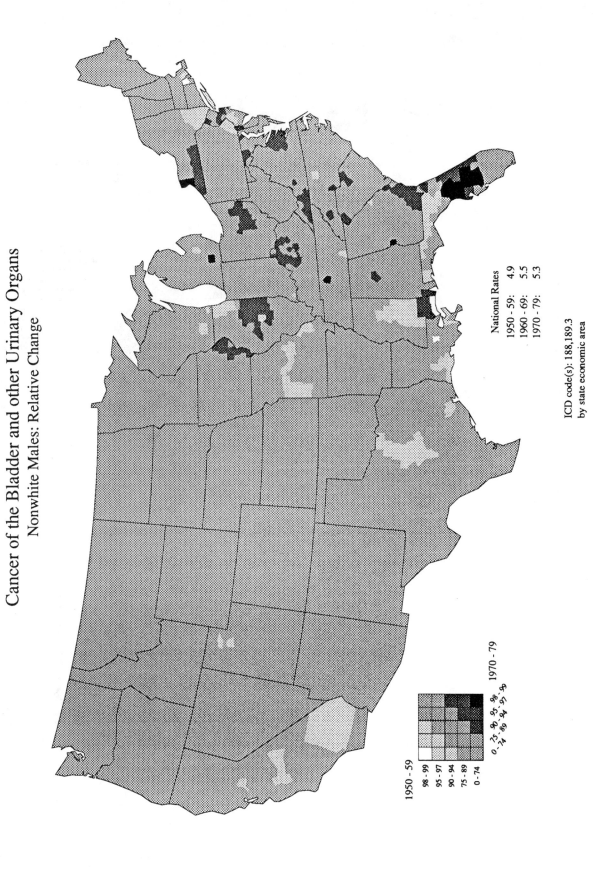

Cancer of the Bladder and other Urinary Organs
Nonwhite Males: Relative Change

National Rates

1950 - 59: 4.9
1960 - 69: 5.5
1970 - 79: 5.3

ICD code(s): 188,189.3
by state economic area

1950 - 59

98 - 99
95 - 97
90 - 94
75 - 89
0 - 74

1970 - 79

0 75 90 95 98 99
   - 74 - 89 - 94 - 97

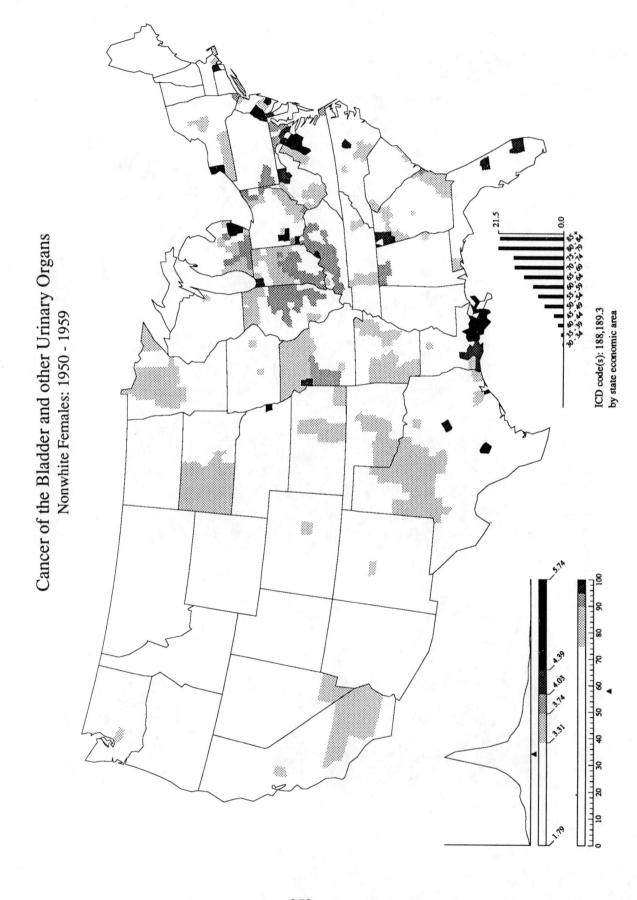

Cancer of the Bladder and other Urinary Organs
Nonwhite Females: 1950 - 1959

ICD code(s): 188,189.3
by state economic area

Cancer of the Bladder and other Urinary Organs
Nonwhite Females: 1960 - 1969

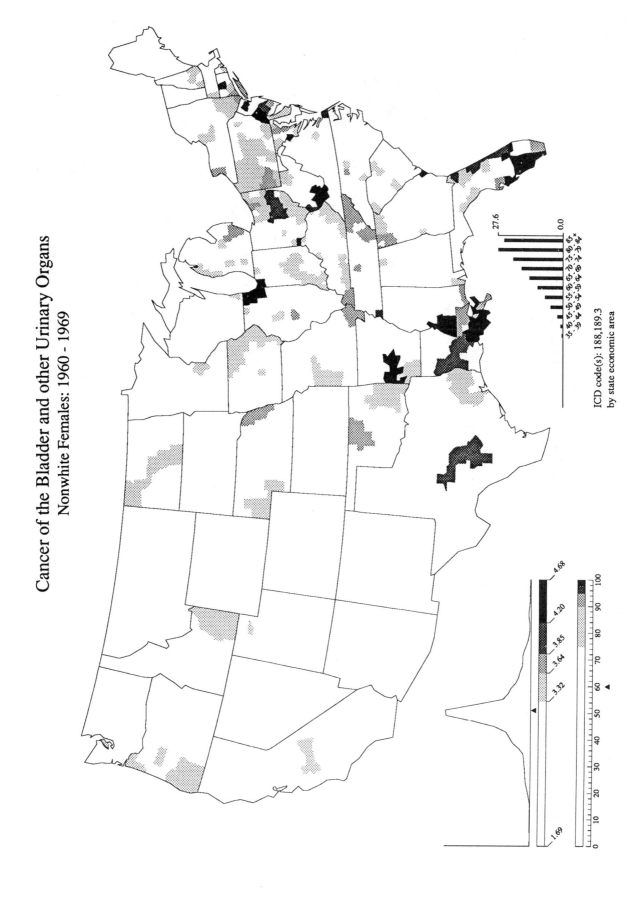

ICD code(s): 188,189.3
by state economic area

Cancer of the Bladder and other Urinary Organs
Nonwhite Females: 1970 - 1979

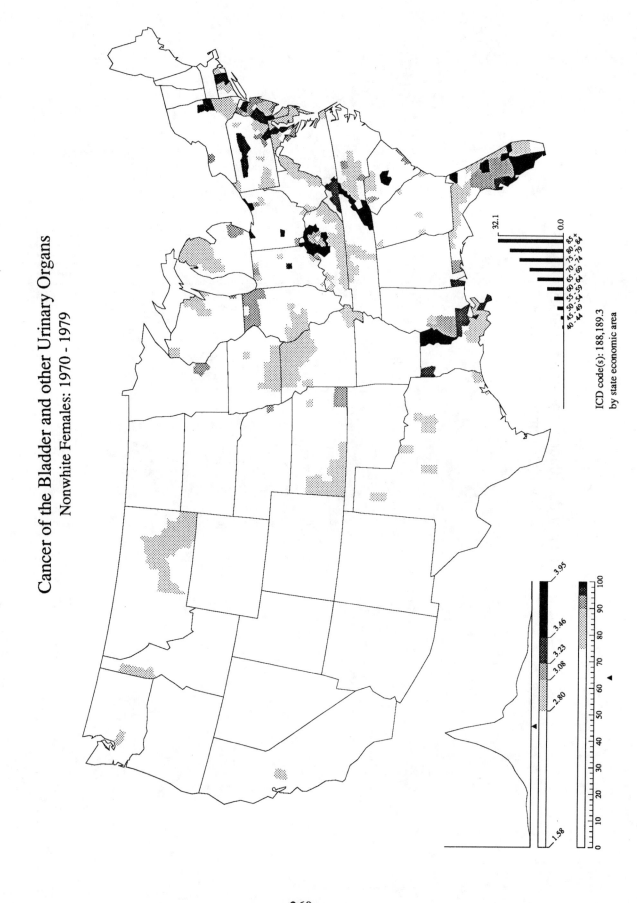

ICD code(s): 188,189.3
by state economic area

Cancer of the Bladder and other Urinary Organs
Nonwhite Females: Relative Change

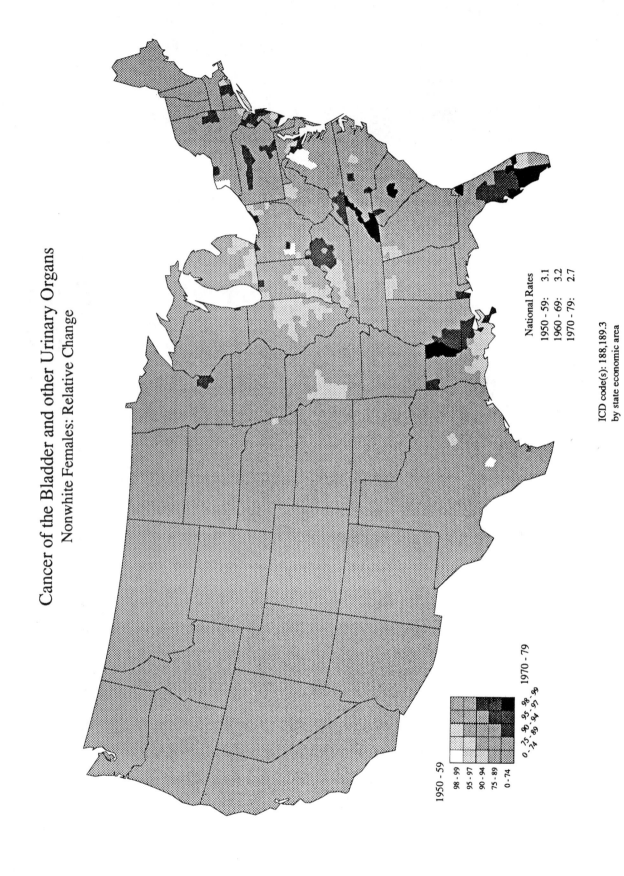

National Rates

1950 - 59:	3.1
1960 - 69:	3.2
1970 - 79:	2.7

ICD code(s): 188,189.3
by state economic area

1950 - 59

98 - 99
95 - 97
90 - 94
75 - 89
0 - 74

1970 - 79

0 - 74 89 94 97 99
75 90 95 98 99

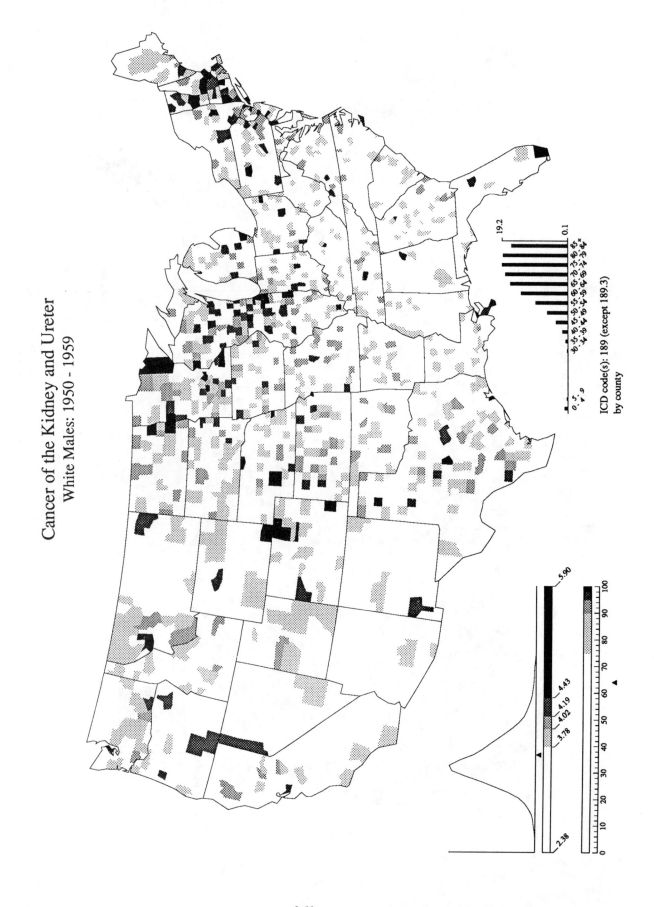

Cancer of the Kidney and Ureter
White Males: 1950 - 1959

ICD code(s): 189 (except 189.3)
by county

Cancer of the Kidney and Ureter
White Males: 1960 - 1969

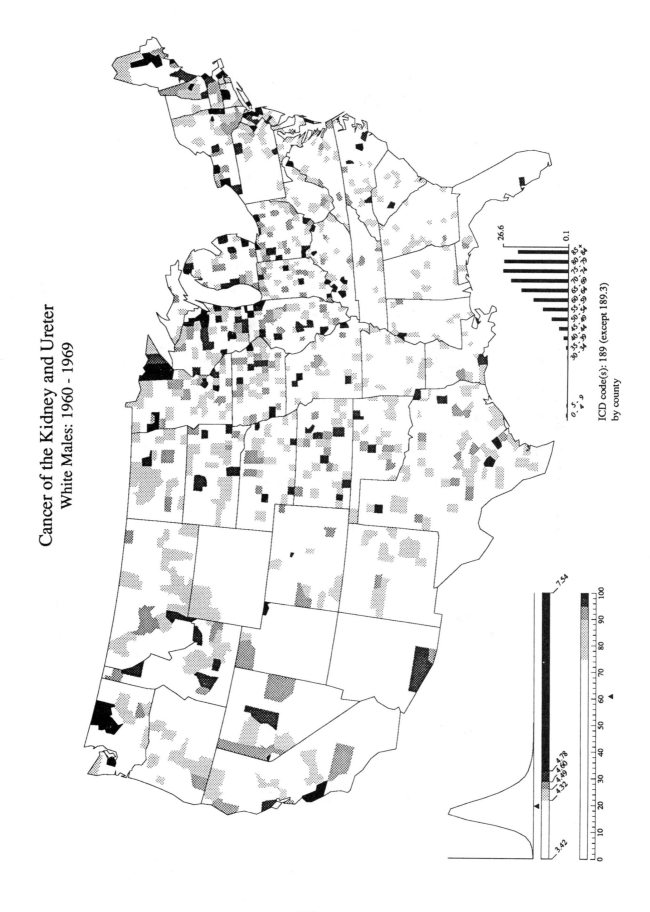

ICD code(s): 189 (except 189.3)
by county

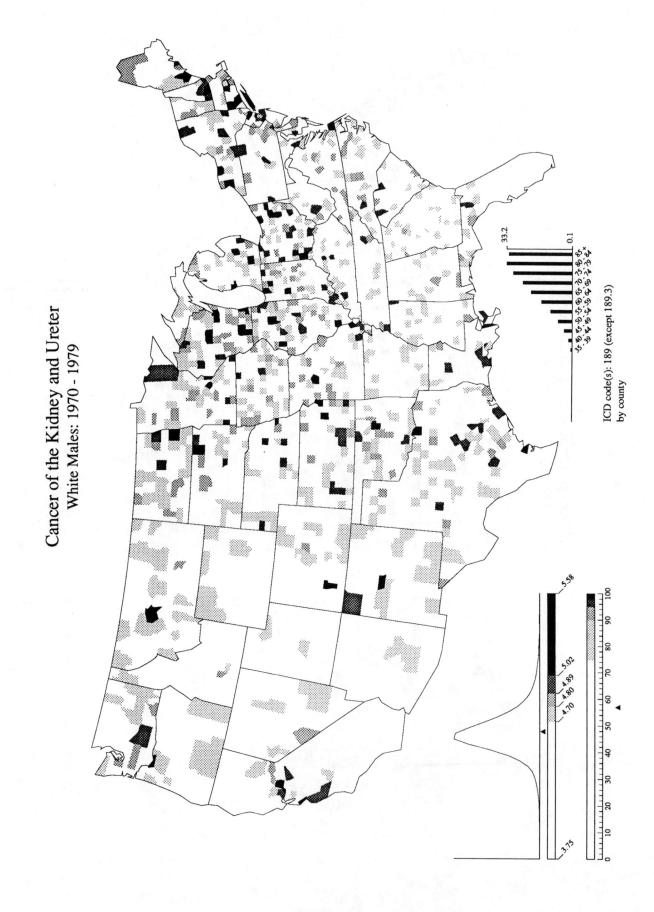

Cancer of the Kidney and Ureter
White Males: 1970 - 1979

ICD code(s): 189 (except 189.3)
by county

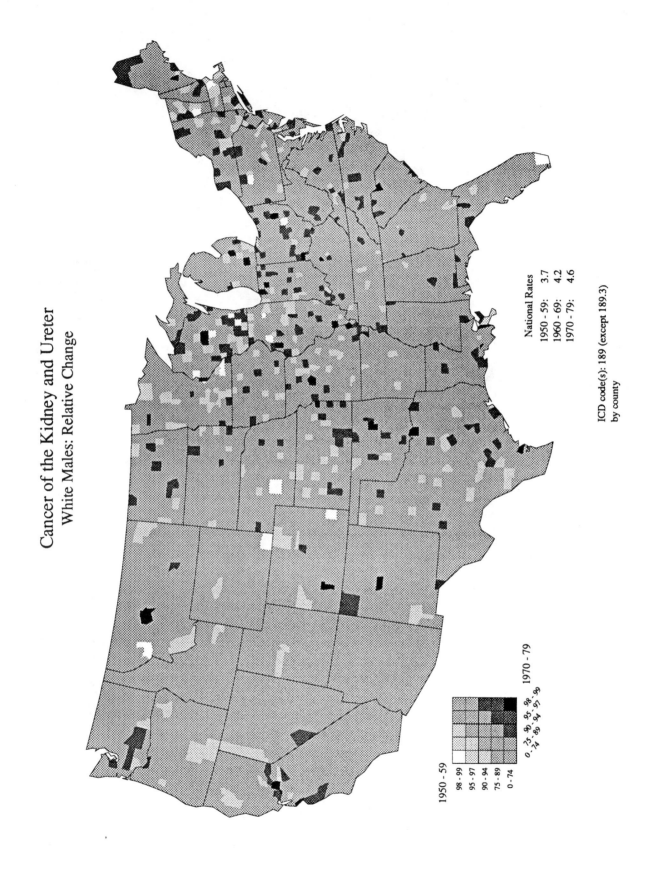

Cancer of the Kidney and Ureter
White Males: Relative Change

National Rates

1950 - 59: 3.7
1960 - 69: 4.2
1970 - 79: 4.6

ICD code(s): 189 (except 189.3)
by county

1950 - 59

98 - 99
95 - 97
90 - 94
75 - 89
0 - 74

1970 - 79

0 - 74 75 - 89 90 - 94 95 - 97 98 - 99

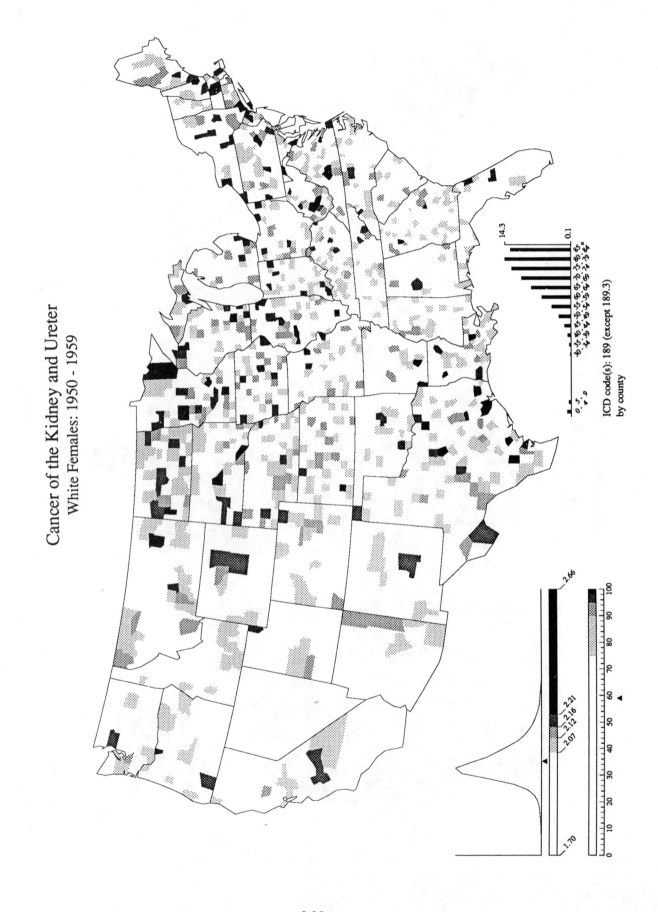

Cancer of the Kidney and Ureter
White Females: 1950 - 1959

ICD code(s): 189 (except 189.3)
by county

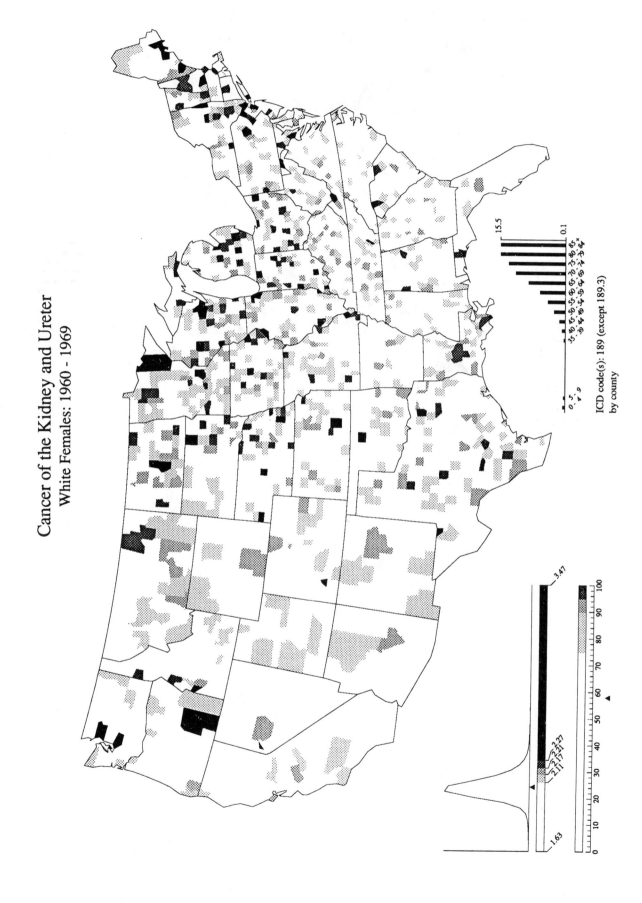

Cancer of the Kidney and Ureter
White Females: 1960 - 1969

ICD code(s): 189 (except 189.3)
by county

Cancer of the Kidney and Ureter
White Females: 1970 - 1979

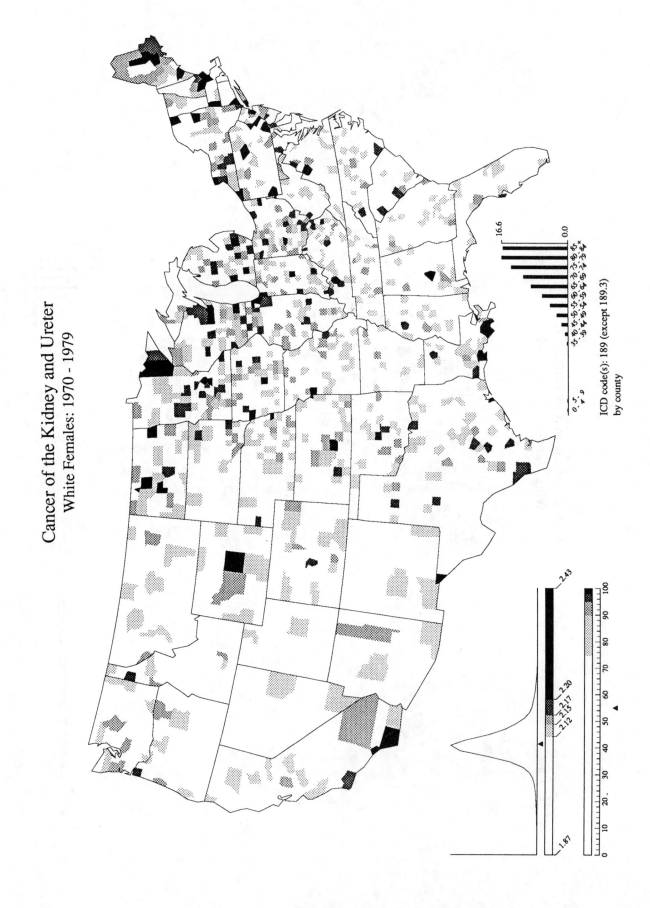

ICD code(s): 189 (except 189.3)
by county

Cancer of the Kidney and Ureter
White Females: Relative Change

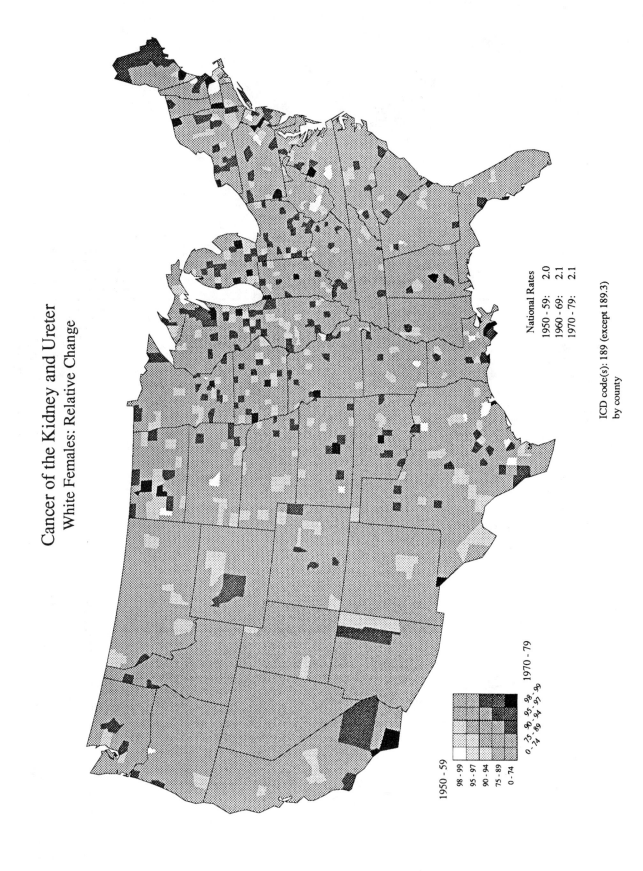

National Rates

1950 - 59:   2.0
1960 - 69:   2.1
1970 - 79:   2.1

ICD code(s): 189 (except 189.3)
by county

1950 - 59

98 - 99
95 - 97
90 - 94
75 - 89
0 - 74

1970 - 79

98 - 99
95 - 97
90 - 94
75 - 89
0 - 74

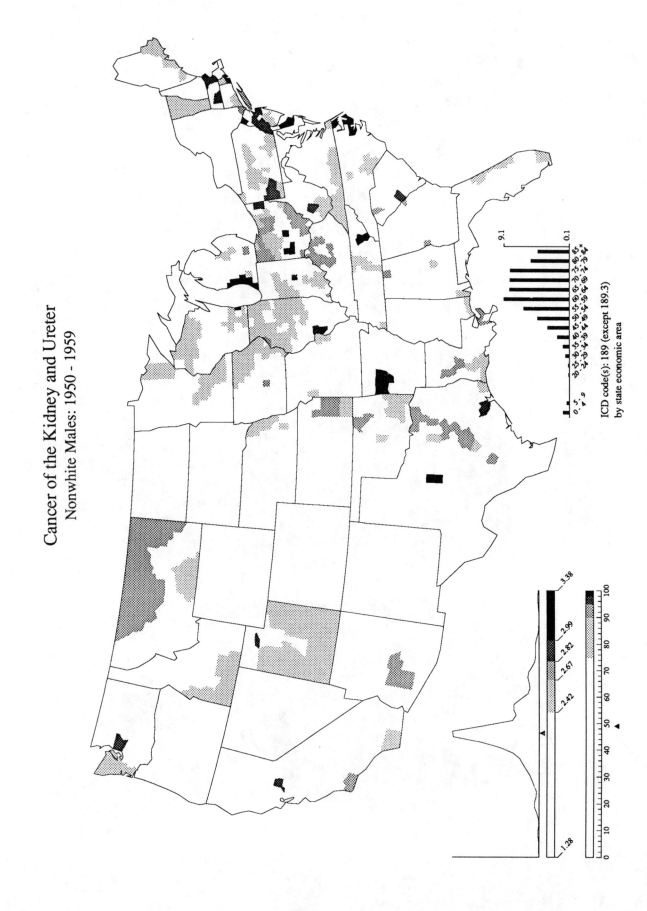

Cancer of the Kidney and Ureter
Nonwhite Males: 1950 - 1959

ICD code(s): 189 (except 189.3)
by state economic area

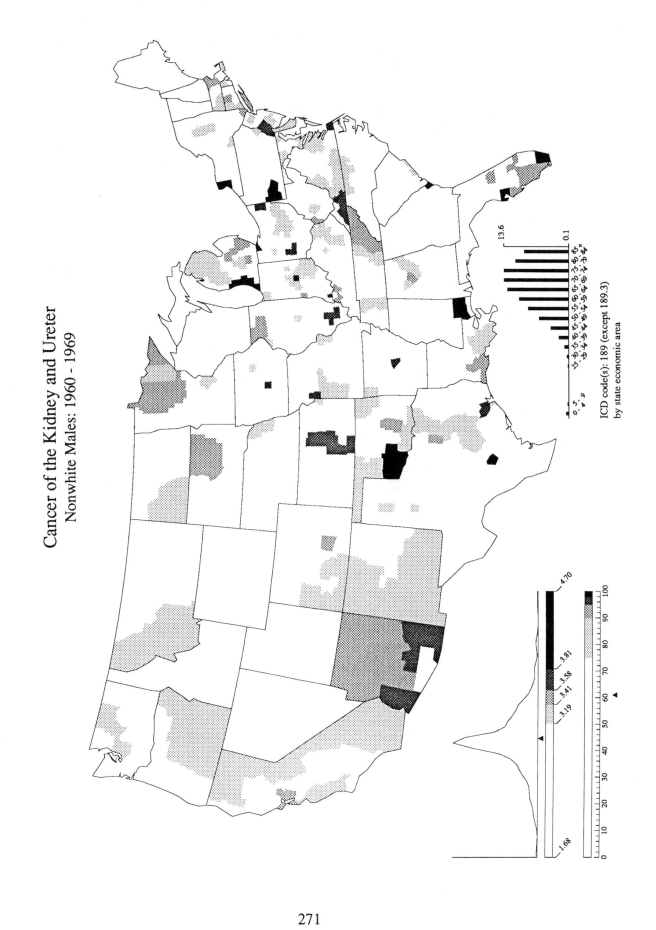

Cancer of the Kidney and Ureter
Nonwhite Males: 1960 - 1969

ICD code(s): 189 (except 189.3)
by state economic area

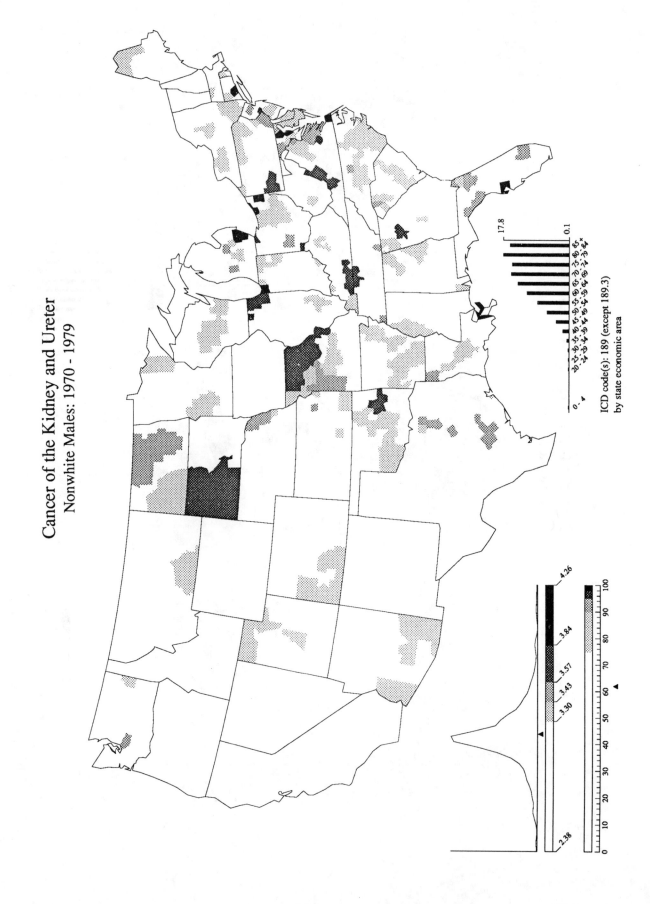

Cancer of the Kidney and Ureter
Nonwhite Males: 1970 - 1979

ICD code(s): 189 (except 189.3)
by state economic area

Cancer of the Kidney and Ureter
Nonwhite Males: Relative Change

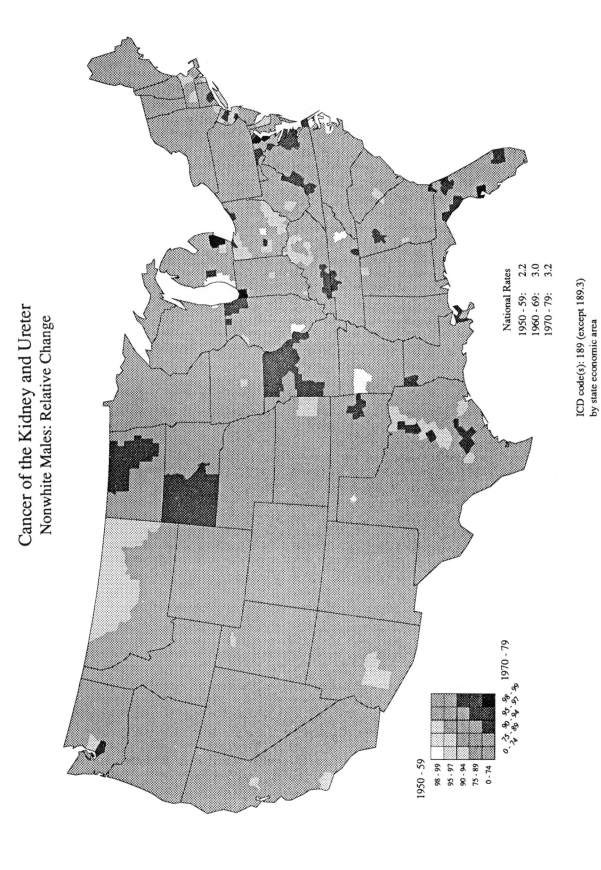

National Rates

1950 - 59:	2.2
1960 - 69:	3.0
1970 - 79:	3.2

ICD code(s): 189 (except 189.3)
by state economic area

1950 - 59

| 98 - 99 |
| 95 - 97 |
| 90 - 94 |
| 75 - 89 |
| 0 - 74 |

1970 - 79

98 - 99
95 - 97
90 - 94
75 - 89
0 - 74

Cancer of the Brain and other parts of the Nervous System
White Males: 1950 - 1959

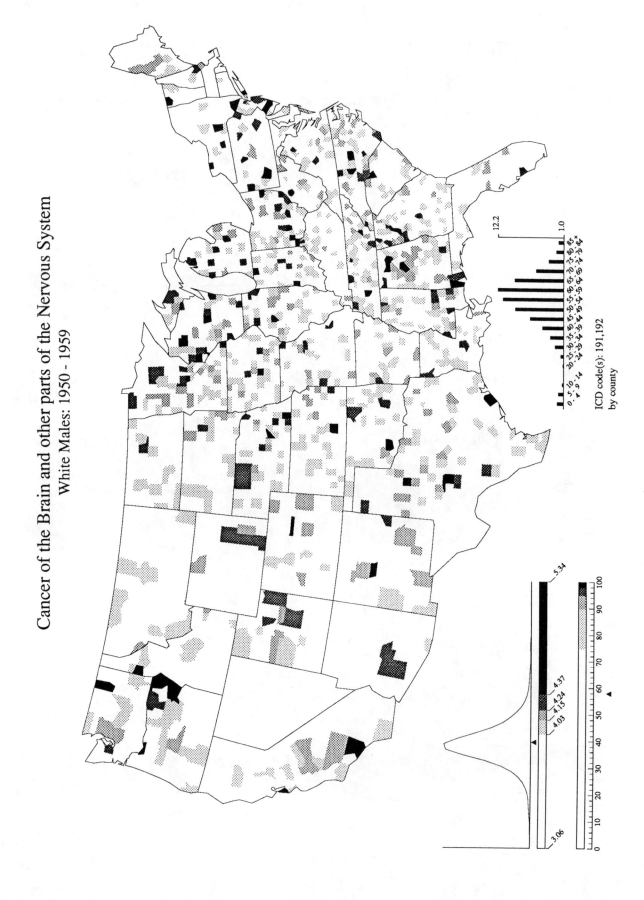

ICD code(s): 191,192
by county

274

Cancer of the Brain and other parts of the Nervous System
White Males: 1960 - 1969

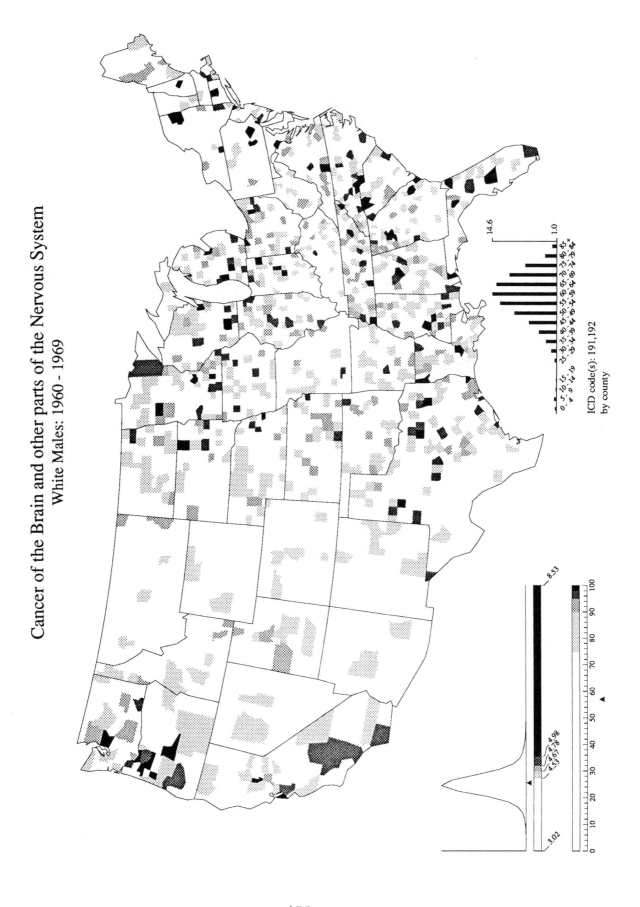

ICD code(s): 191,192
by county

Cancer of the Brain and other parts of the Nervous System
White Males: 1970 - 1979

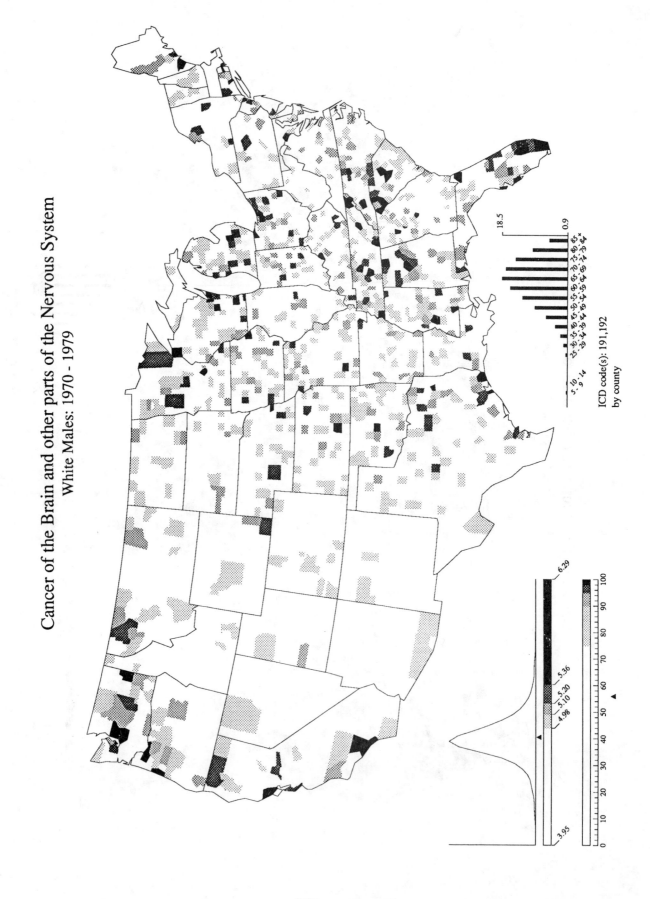

ICD code(s): 191,192
by county

Cancer of the Brain and other parts of the Nervous System
White Males: Relative Change

National Rates

1950 - 59:	4.0
1960 - 69:	4.4
1970 - 79:	4.9

ICD code(s): 191,192
by county

1950 - 59

1970 - 79

98 - 99
95 - 97
90 - 94
75 - 89
0 - 74

0 - 74   75 - 89   90 - 94   95 - 97   98 - 99

Cancer of the Brain and other parts of the Nervous System
White Females: 1950 - 1959

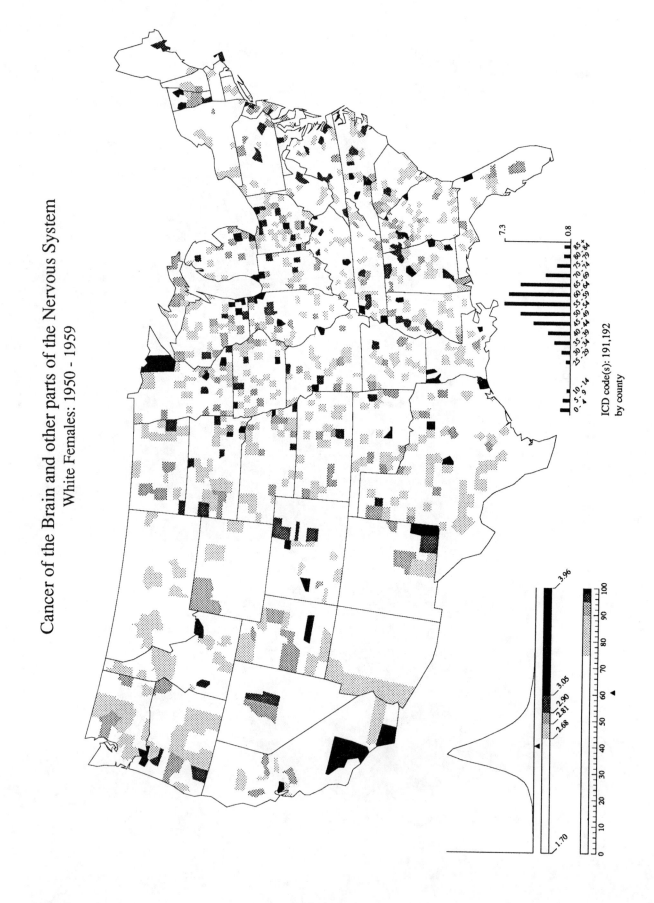

ICD code(s): 191,192
by county

Cancer of the Brain and other parts of the Nervous System
White Females: 1960 - 1969

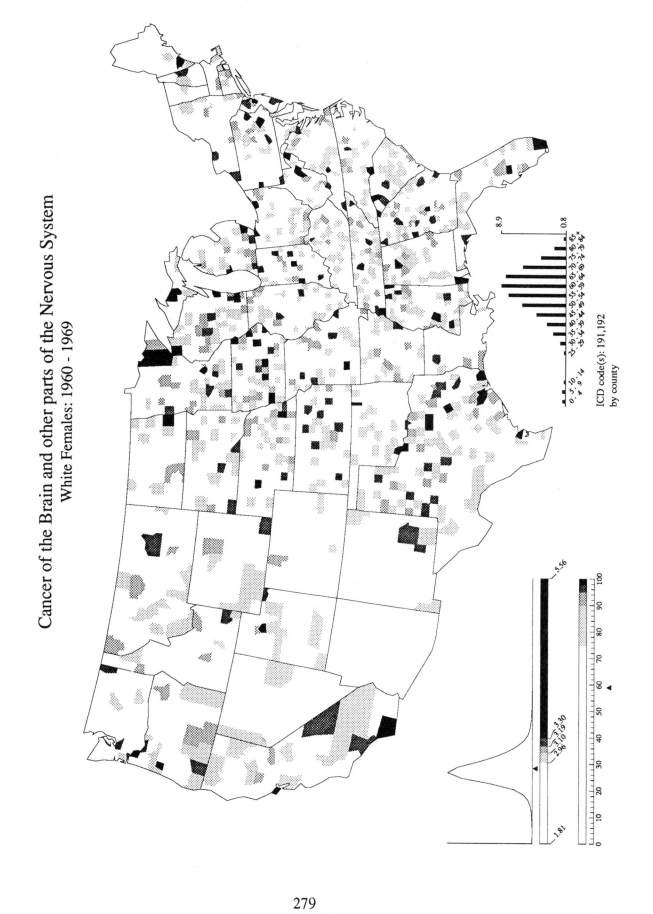

ICD code(s): 191,192
by county

279

Cancer of the Brain and other parts of the Nervous System
White Females: 1970 - 1979

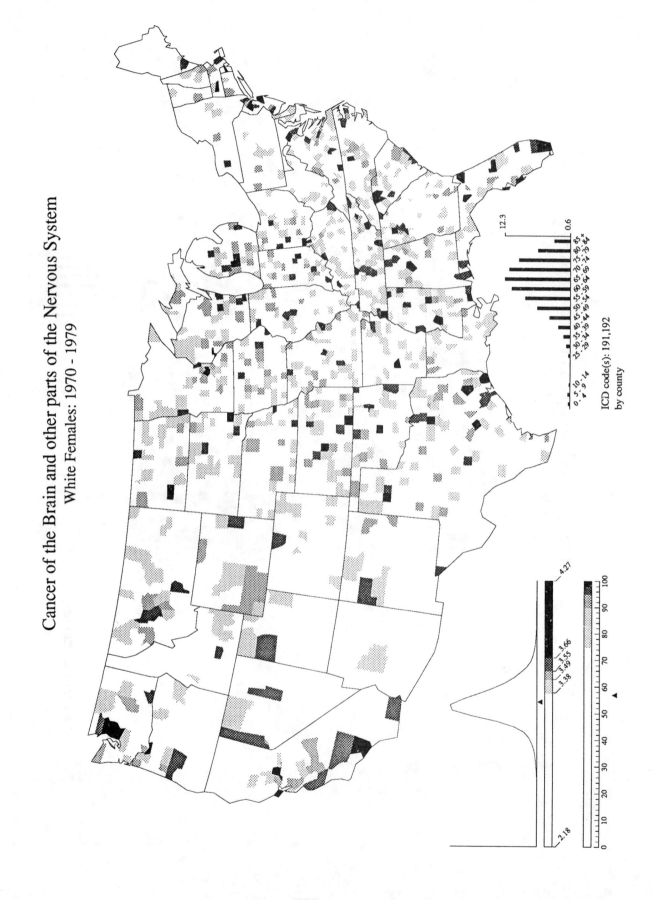

ICD code(s): 191,192
by county

Cancer of the Brain and other parts of the Nervous System
White Females: Relative Change

National Rates

1950 - 59:	2.6
1960 - 69:	2.9
1970 - 79:	3.3

ICD code(s): 191,192
by county

1950 - 59

98 - 99
95 - 97
90 - 94
75 - 89
0 - 74

1970 - 79

0 - 74 75 - 89 90 - 94 95 - 97 98 - 99

Cancer of the Brain and other parts of the Nervous System
Nonwhite Males: 1950 - 1959

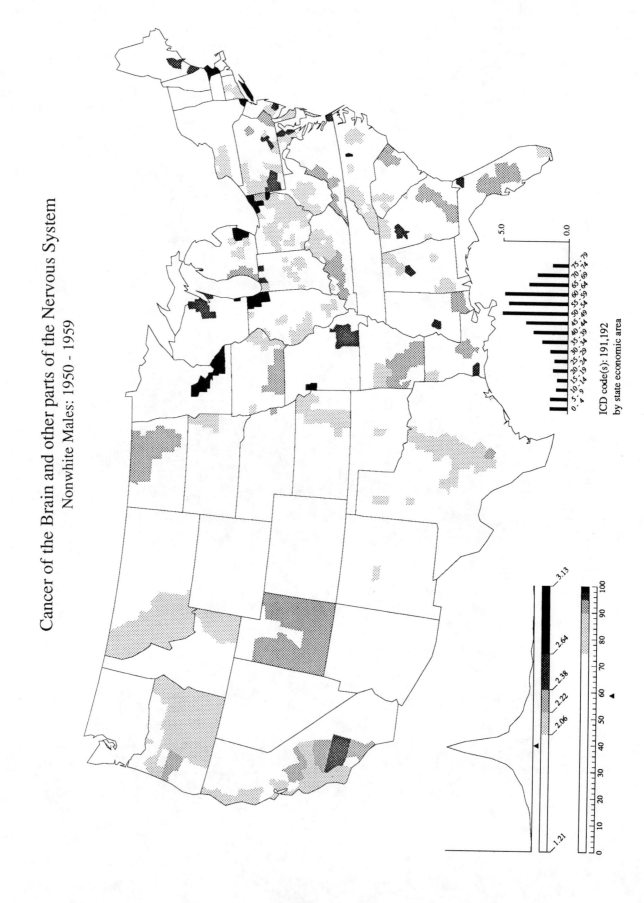

ICD code(s): 191,192
by state economic area

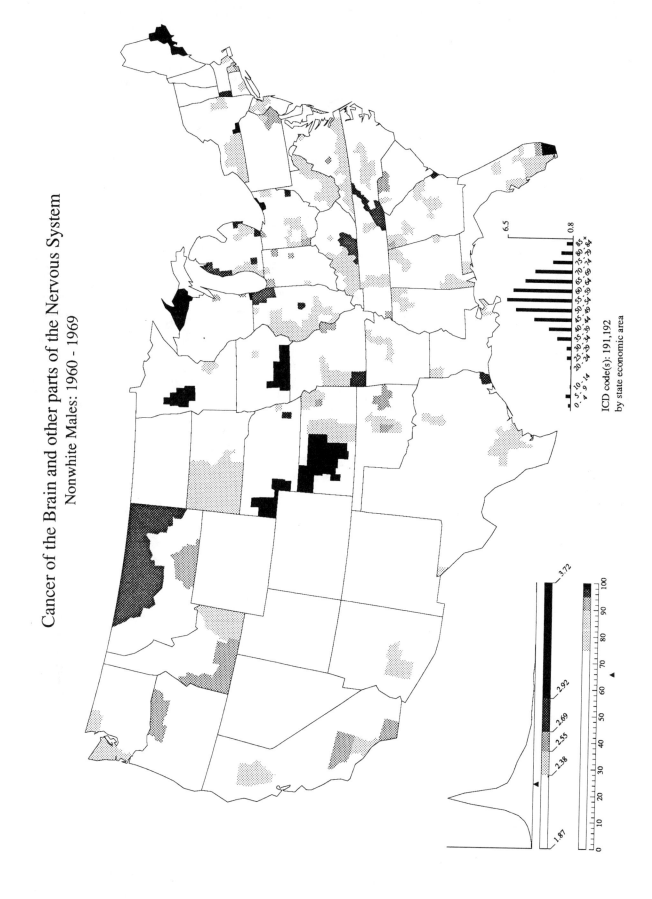

Cancer of the Brain and other parts of the Nervous System
Nonwhite Males: 1960 - 1969

ICD code(s): 191,192
by state economic area

Cancer of the Brain and other parts of the Nervous System
Nonwhite Males: 1970 - 1979

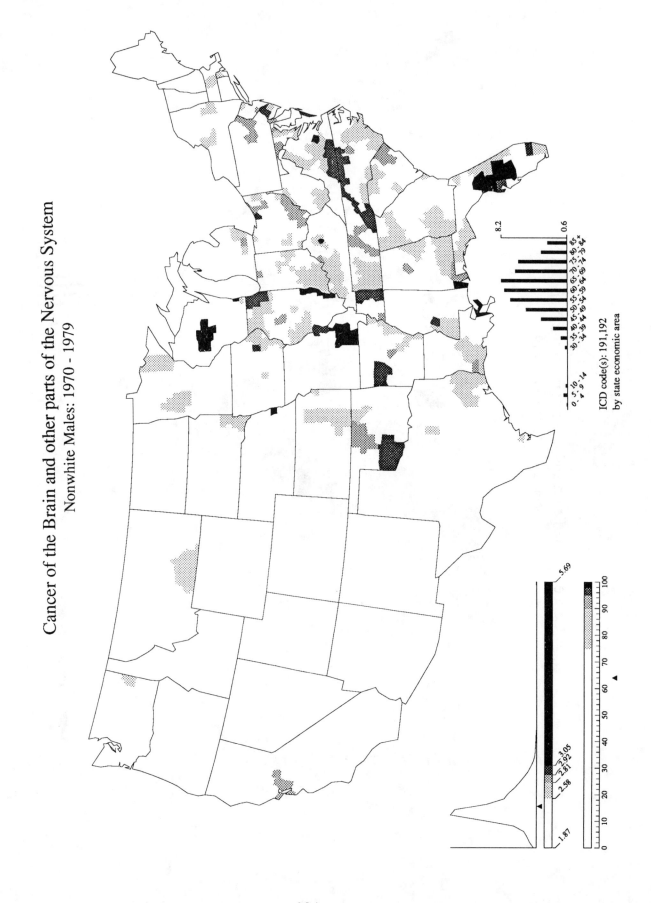

ICD code(s): 191,192
by state economic area

Cancer of the Brain and other parts of the Nervous System
Nonwhite Males: Relative Change

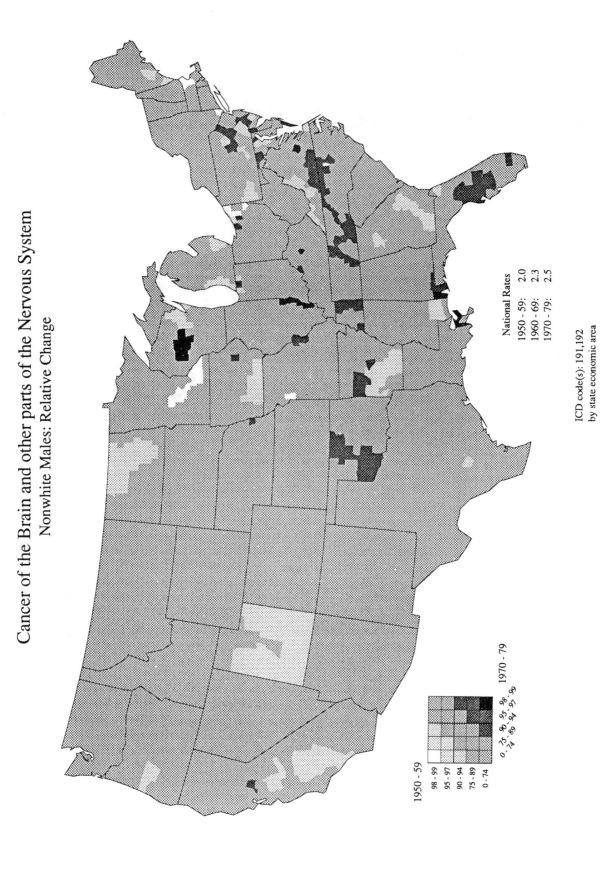

National Rates

1950 - 59:	2.0
1960 - 69:	2.3
1970 - 79:	2.5

ICD code(s): 191,192
by state economic area

1950 - 59

98 - 99
95 - 97
90 - 94
75 - 89
0 - 74

1970 - 79

0 - 74 75 - 89 90 - 94 95 - 97 98 - 99

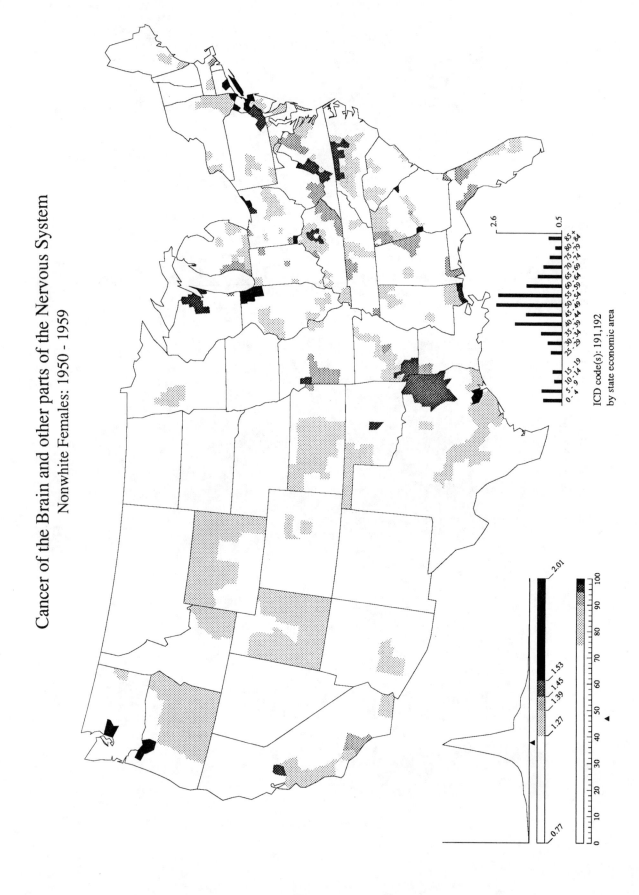

Cancer of the Brain and other parts of the Nervous System
Nonwhite Females: 1950 - 1959

ICD code(s): 191,192
by state economic area

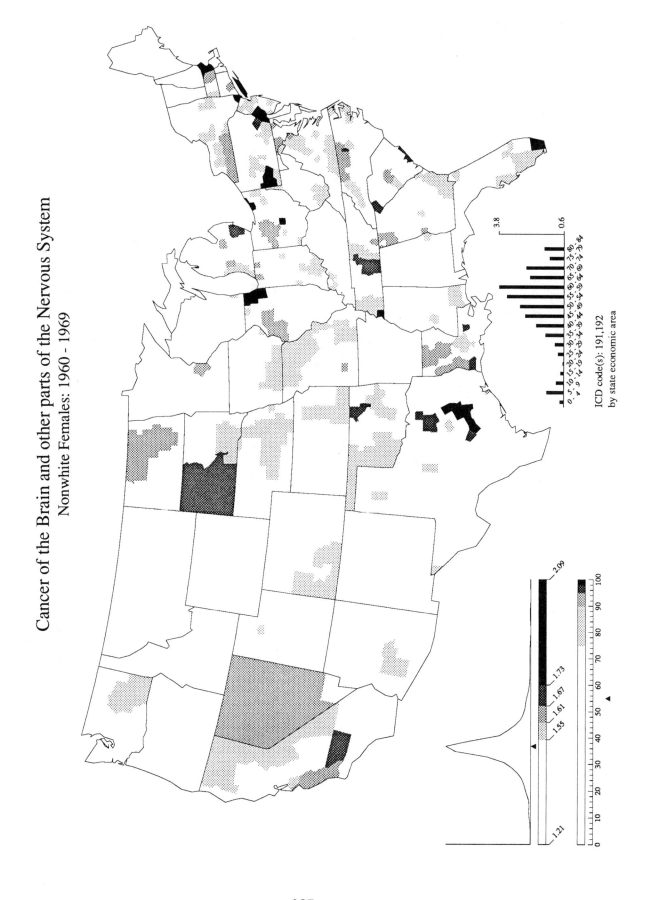

Cancer of the Brain and other parts of the Nervous System
Nonwhite Females: 1960 - 1969

ICD code(s): 191,192
by state economic area

287

Cancer of the Brain and other parts of the Nervous System
Nonwhite Females: 1970 - 1979

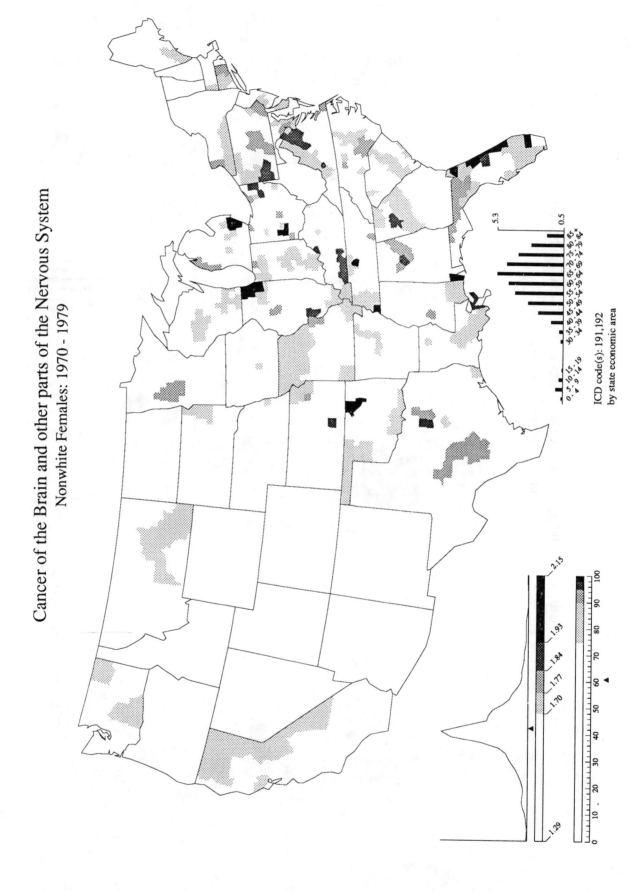

ICD code(s): 191,192
by state economic area

Cancer of the Brain and other parts of the Nervous System
Nonwhite Females: Relative Change

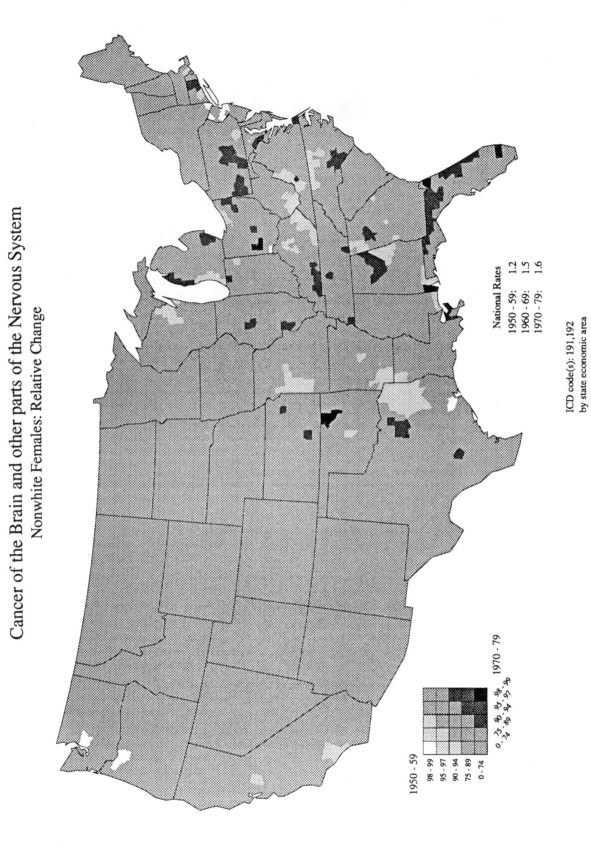

National Rates

1950 - 59:	1.2
1960 - 69:	1.5
1970 - 79:	1.6

ICD code(s): 191,192
by state economic area

1950 - 59

98 - 99
95 - 97
90 - 94
75 - 89
0 - 74

0 - 74 75 - 89 90 - 94 95 - 97 98 - 99

1970 - 79

289

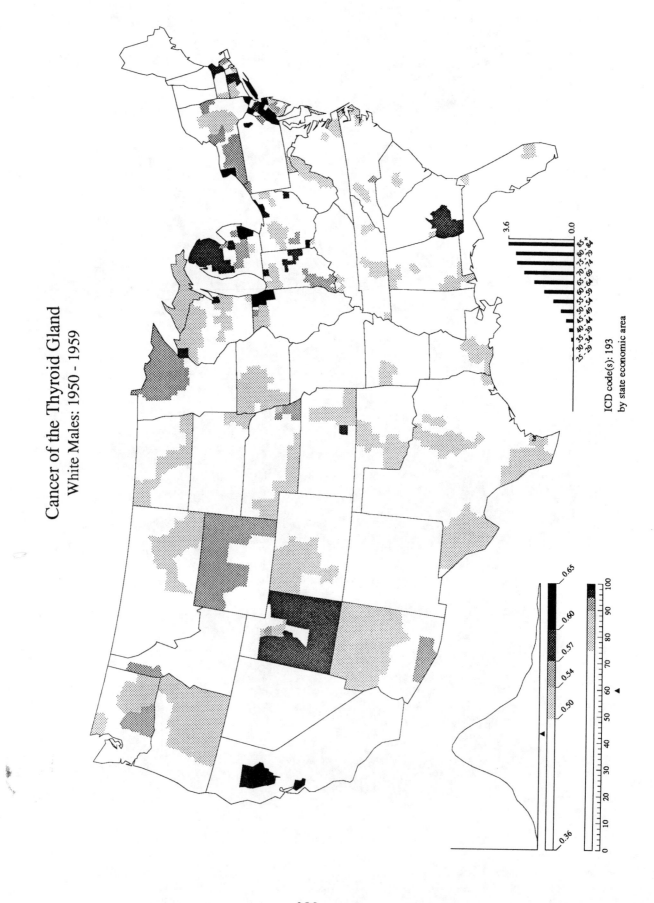

Cancer of the Thyroid Gland
White Males: 1950 - 1959

ICD code(s): 193
by state economic area

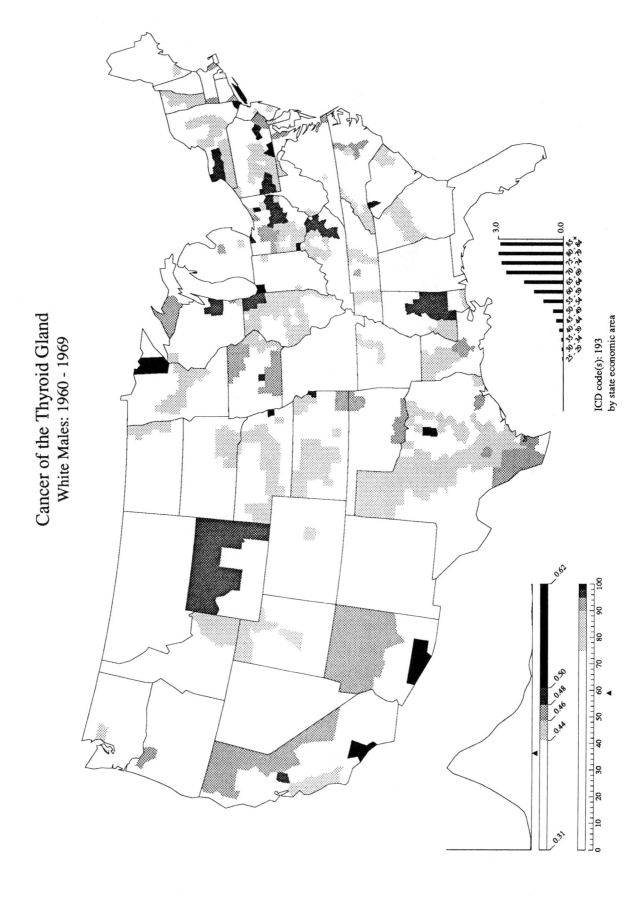

Cancer of the Thyroid Gland
White Males: 1960 - 1969

ICD code(s): 193
by state economic area

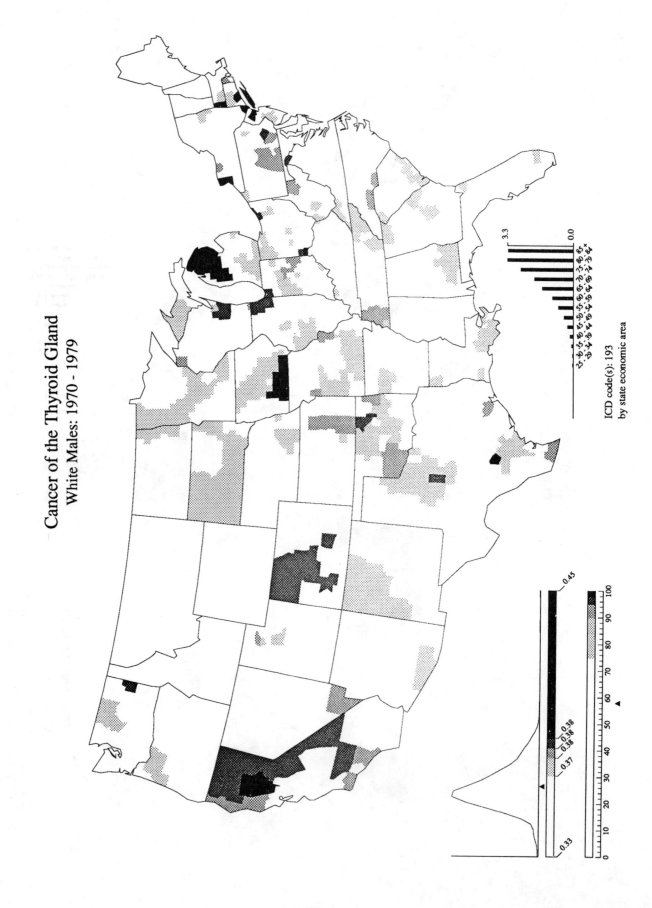

Cancer of the Thyroid Gland
White Males: 1970 - 1979

ICD code(s): 193
by state economic area

Cancer of the Thyroid Gland
White Males: Relative Change

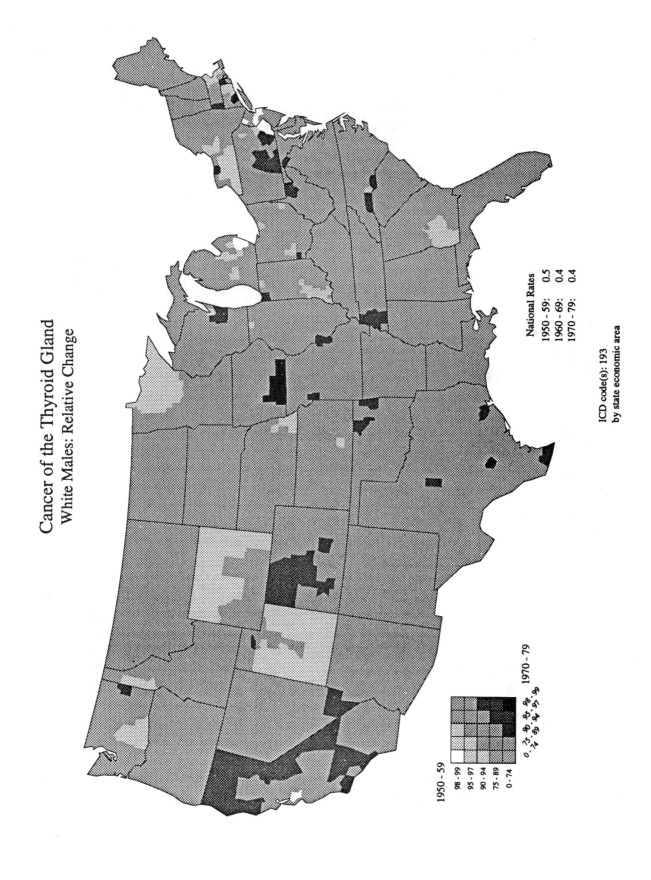

National Rates

1950 - 59:   0.5
1960 - 69:   0.4
1970 - 79:   0.4

ICD code(s): 193
by state economic area

1950 - 59

98 - 99
95 - 97
90 - 94
75 - 89
0 - 74

1970 - 79

0 - 74 75 - 89 90 - 94 95 - 97 98 - 99

Cancer of the Thyroid Gland
White Females: 1950 - 1959

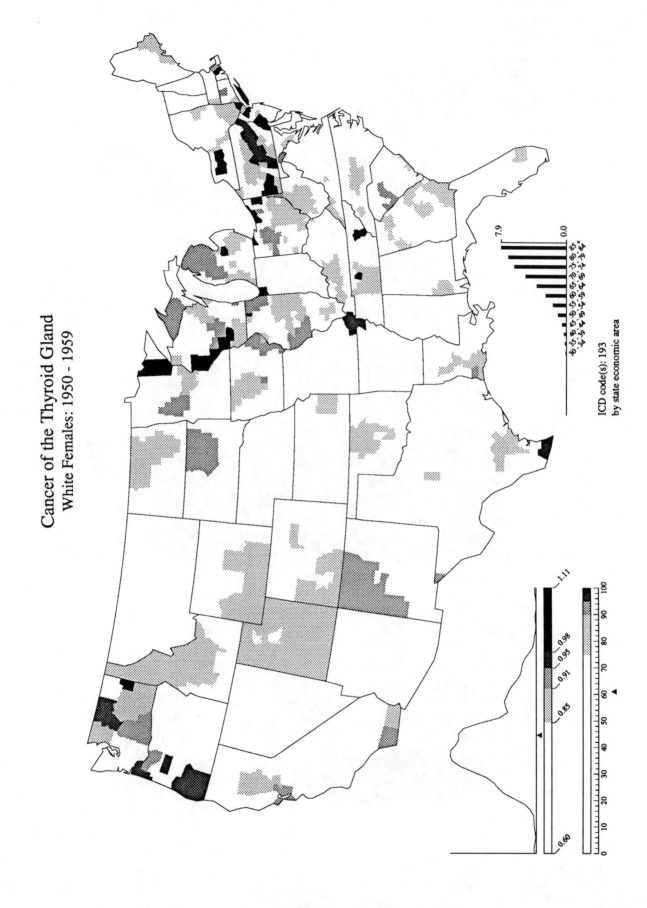

ICD code(s): 193
by state economic area

294

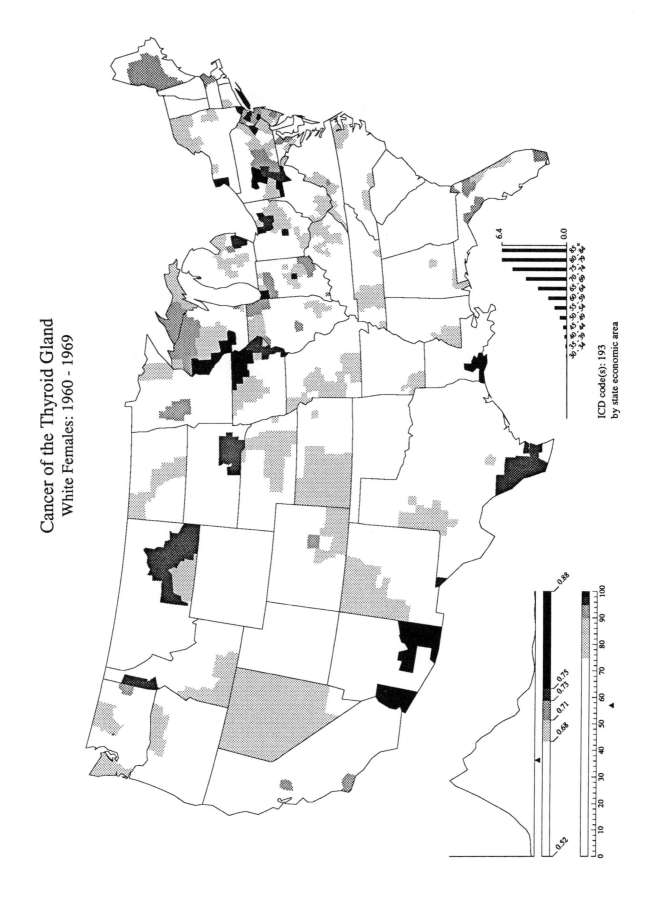

Cancer of the Thyroid Gland
White Females: 1960 - 1969

ICD code(s): 193
by state economic area

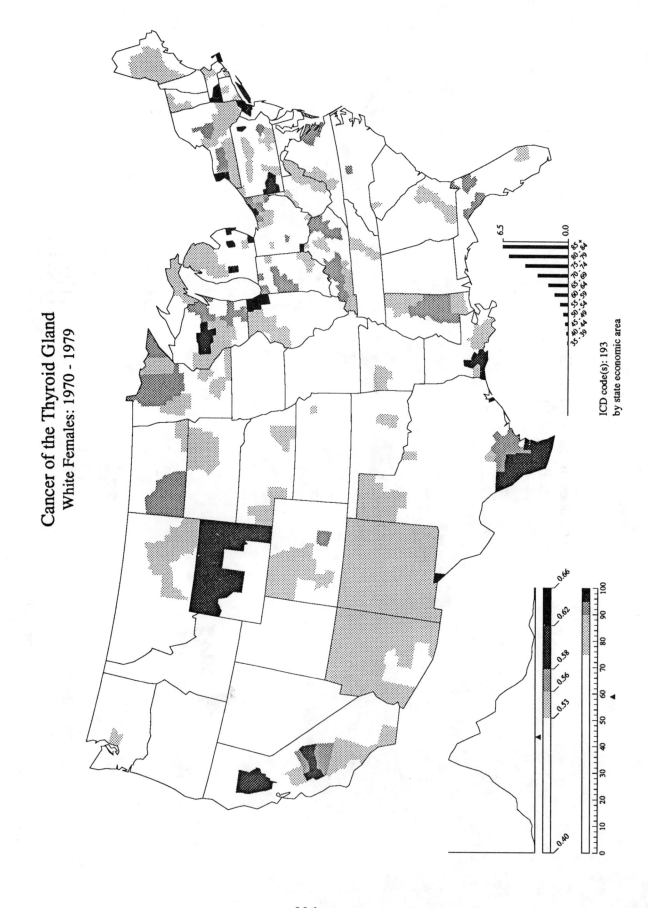

Cancer of the Thyroid Gland
White Females: 1970 - 1979

ICD code(s): 193
by state economic area

Cancer of the Thyroid Gland
White Females: Relative Change

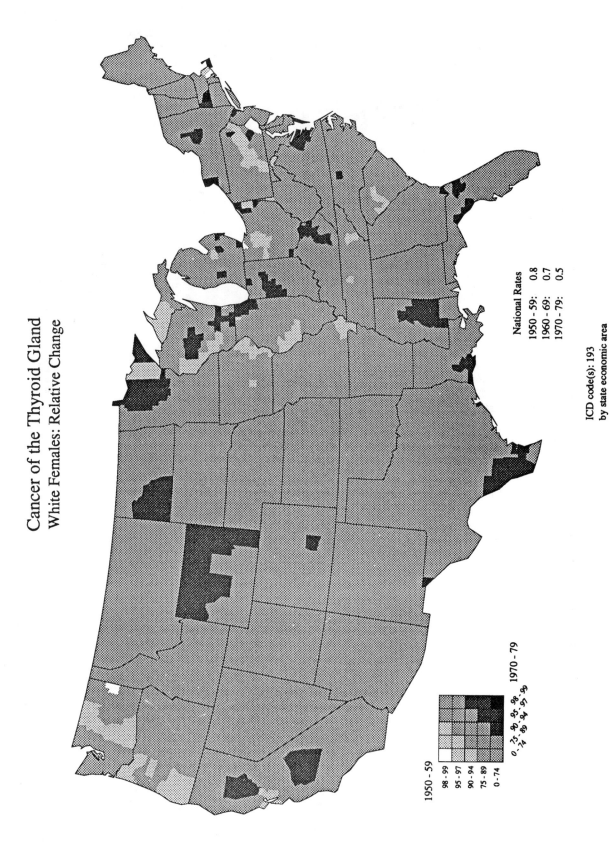

National Rates

1950 - 59: 0.8
1960 - 69: 0.7
1970 - 79: 0.5

ICD code(s): 193
by state economic area

1950 - 59

98 - 99
95 - 97
90 - 94
75 - 89
0 - 74

1970 - 79

0 - 74 75 - 89 90 - 94 95 - 97 98 - 99

Lymphosarcoma and Reticulum Cell Sarcoma including other Lymphomas
White Males: 1950 - 1959

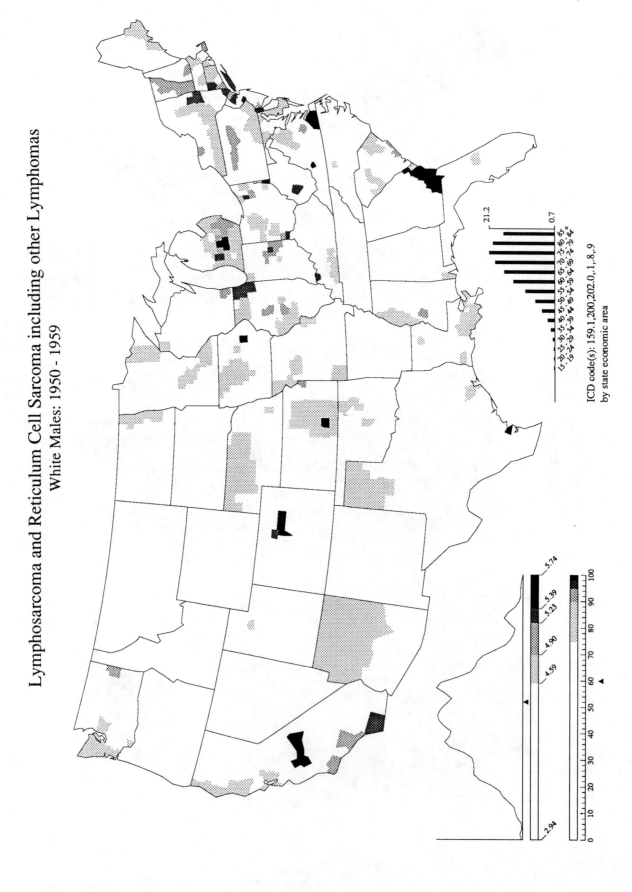

ICD code(s): 159.1,200,202.0,.1,.8,.9
by state economic area

298

Lymphosarcoma and Reticulum Cell Sarcoma including other Lymphomas
White Males: 1960 - 1969

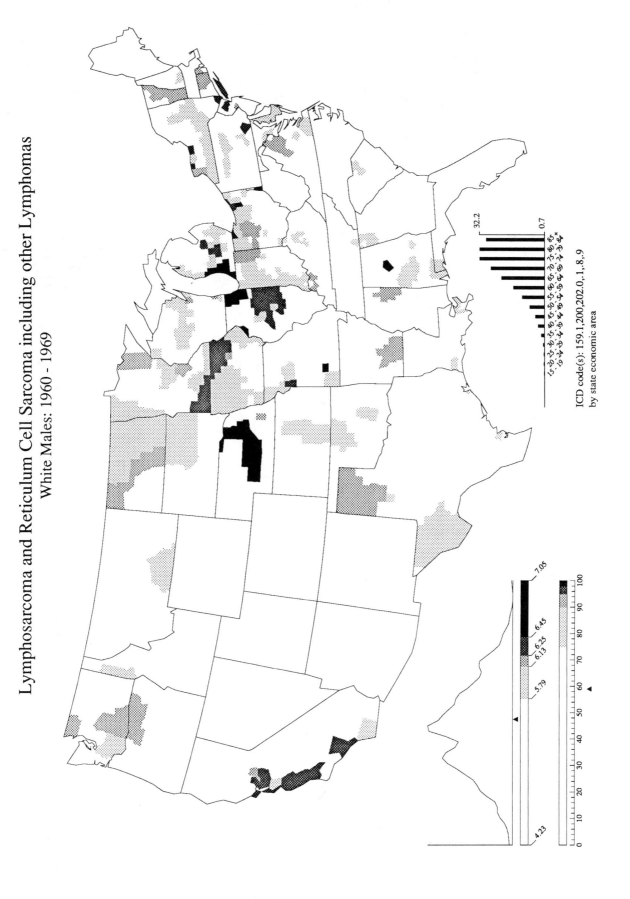

ICD code(s): 159.1,200,202.0.,1.,8.,9
by state economic area

Lymphosarcoma and Reticulum Cell Sarcoma including other Lymphomas
White Males: 1970 - 1979

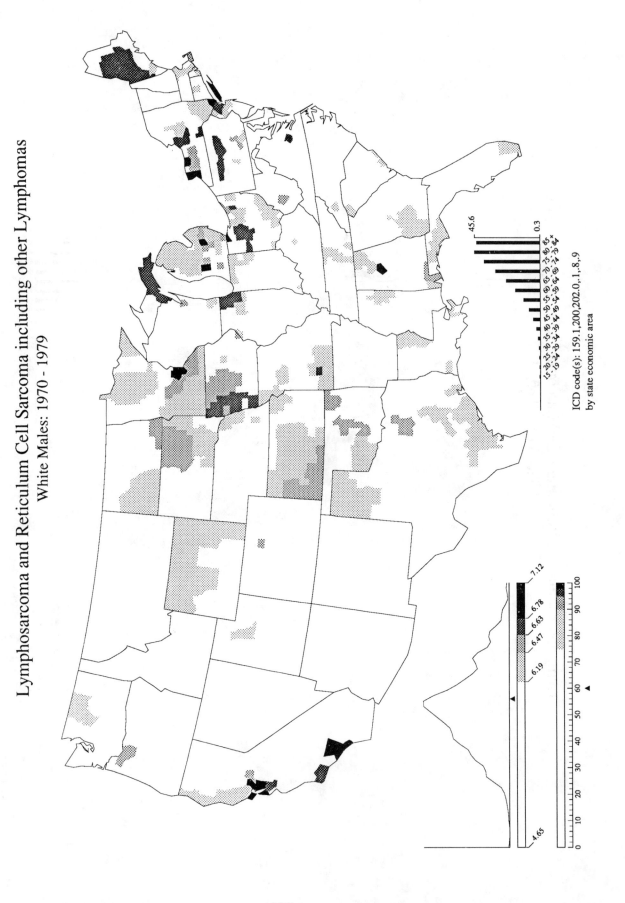

ICD code(s): 159.1,200,202.0,.1,.8,.9
by state economic area

Lymphosarcoma and Reticulum Cell Sarcoma including other Lymphomas
White Males: Relative Change

National Rates

1950 - 59: 4.4
1960 - 69: 5.6
1970 - 79: 6.0

ICD code(s): 159.1,200,202.0,.1,.8,.9
by state economic area

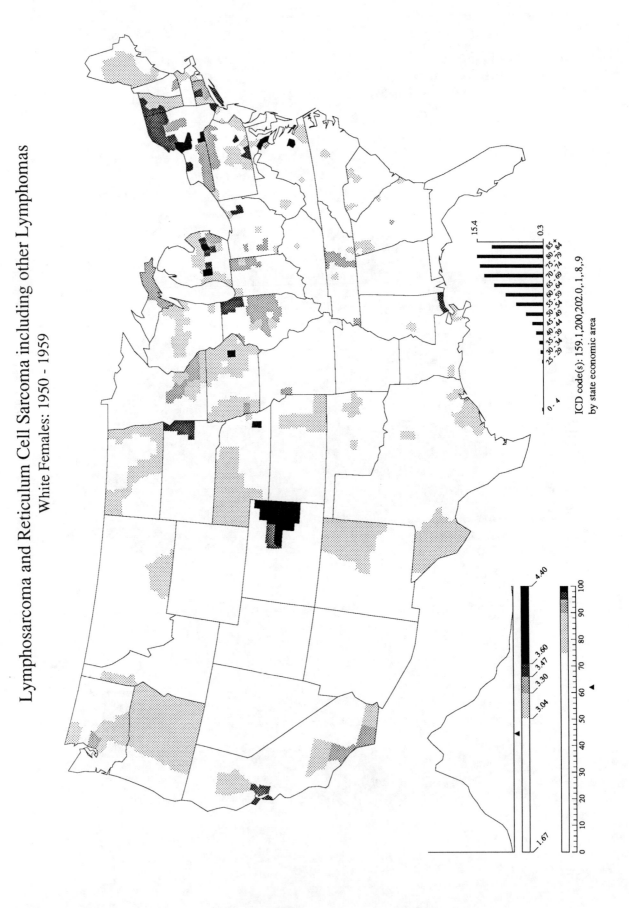

Lymphosarcoma and Reticulum Cell Sarcoma including other Lymphomas
White Females: 1950 - 1959

ICD code(s): 159.1,200,202.0,.1,.8,.9
by state economic area

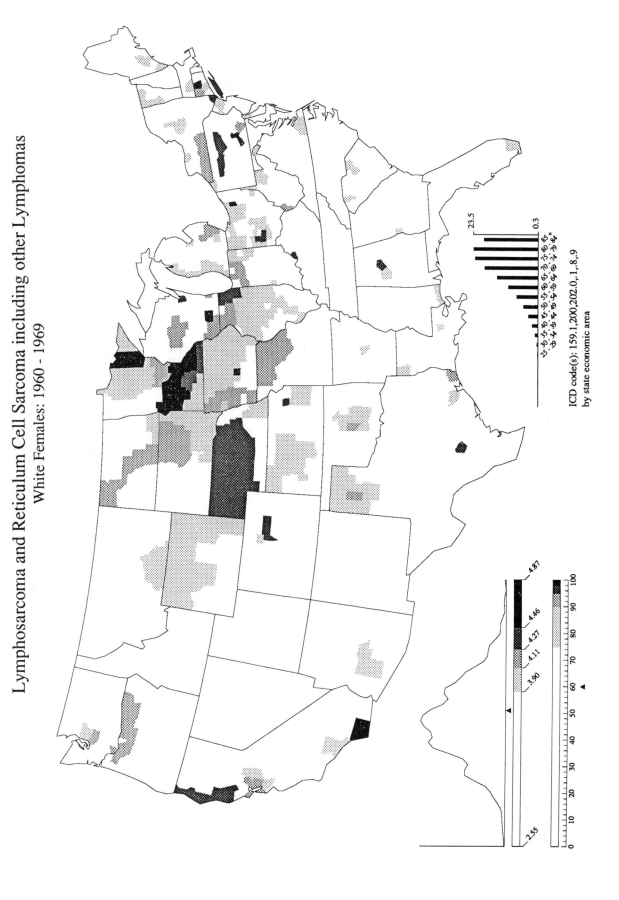

Lymphosarcoma and Reticulum Cell Sarcoma including other Lymphomas
White Females: 1960 - 1969

ICD code(s): 159.1,200,202.0,.1,.8,.9
by state economic area

Lymphosarcoma and Reticulum Cell Sarcoma including other Lymphomas
White Females: 1970 - 1979

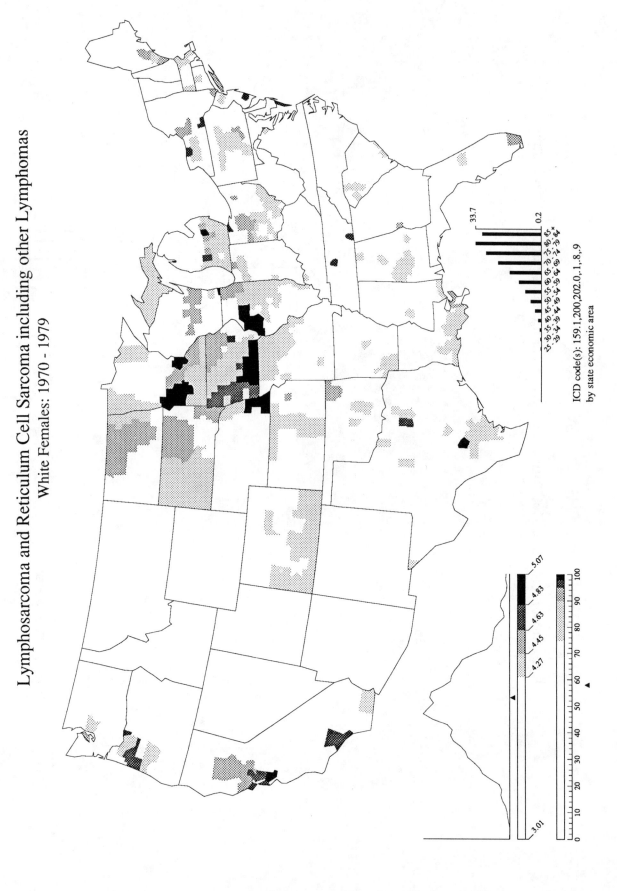

ICD code(s): 159.1,200,202.0,.1,.8,.9
by state economic area

Lymphosarcoma and Reticulum Cell Sarcoma including other Lymphomas
White Females: Relative Change

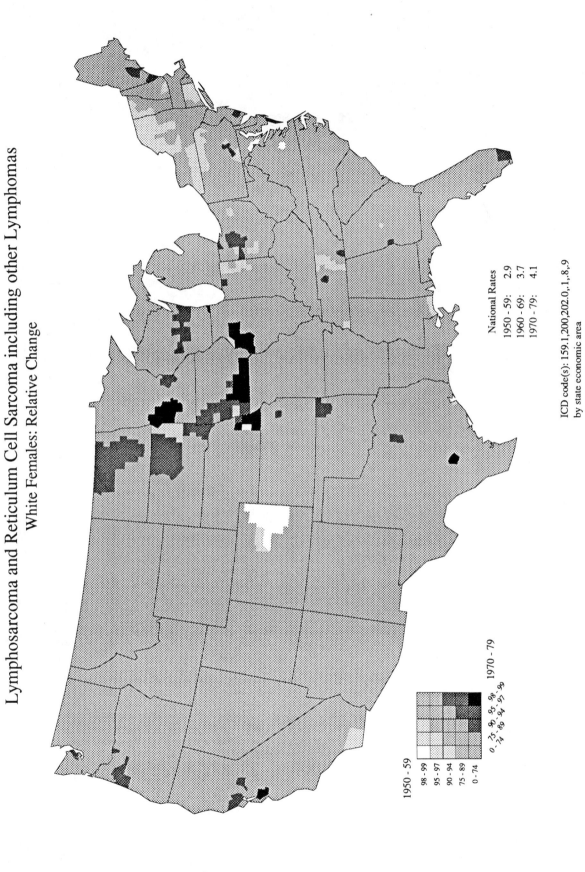

National Rates

1950 - 59:	2.9
1960 - 69:	3.7
1970 - 79:	4.1

ICD code(s): 159.1,200,202.0,.1,.8,.9
by state economic area

1950 - 59

98 - 99
95 - 97
90 - 94
75 - 89
0 - 74

1970 - 79

0 - 74 75 - 89 90 - 94 95 - 97 98 - 99

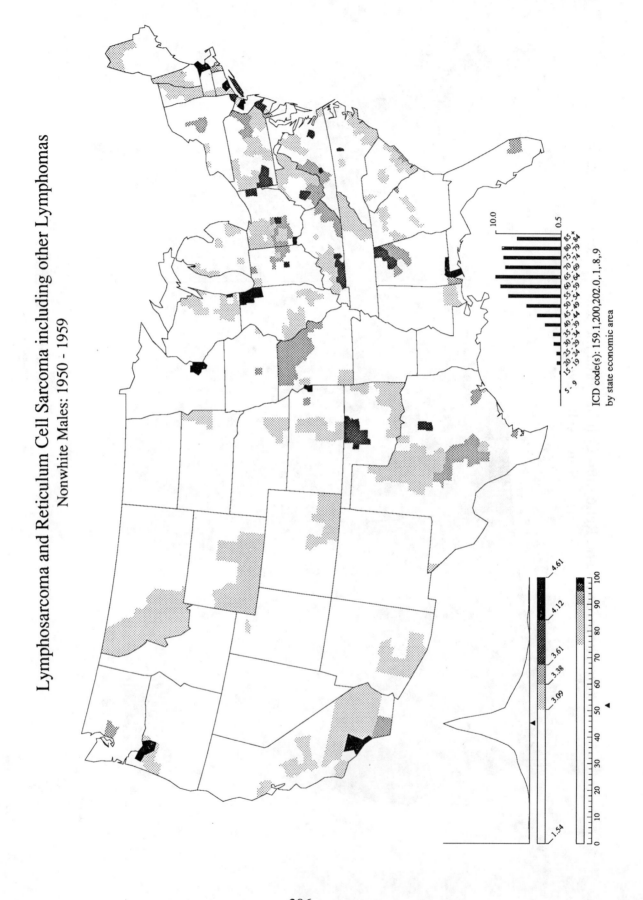

Lymphosarcoma and Reticulum Cell Sarcoma including other Lymphomas
Nonwhite Males: 1950 - 1959

ICD code(s): 159.1,200,202.0,.1,.8,.9
by state economic area

Lymphosarcoma and Reticulum Cell Sarcoma including other Lymphomas
Nonwhite Males: 1960 - 1969

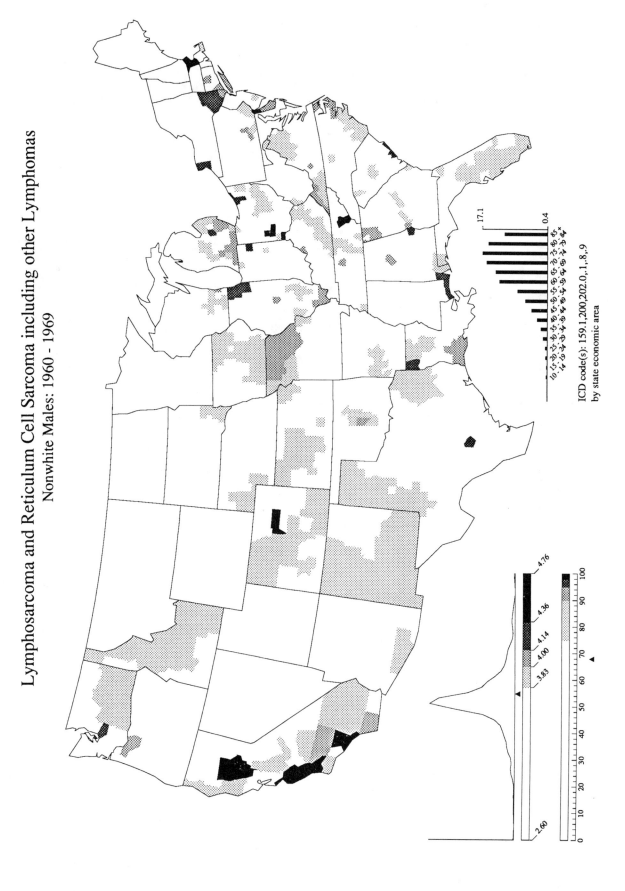

ICD code(s): 159.1,200,202.0,.1,.8,.9
by state economic area

307

Lymphosarcoma and Reticulum Cell Sarcoma including other Lymphomas
Nonwhite Males: 1970 - 1979

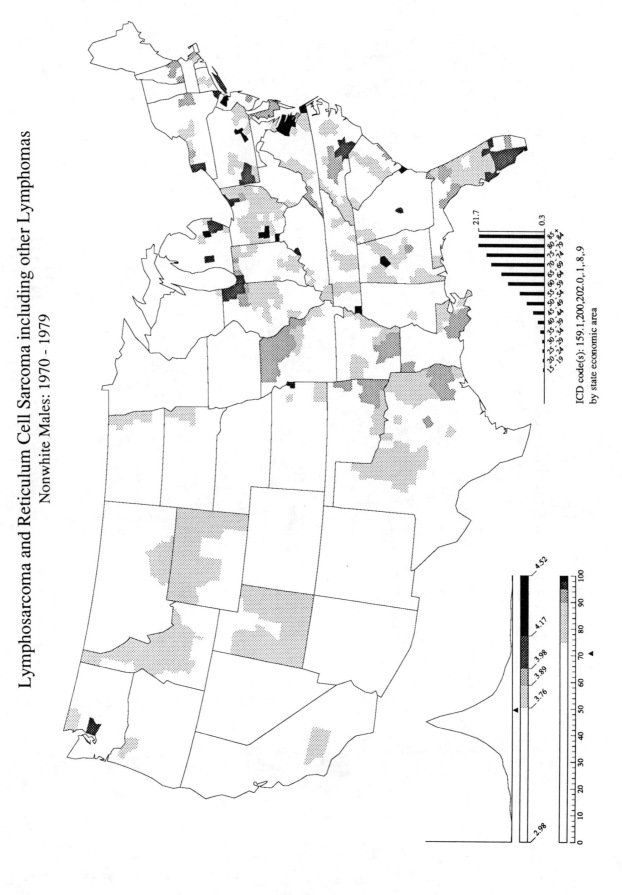

ICD code(s): 159.1,200,202.0,.1,.8,.9
by state economic area

Lymphosarcoma and Reticulum Cell Sarcoma including other Lymphomas
Nonwhite Males: Relative Change

National Rates

1950 - 59:	2.9
1960 - 69:	3.8
1970 - 79:	3.8

ICD code(s): 159.1,200,202.0,.1,.8,.9
by state economic area

1950 - 59

98 - 99
95 - 97
90 - 94
75 - 89
0 - 74

1970 - 79

0 - 74 75 - 89 90 - 94 95 - 97 98 - 99

309

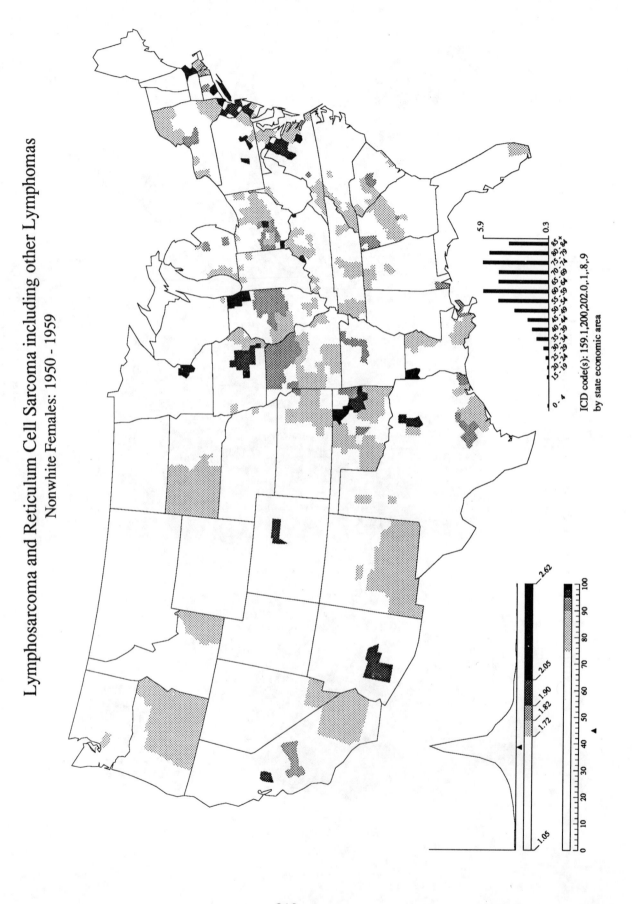

Lymphosarcoma and Reticulum Cell Sarcoma including other Lymphomas
Nonwhite Females: 1950 - 1959

ICD code(s): 159.1,200,202.0,.1,.8,.9
by state economic area

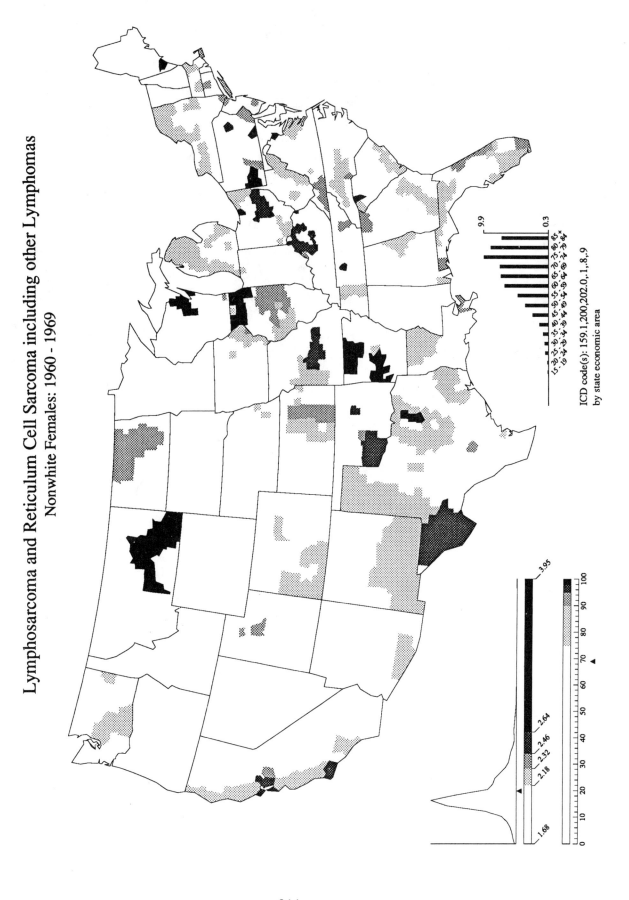

Lymphosarcoma and Reticulum Cell Sarcoma including other Lymphomas
Nonwhite Females: 1960 - 1969

ICD code(s): 159.1,200,202.0,.1,.8,.9
by state economic area

Lymphosarcoma and Reticulum Cell Sarcoma including other Lymphomas
Nonwhite Females: 1970 - 1979

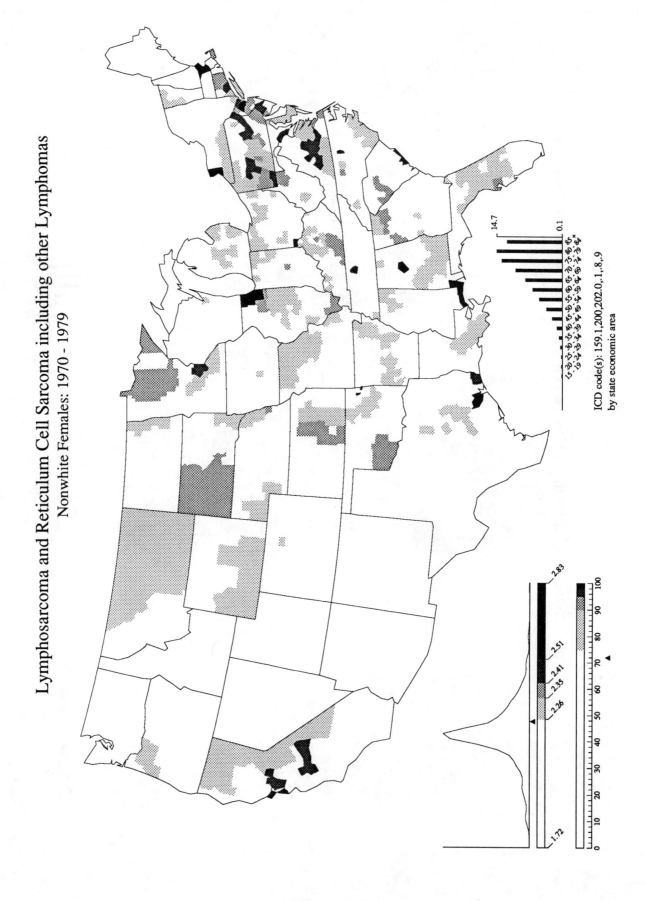

ICD code(s): 159.1,200,202.0,.1,.8,.9
by state economic area

Lymphosarcoma and Reticulum Cell Sarcoma including other Lymphomas
Nonwhite Females: Relative Change

National Rates
1950 - 59:   1.6
1960 - 69:   2.1
1970 - 79:   2.2

ICD code(s): 159.1,200,202.0,.1,.8,.9
by state economic area

1950 - 59

98 - 99
95 - 97
90 - 94
75 - 89
0 - 74

1970 - 79
0 . 75 . 90 . 95 . 98 . 99
. 74 . 89 . 94 . 97 . 99

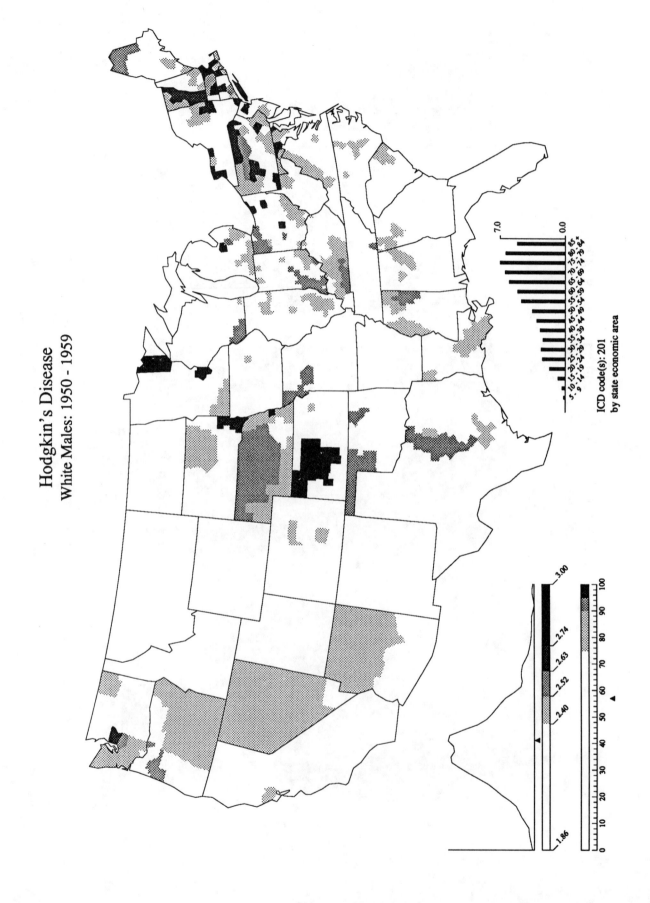

Hodgkin's Disease
White Males: 1950 - 1959

ICD code(s): 201
by state economic area

314

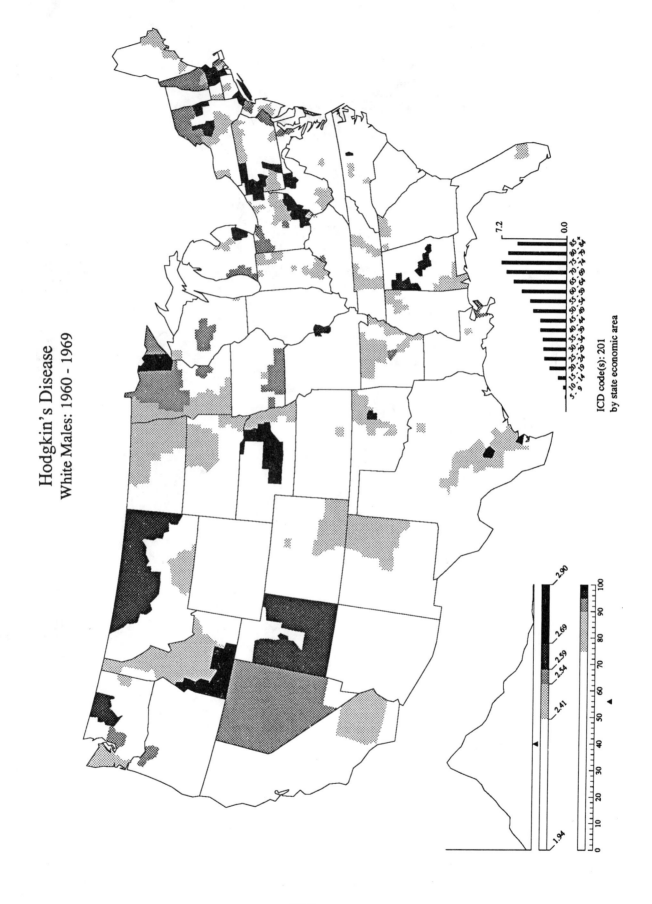

Hodgkin's Disease
White Males: 1960 - 1969

ICD code(s): 201
by state economic area

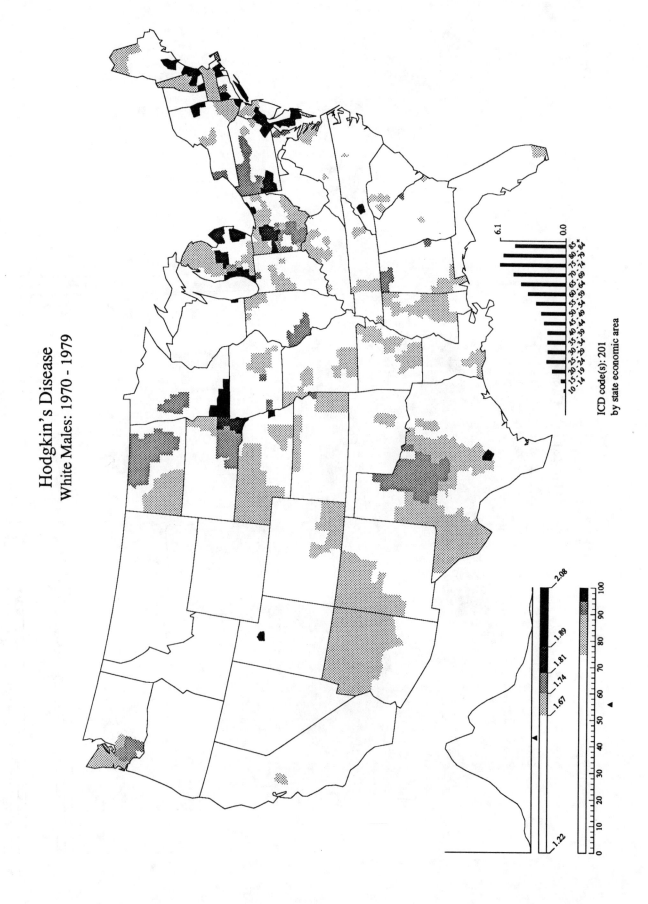

Hodgkin's Disease
White Males: 1970 - 1979

ICD code(s): 201
by state economic area

Hodgkin's Disease
White Males: Relative Change

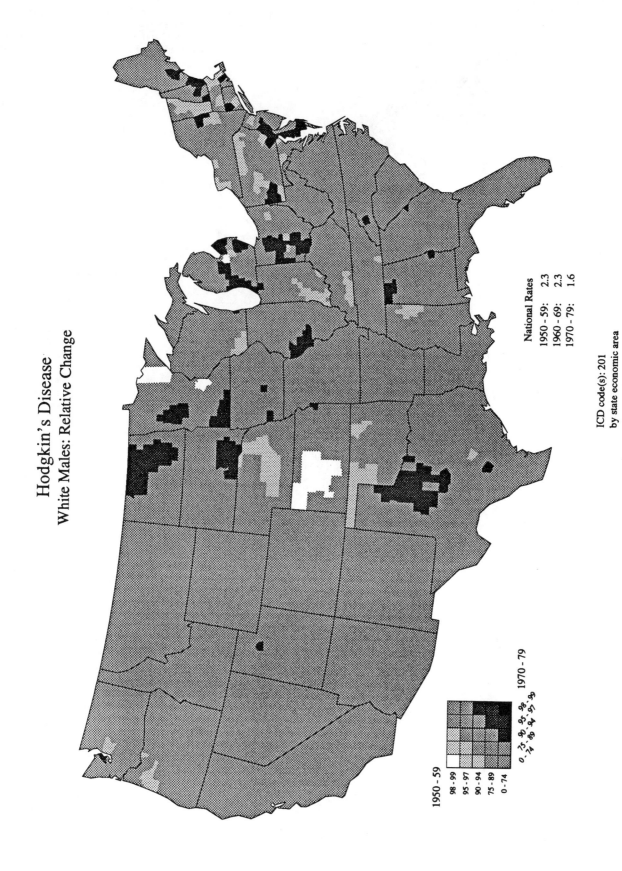

National Rates
1950 - 59:   2.3
1960 - 69:   2.3
1970 - 79:   1.6

ICD code(s): 201
by state economic area

Hodgkin's Disease
White Females: 1950 - 1959

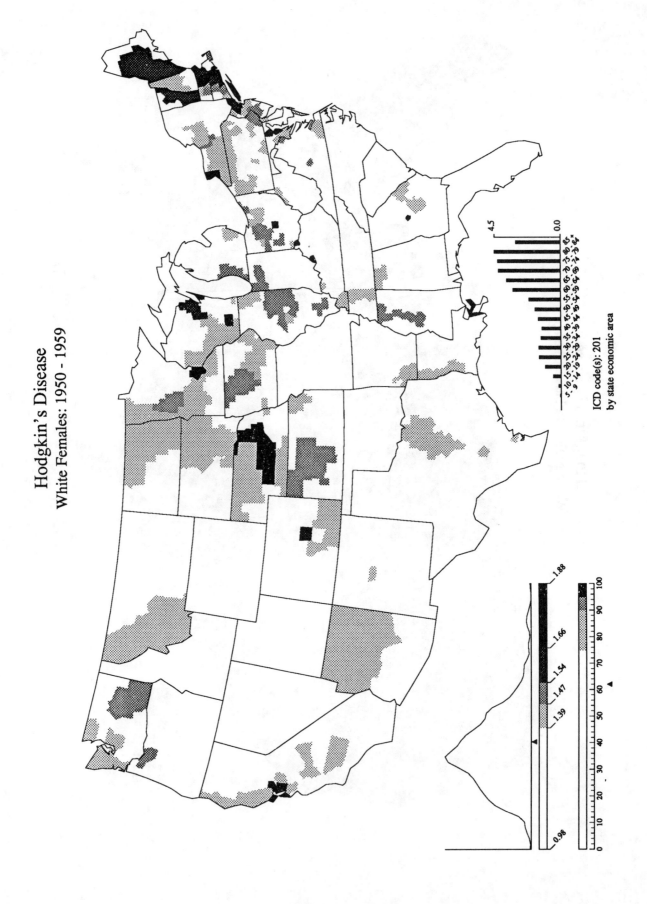

ICD code(s): 201
by state economic area

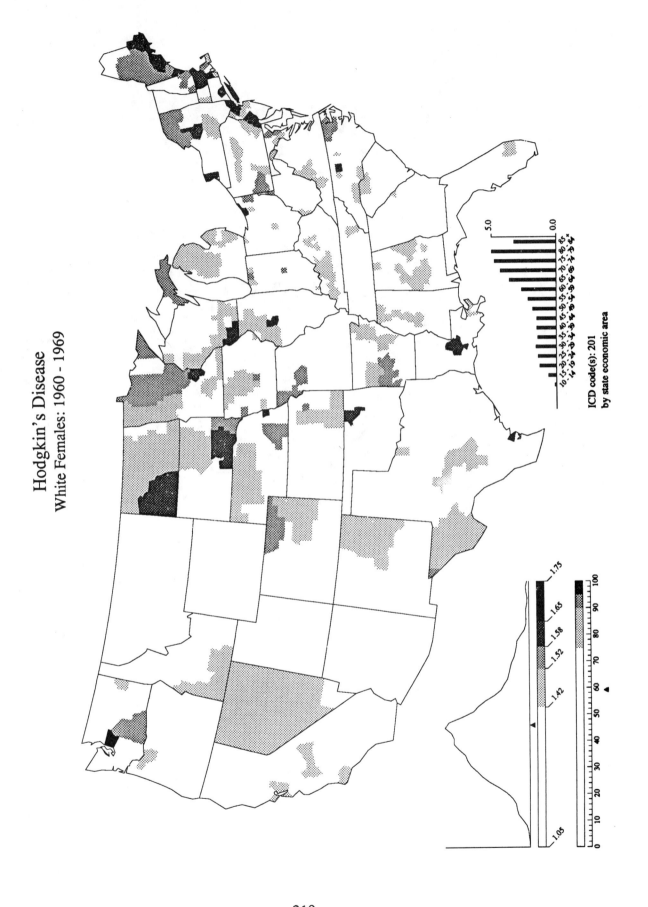

Hodgkin's Disease
White Females: 1960 - 1969

ICD code(s): 201
by state economic area

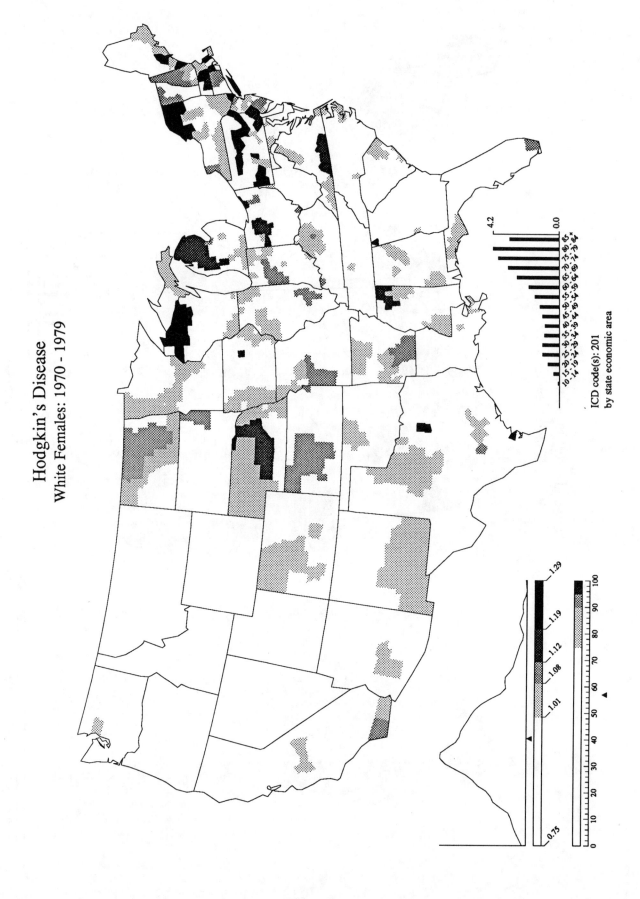

Hodgkin's Disease
White Females: 1970 - 1979

ICD code(s): 201
by state economic area

Hodgkin's Disease
White Females: Relative Change

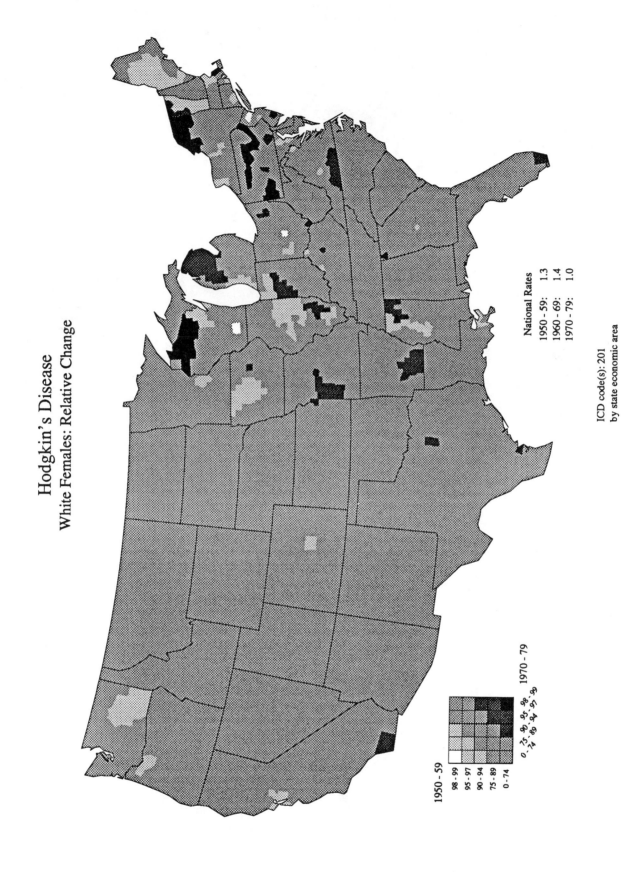

National Rates

1950 - 59:	1.3
1960 - 69:	1.4
1970 - 79:	1.0

ICD code(s): 201
by state economic area

1950 - 59

| 98 - 99 |
| 95 - 97 |
| 90 - 94 |
| 75 - 89 |
| 0 - 74 |

0 75 90 95 98 99
  74 89 94 97 99

1970 - 79

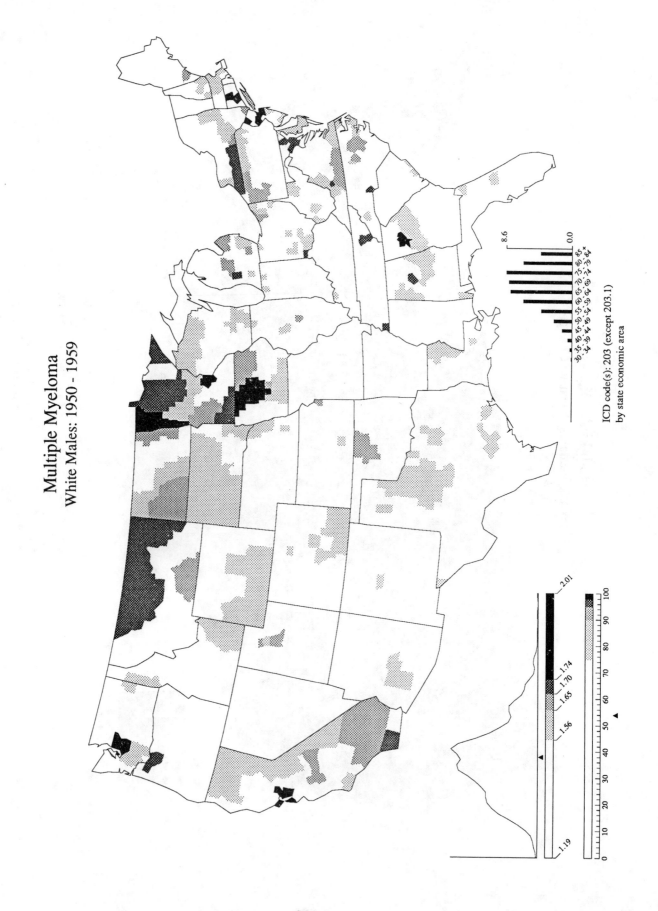

Multiple Myeloma
White Males: 1950 - 1959

ICD code(s): 203 (except 203.1)
by state economic area

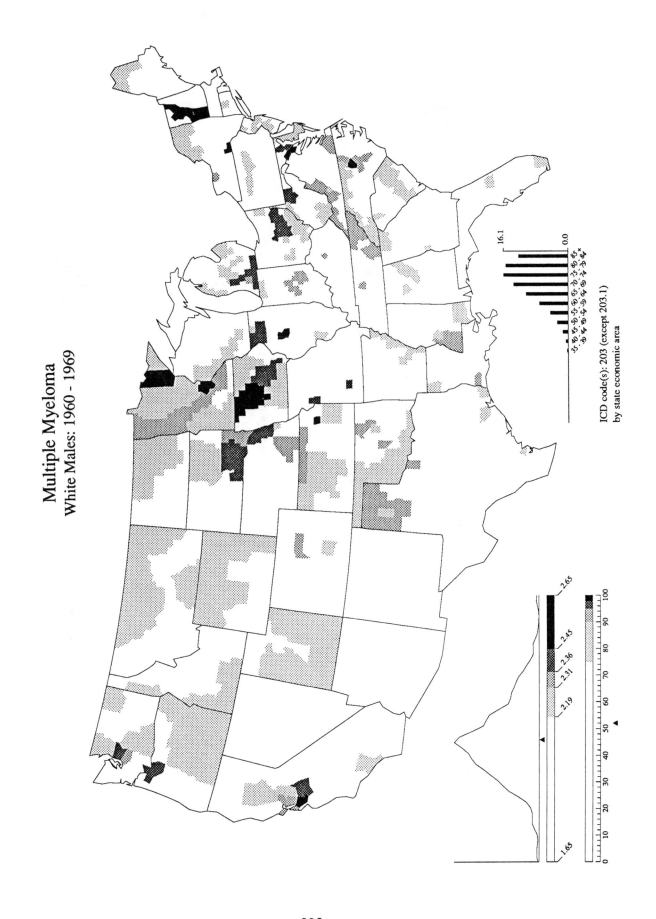

Multiple Myeloma
White Males: 1960 - 1969

ICD code(s): 203 (except 203.1)
by state economic area

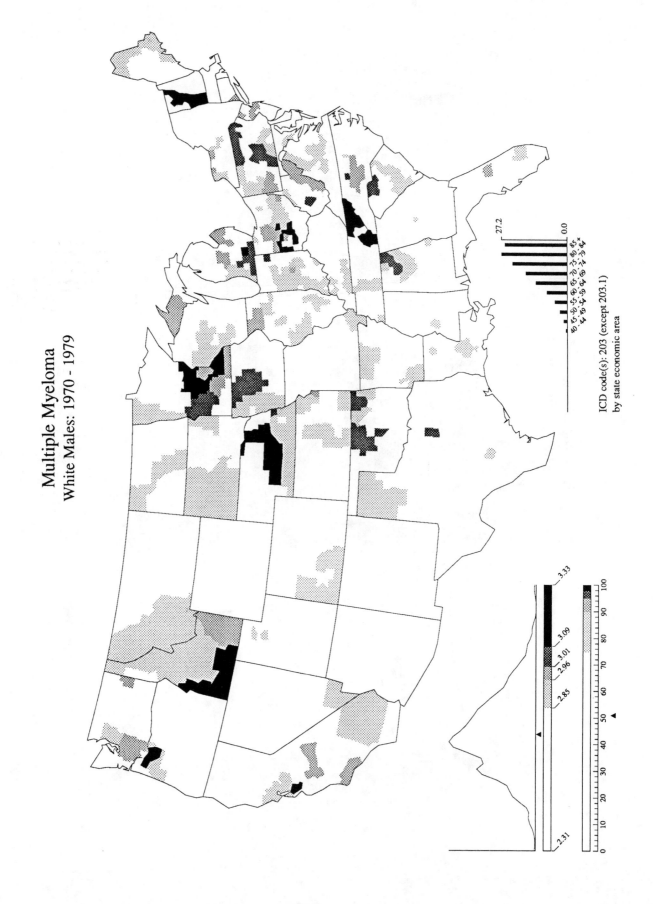

Multiple Myeloma
White Males: 1970 - 1979

ICD code(s): 203 (except 203.1)
by state economic area

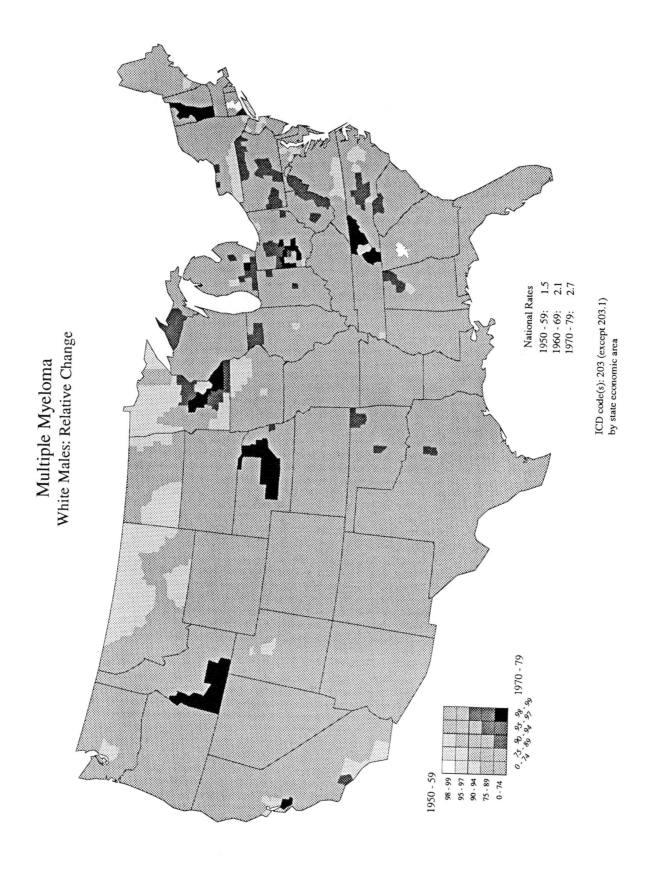

Multiple Myeloma
White Males: Relative Change

National Rates

1950 - 59:   1.5
1960 - 69:   2.1
1970 - 79:   2.7

ICD code(s): 203 (except 203.1)
by state economic area

1950 - 59

1970 - 79

98 - 99
95 - 97
90 - 94
75 - 89
0 - 74

0 - 74   75 - 89   90 - 94   95 - 97   98 - 99

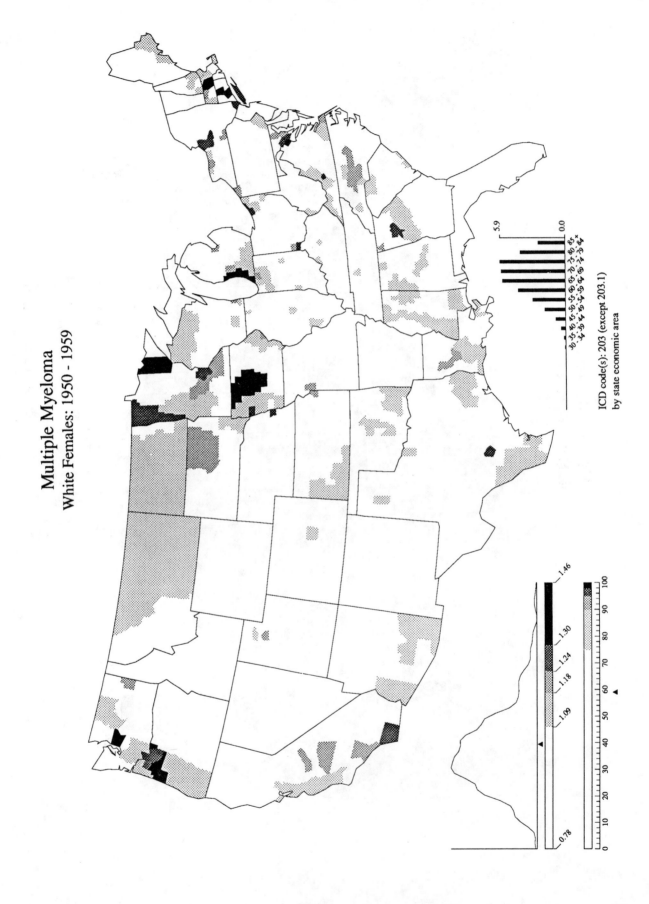

Multiple Myeloma
White Females: 1950 - 1959

ICD code(s): 203 (except 203.1)
by state economic area

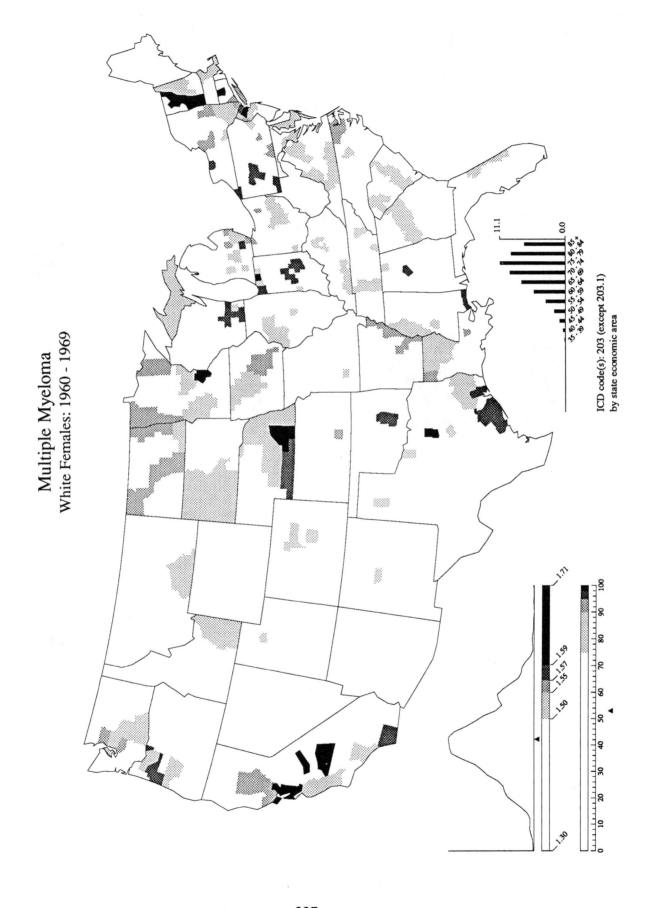

Multiple Myeloma
White Females: 1960 - 1969

ICD code(s): 203 (except 203.1)
by state economic area

327

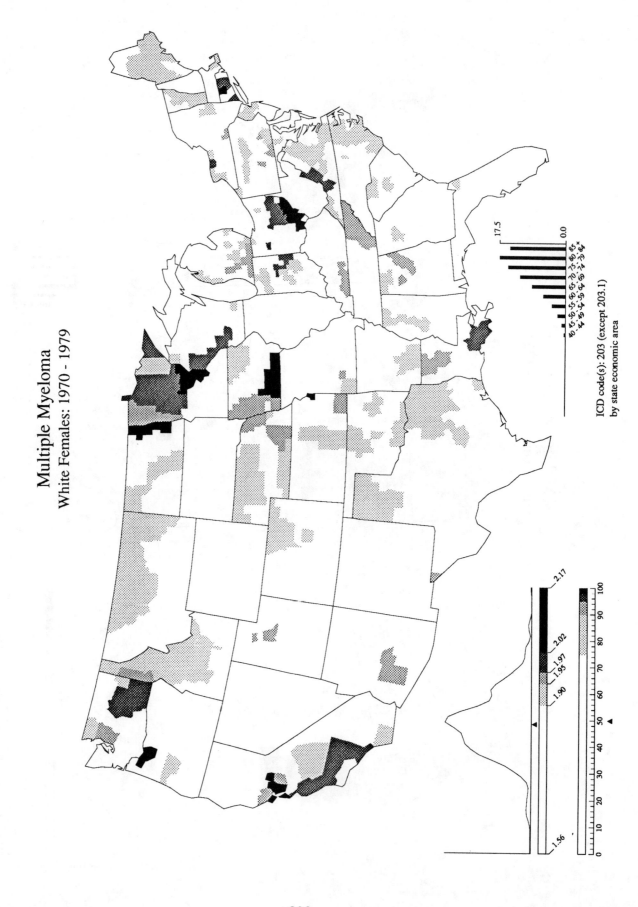

Multiple Myeloma
White Females: 1970 - 1979

ICD code(s): 203 (except 203.1)
by state economic area

328

Multiple Myeloma
White Females: Relative Change

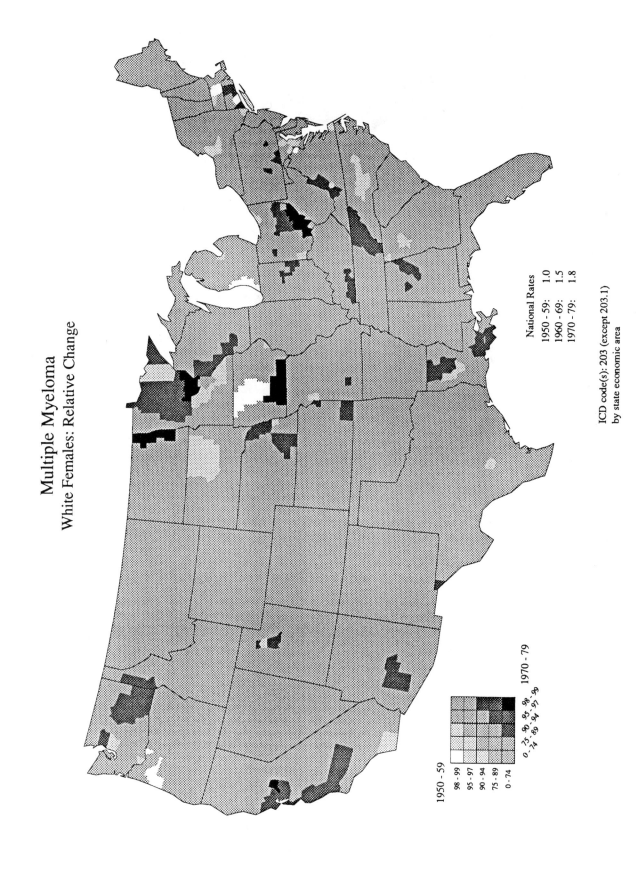

National Rates

1950 - 59: 1.0
1960 - 69: 1.5
1970 - 79: 1.8

ICD code(s): 203 (except 203.1)
by state economic area

1950 - 59

98 - 99
95 - 97
90 - 94
75 - 89
0 - 74

1970 - 79

0 - 74 89 94 97 99

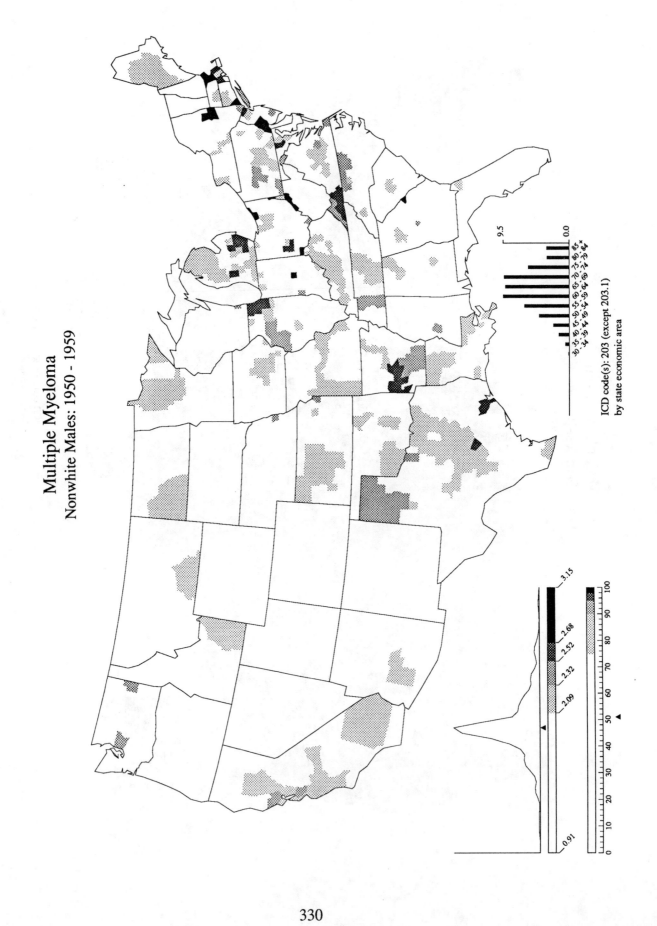

Multiple Myeloma
Nonwhite Males: 1950 - 1959

ICD code(s): 203 (except 203.1)
by state economic area

330

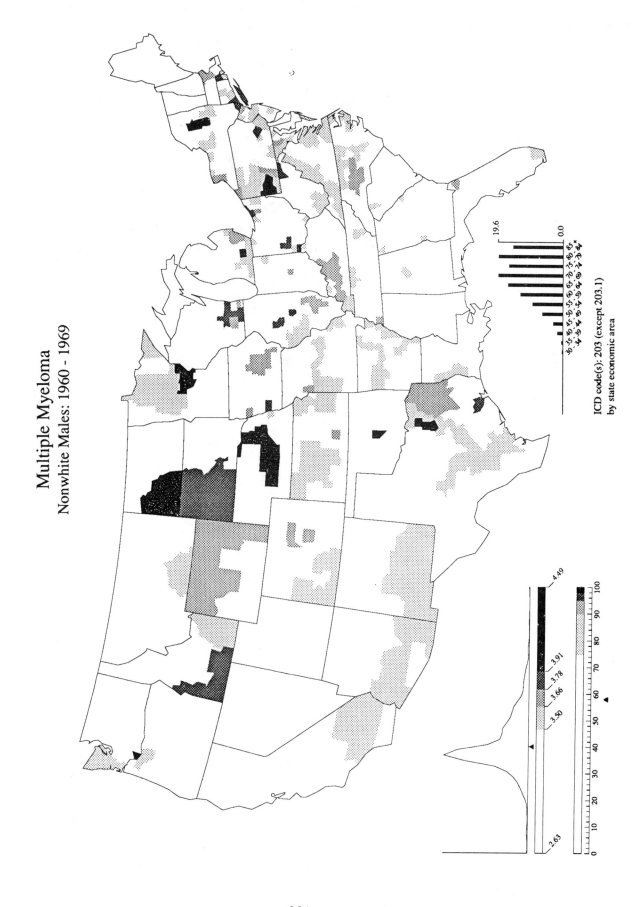

Multiple Myeloma
Nonwhite Males: 1960 - 1969

ICD code(s): 203 (except 203.1)
by state economic area

Multiple Myeloma
Nonwhite Males: 1970 - 1979

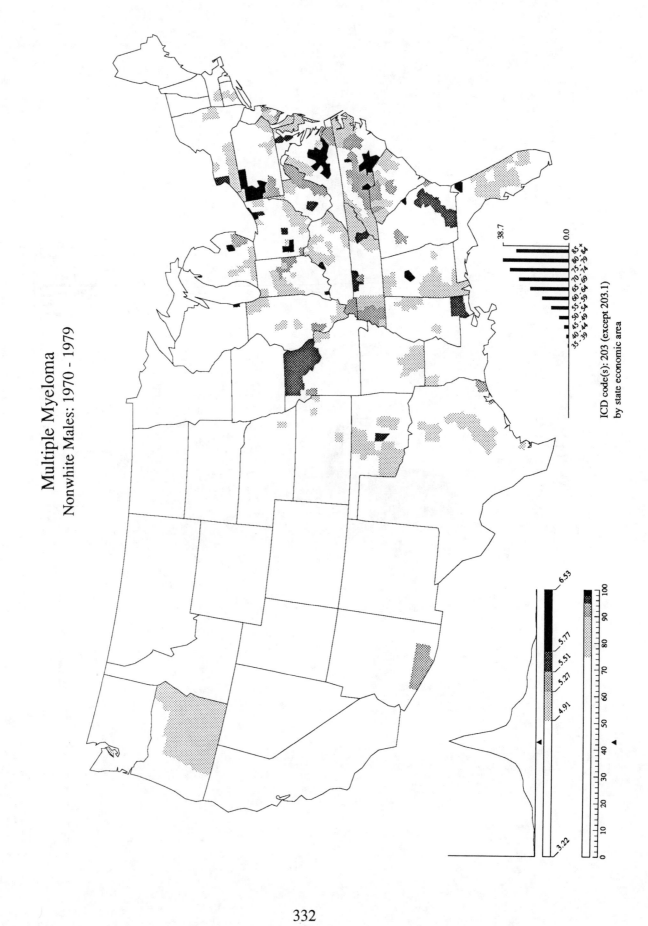

ICD code(s): 203 (except 203.1)
by state economic area

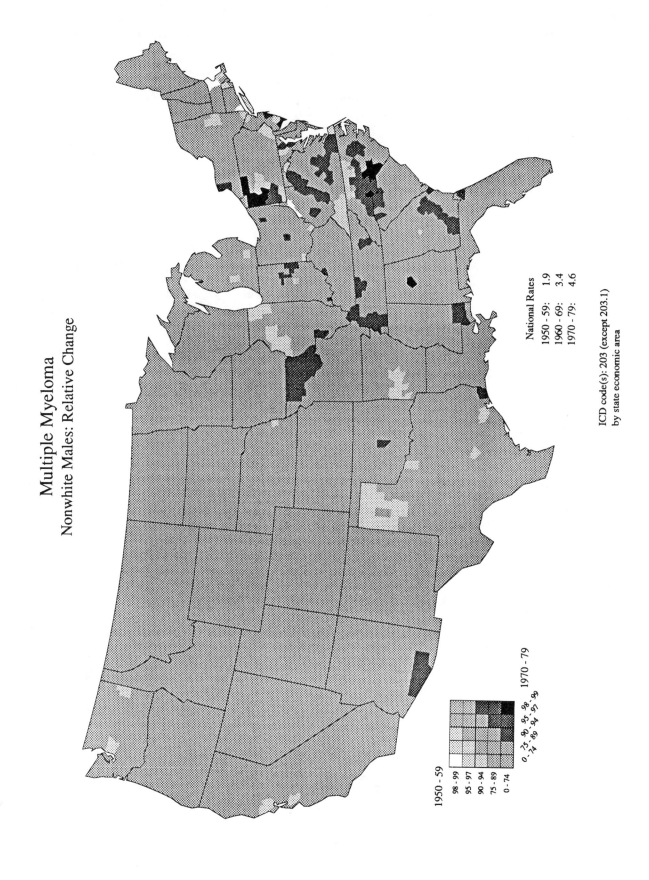

Multiple Myeloma
Nonwhite Males: Relative Change

National Rates

1950 - 59:   1.9
1960 - 69:   3.4
1970 - 79:   4.6

ICD code(s): 203 (except 203.1)
by state economic area

1950 - 59

98 - 99
95 - 97
90 - 94
75 - 89
0 - 74

1970 - 79

0 - 74 90 95 98 - 99
      75 - 89 94 97

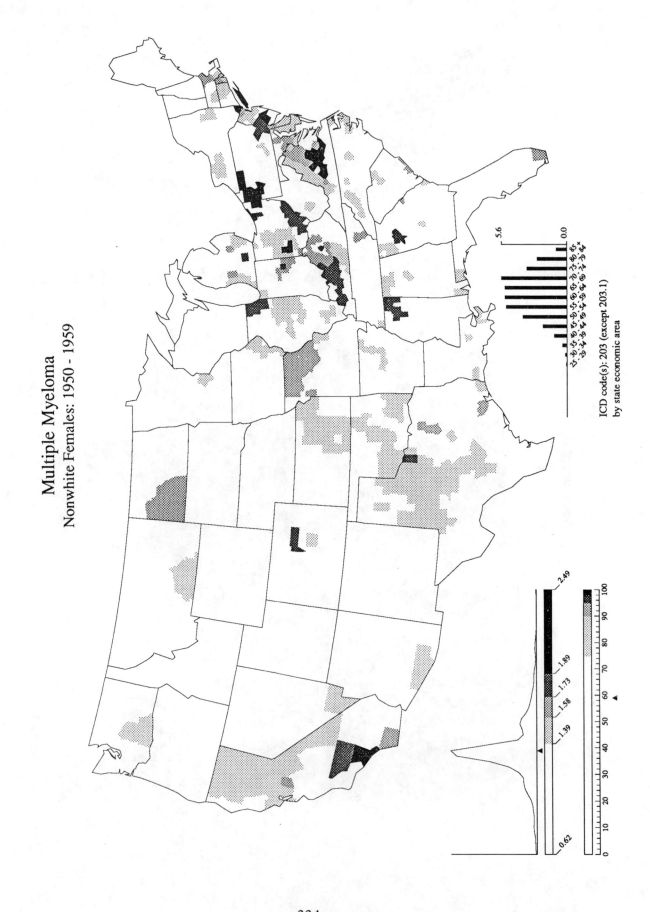

Multiple Myeloma
Nonwhite Females: 1950 - 1959

ICD code(s): 203 (except 203.1)
by state economic area

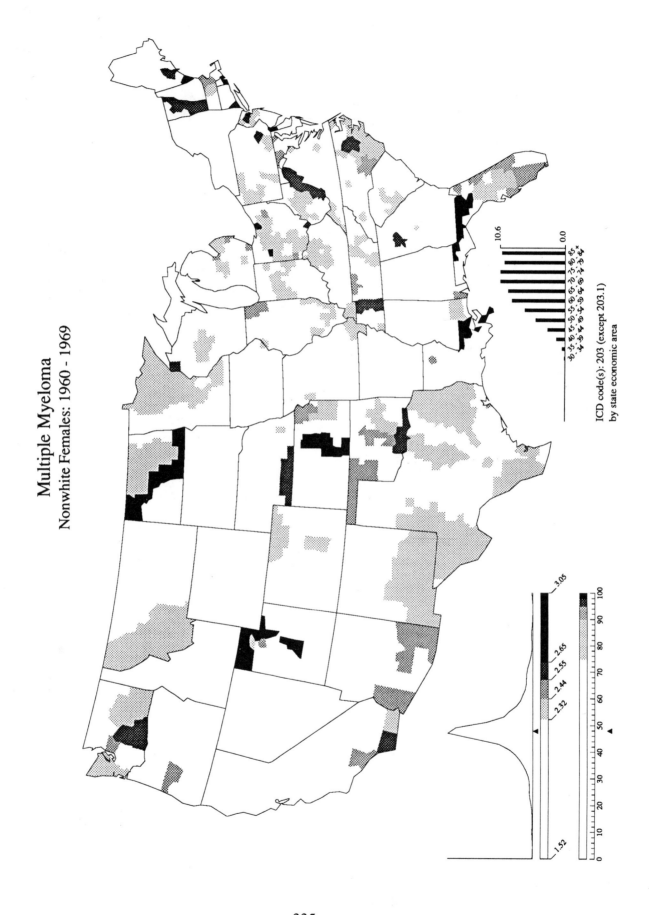

Multiple Myeloma
Nonwhite Females: 1960 - 1969

ICD code(s): 203 (except 203.1)
by state economic area

Multiple Myeloma
Nonwhite Females: 1970 - 1979

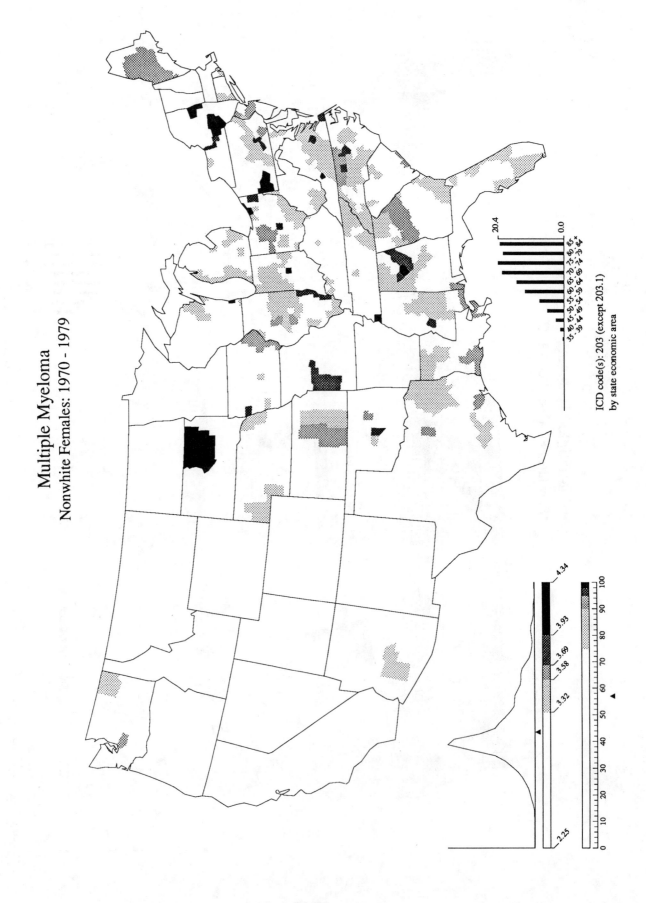

ICD code(s): 203 (except 203.1)
by state economic area

Multiple Myeloma
Nonwhite Females: Relative Change

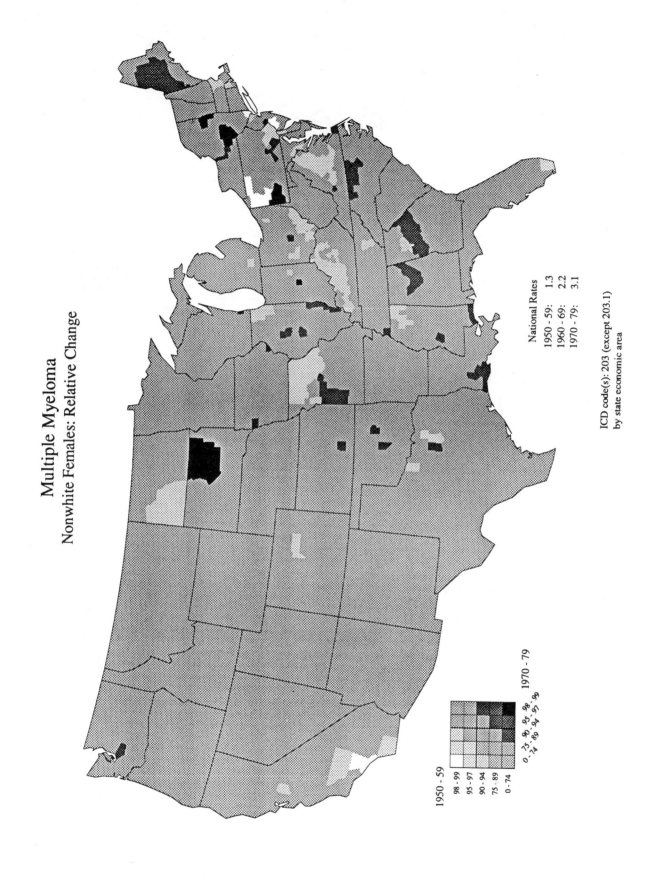

National Rates

1950 - 59:	1.3
1960 - 69:	2.2
1970 - 79:	3.1

ICD code(s): 203 (except 203.1)
by state economic area

1970 - 79

1950 - 59
98 - 99
95 - 97
90 - 94
75 - 89
0 - 74

98 - 99   95   95   98 - 99
0 - 74   89   94   97

337

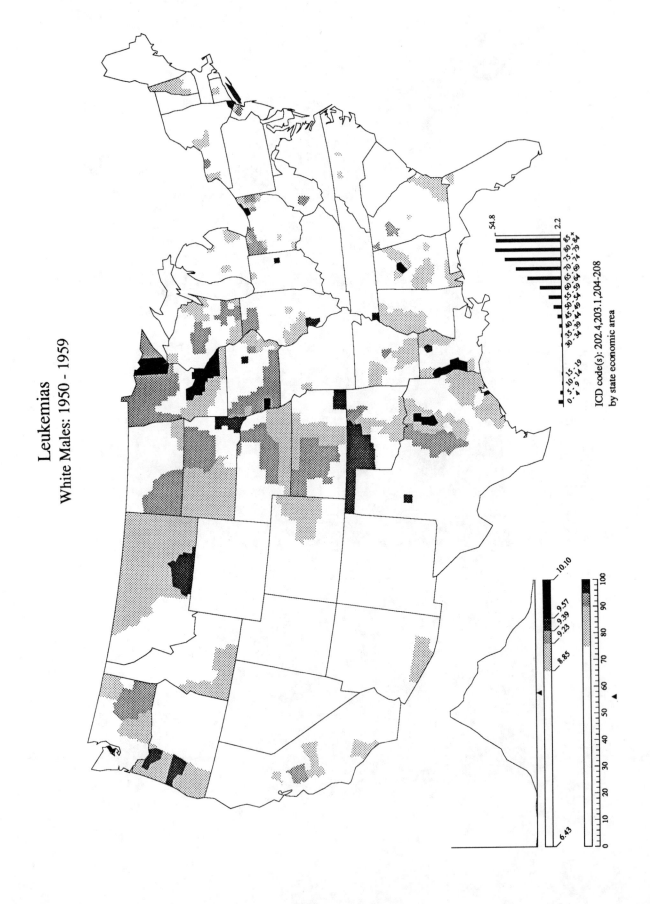

Leukemias
White Males: 1950 - 1959

ICD code(s): 202.4,203.1,204-208
by state economic area

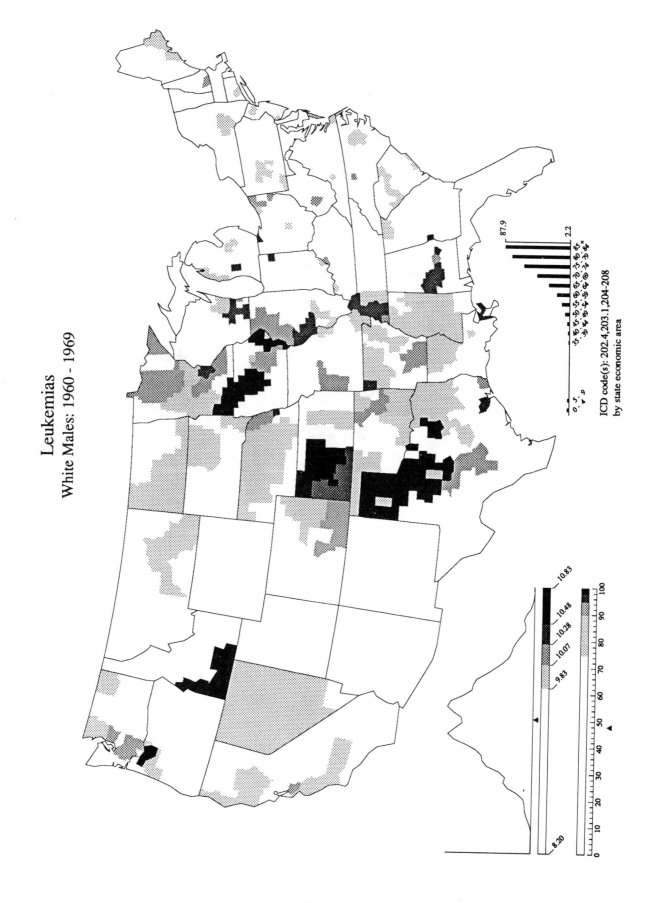

Leukemias
White Males: 1960 - 1969

ICD code(s): 202.4,203.1,204-208
by state economic area

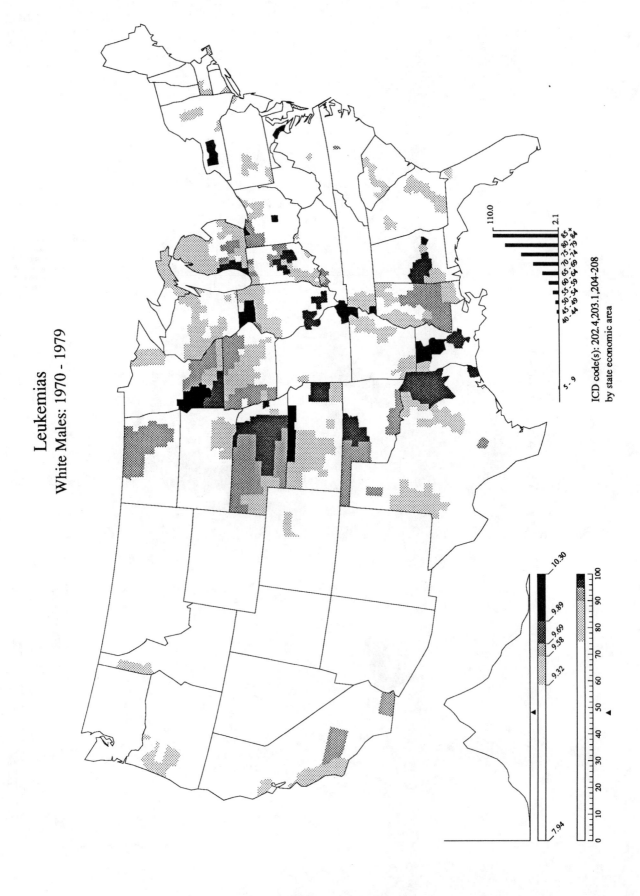

Leukemias
White Males: 1970 - 1979

ICD code(s): 202.4,203.1,204-208
by state economic area

Leukemias
White Males: Relative Change

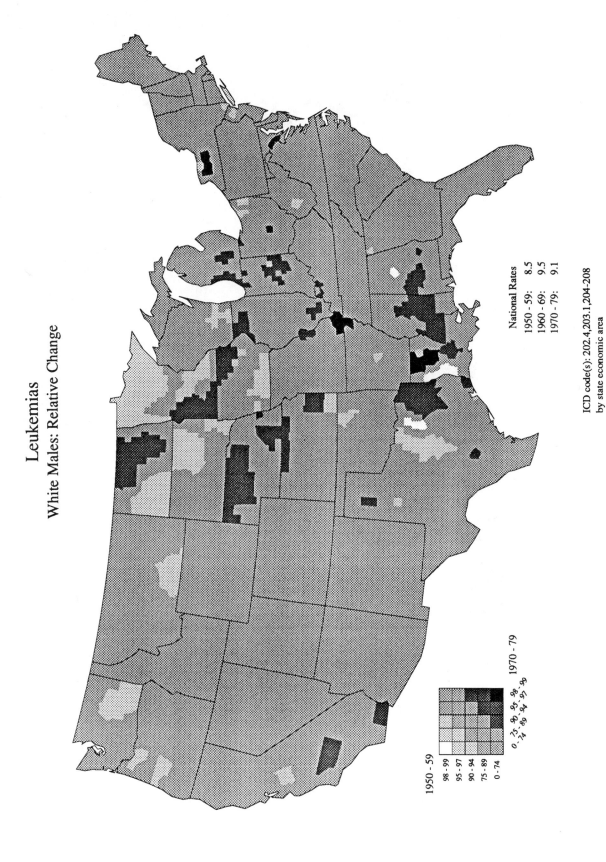

National Rates
1950 - 59:   8.5
1960 - 69:   9.5
1970 - 79:   9.1

ICD code(s): 202.4,203.1,204-208
by state economic area

1950 - 59

| 98 - 99 |
| 95 - 97 |
| 90 - 94 |
| 75 - 89 |
| 0 - 74 |

1970 - 79

0 - 75 - 90 - 95 - 98 - 99
74 - 89 - 94 - 97 - 99

341

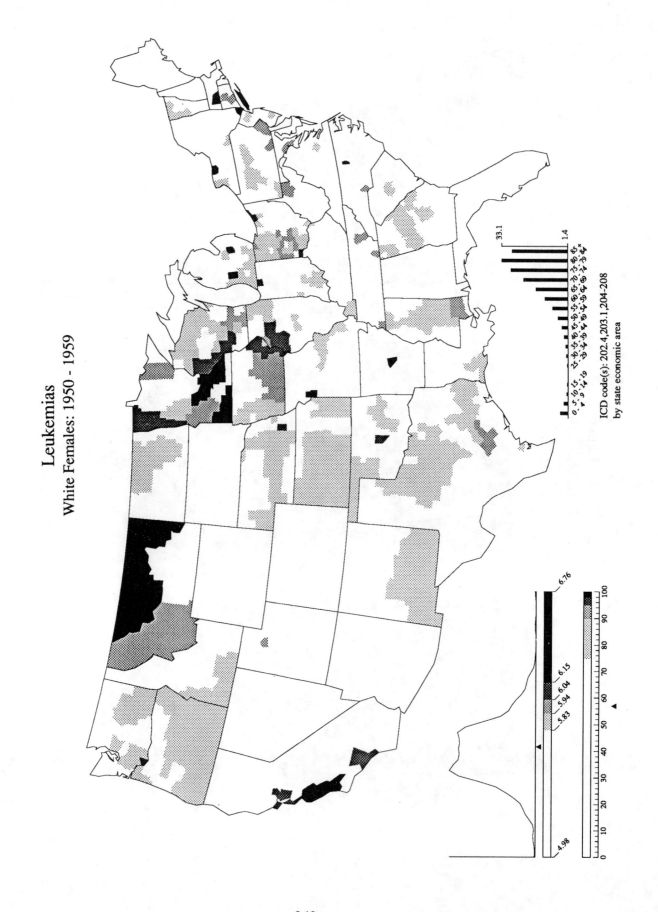

Leukemias
White Females: 1950 - 1959

ICD code(s): 202.4,203.1,204-208
by state economic area

Leukemias
White Females: 1960 - 1969

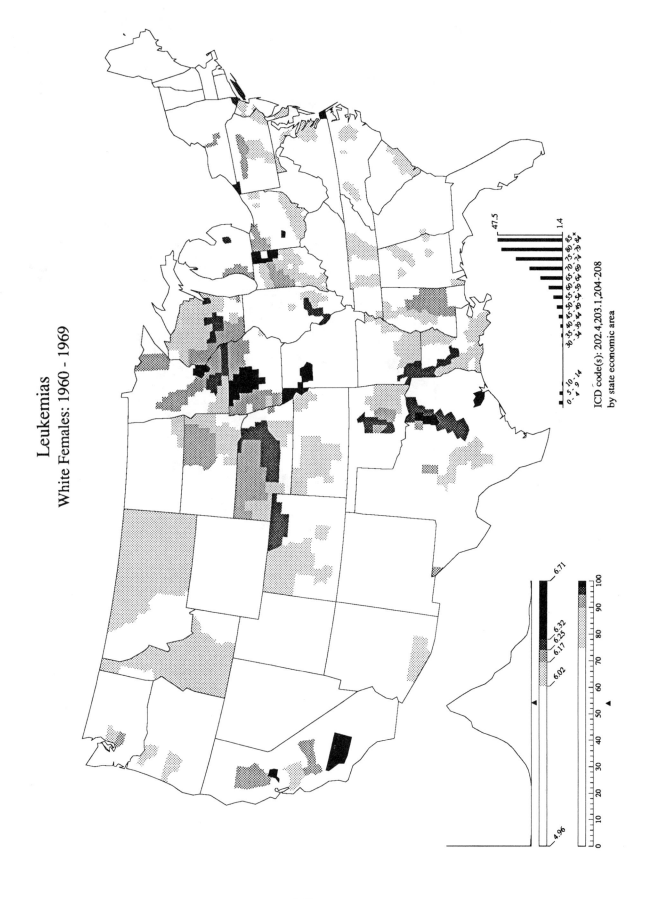

ICD code(s): 202.4,203.1,204-208
by state economic area

343

Leukemias
White Females: 1970 - 1979

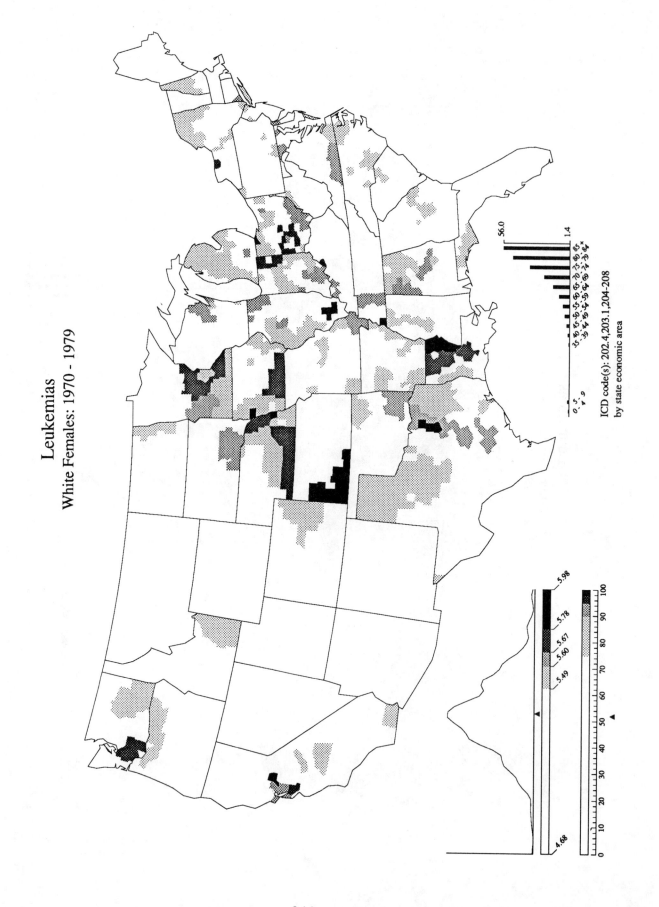

ICD code(s): 202.4,203.1,204-208
by state economic area

344

Leukemias
White Females: Relative Change

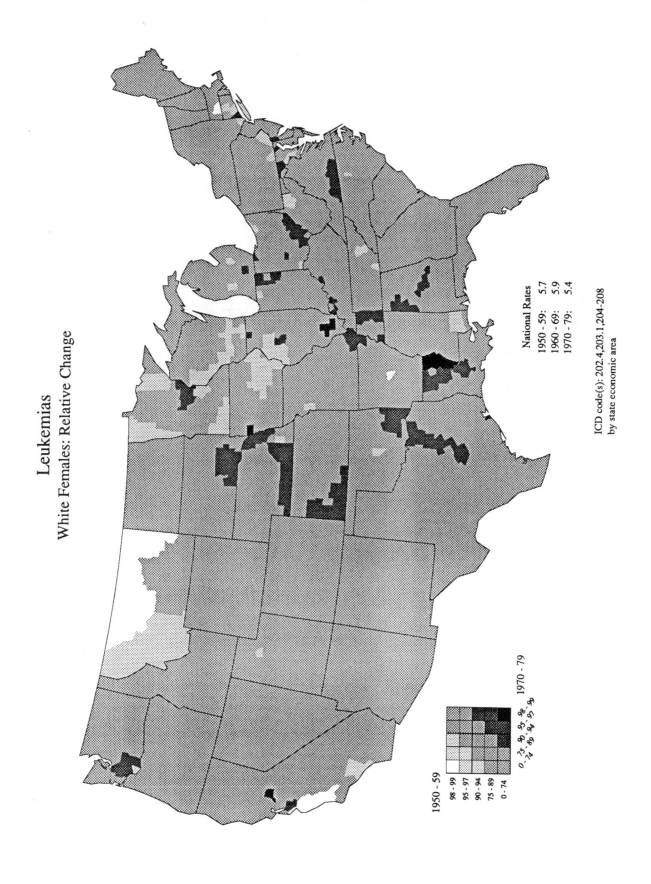

National Rates
1950 - 59:   5.7
1960 - 69:   5.9
1970 - 79:   5.4

ICD code(s): 202.4,203.1,204-208
by state economic area

345

Secondary, Site Unspecified and Not Previously Listed Cancers
White Males: 1950 - 1959

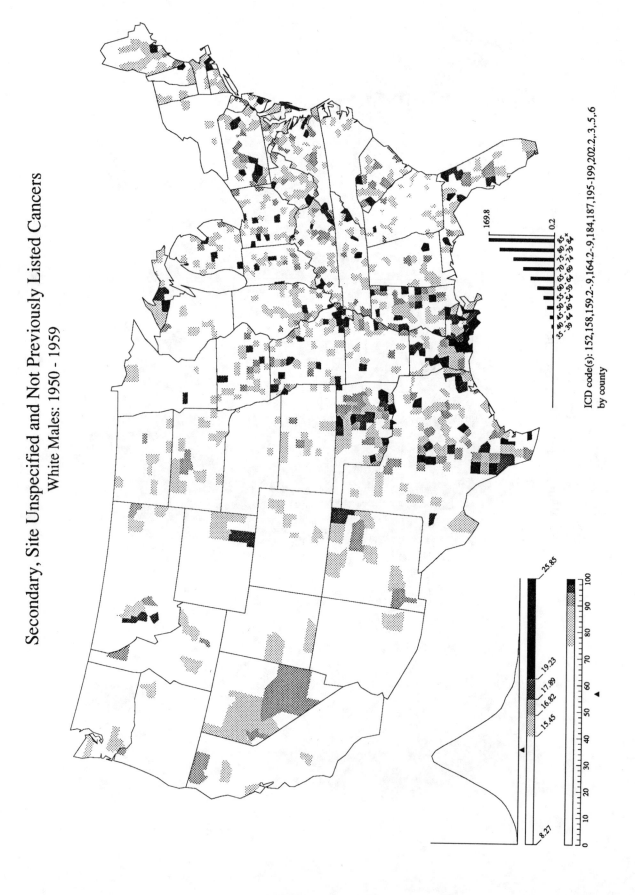

ICD code(s): 152,158,159.2-.9,164.2-.9,184,187,195-199,202.2,.3,..5,.6
by county

Secondary, Site Unspecified and Not Previously Listed Cancers
White Males: 1960 - 1969

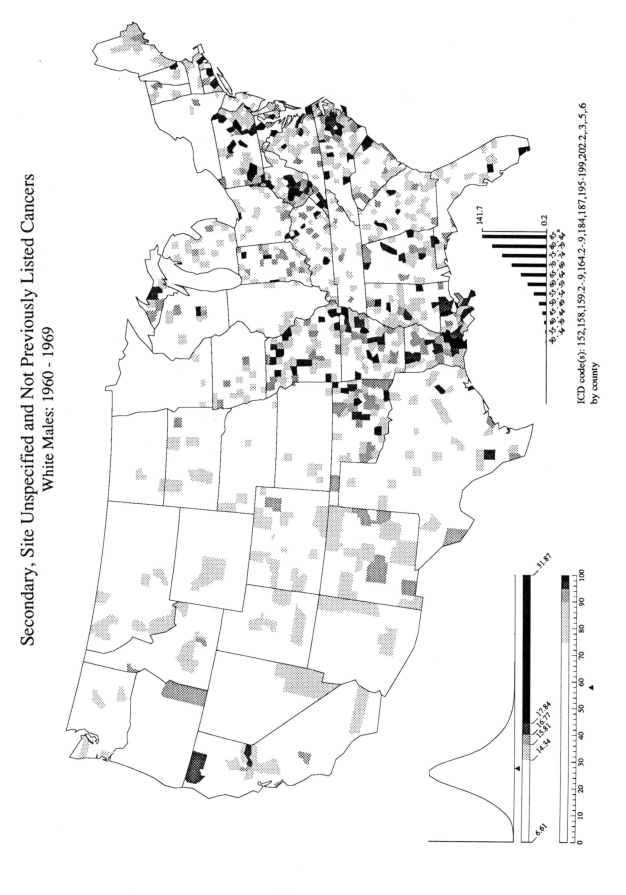

ICD code(s): 152,158,159.2-.9,164.2-.9,184,187,195-199,202.2,.3,.5,.6
by county

347

Secondary, Site Unspecified and Not Previously Listed Cancers
White Males: 1970 - 1979

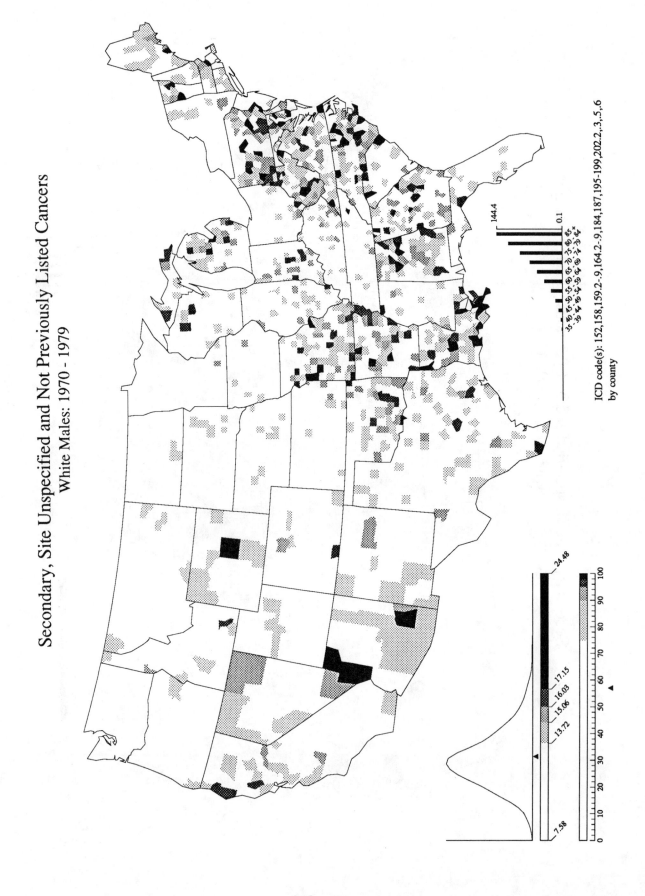

ICD code(s): 152,158,159.2-.9,164.2-.9,184,187,195-199,202.2,.3,.5,.6
by county

Secondary, Site Unspecified and Not Previously Listed Cancers
White Males: Relative Change

National Rates

1950 - 59: 14.5
1960 - 69: 13.6
1970 - 79: 12.8

ICD code(s): 152,158,159.2-.9,164.2-.9,184,187,195-199,202.2,.3,.5,.6
by county

1950 - 59

98 - 99
95 - 97
90 - 94
75 - 89
0 - 74

0 - 74 75 - 89 90 - 94 95 - 97 98 - 99

1970 - 79

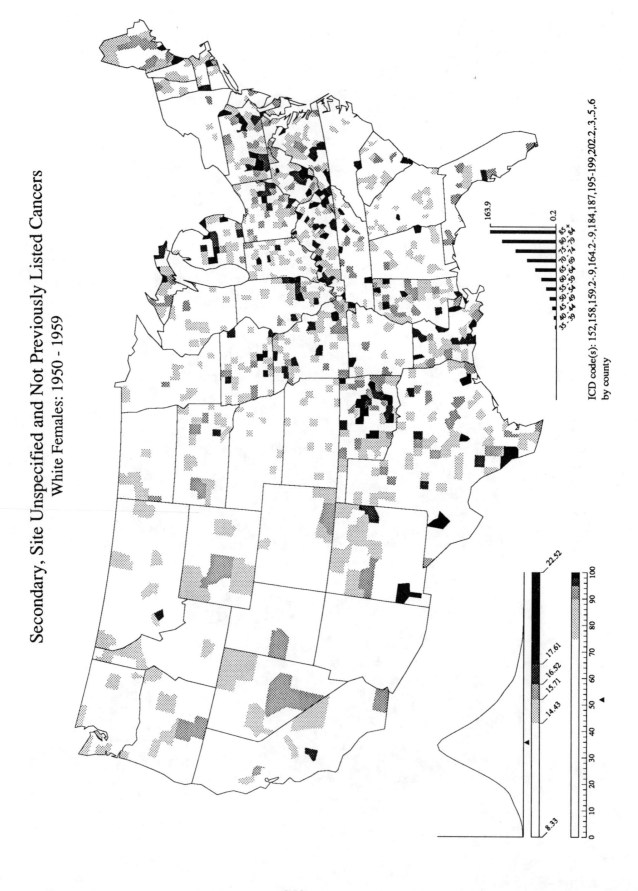

Secondary, Site Unspecified and Not Previously Listed Cancers
White Females: 1950 - 1959

ICD code(s): 152,158,159.2-.9,164.2-.9,184,187,195-199,202.2,.3,.5,.6
by county

Secondary, Site Unspecified and Not Previously Listed Cancers
White Females: 1960 - 1969

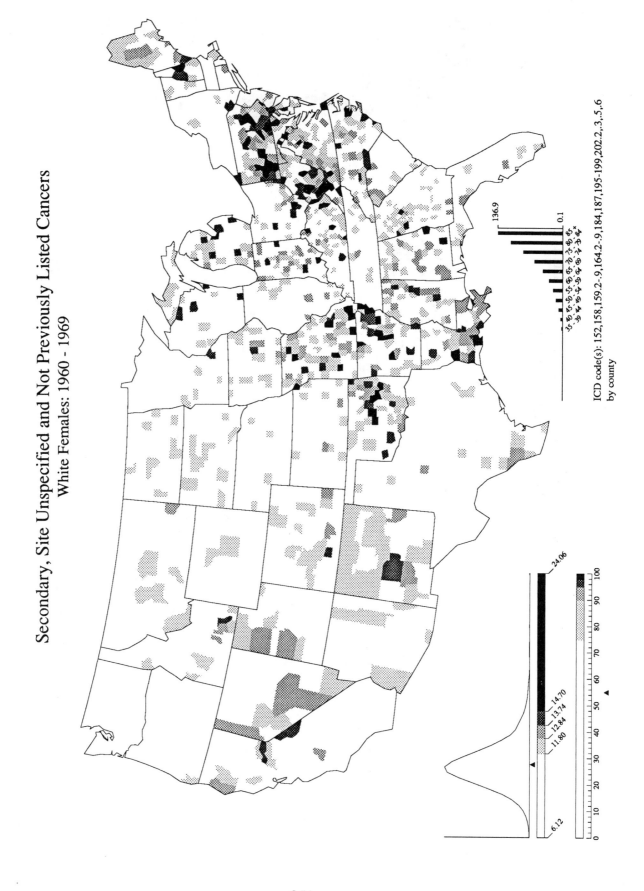

ICD code(s): 152,158,159.2-.9,164.2-.9,184,187,195-199,202.2,.3,.5,.6
by county

Secondary, Site Unspecified and Not Previously Listed Cancers
White Females: 1970 - 1979

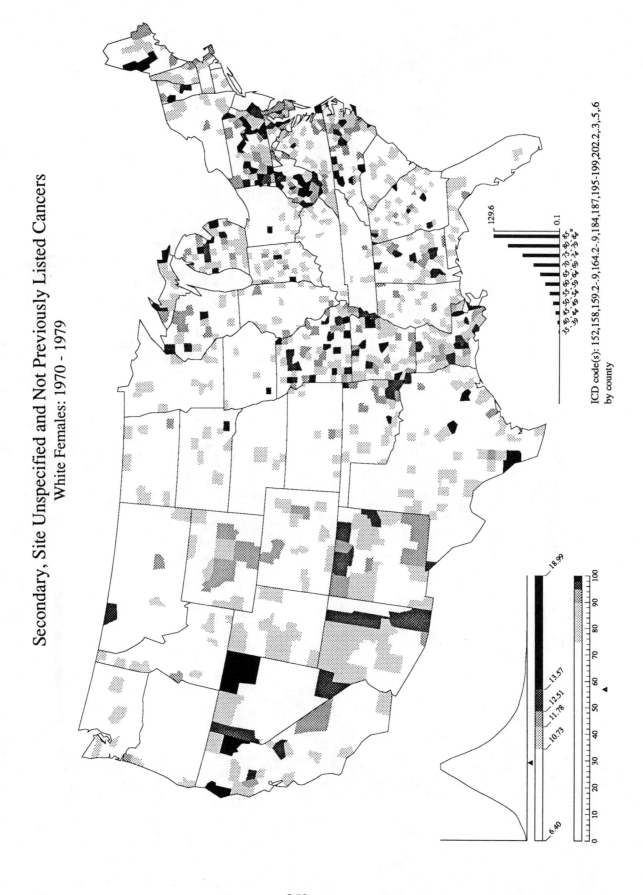

ICD code(s): 152,158,159.2-.9,164.2-.9,184,187,195-199,202.2,.3,.5,.6
by county

Secondary, Site Unspecified and Not Previously Listed Cancers
White Females: Relative Change

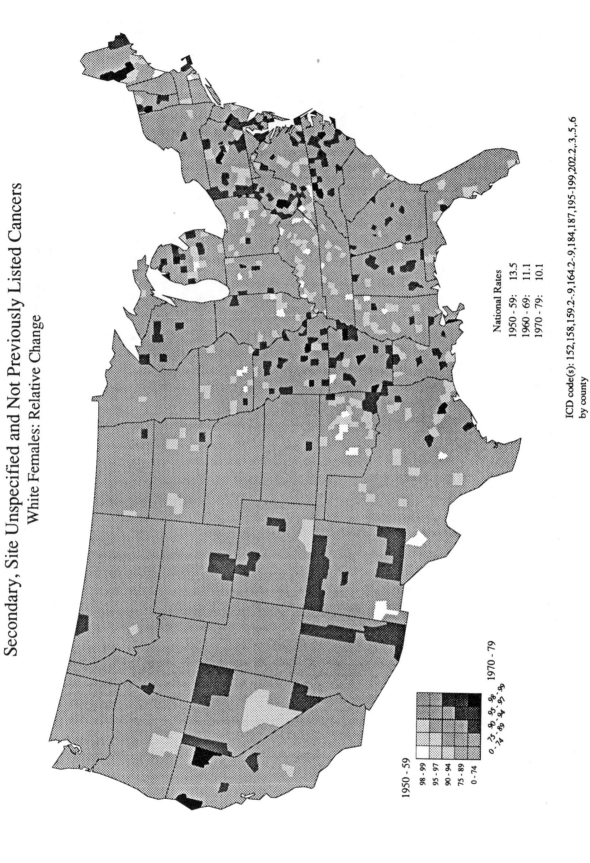

National Rates

1950 - 59:	13.5
1960 - 69:	11.1
1970 - 79:	10.1

ICD code(s): 152,158,159.2-.9,164.2-.9,184,187,195-199,202.2,.3,.5,.6
by county

353

Secondary, Site Unspecified and Not Previously Listed Cancers
Nonwhite Males: 1950 - 1959

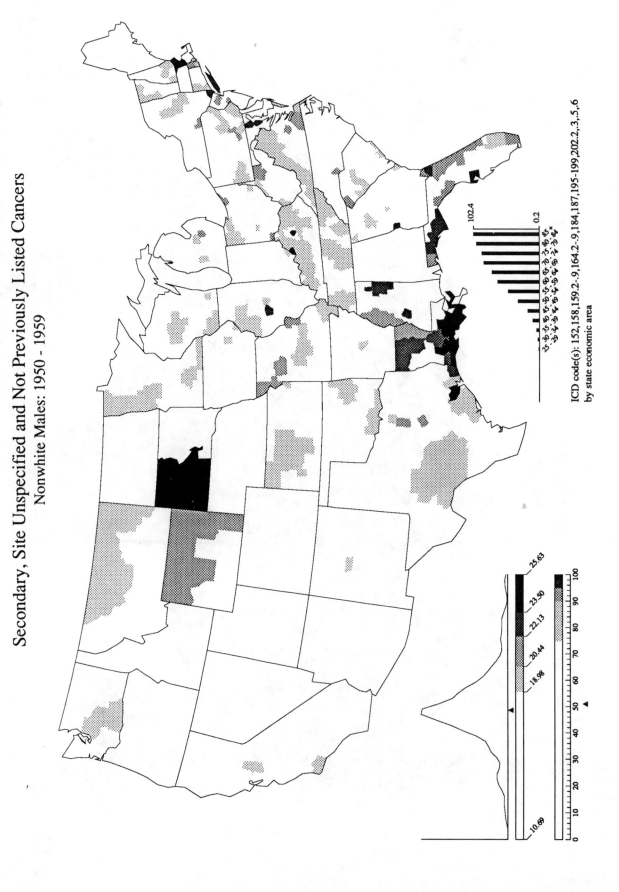

ICD code(s): 152,158,159.2-.9,164.2-.9,184,187,195-199,202.2,.3,.5,.6
by state economic area

Secondary, Site Unspecified and Not Previously Listed Cancers
Nonwhite Males: 1960 - 1969

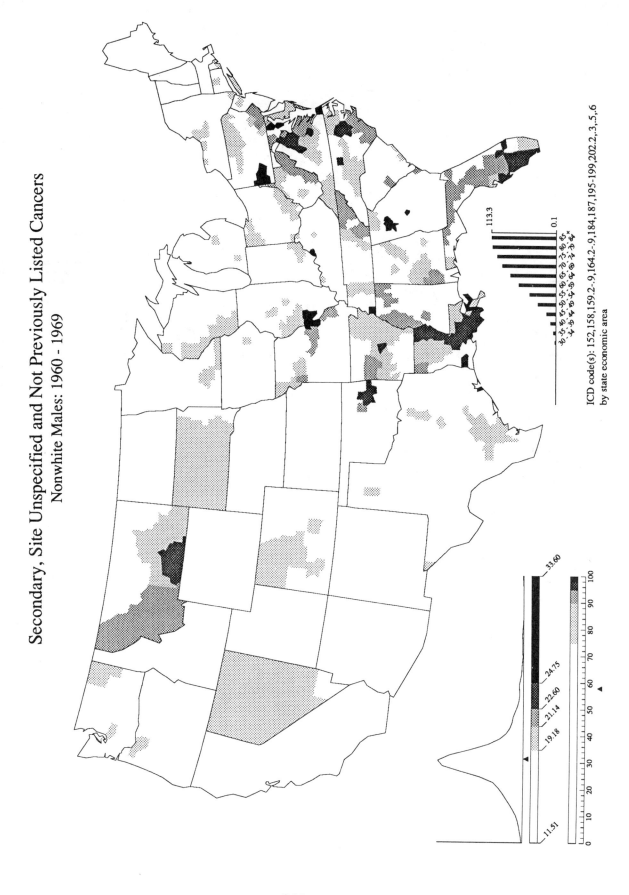

ICD code(s): 152,158,159.2-.9,164.2-.9,184,187,195-199,202.2,.3,.5,.6
by state economic area

Secondary, Site Unspecified and Not Previously Listed Cancers
Nonwhite Males: 1970 - 1979

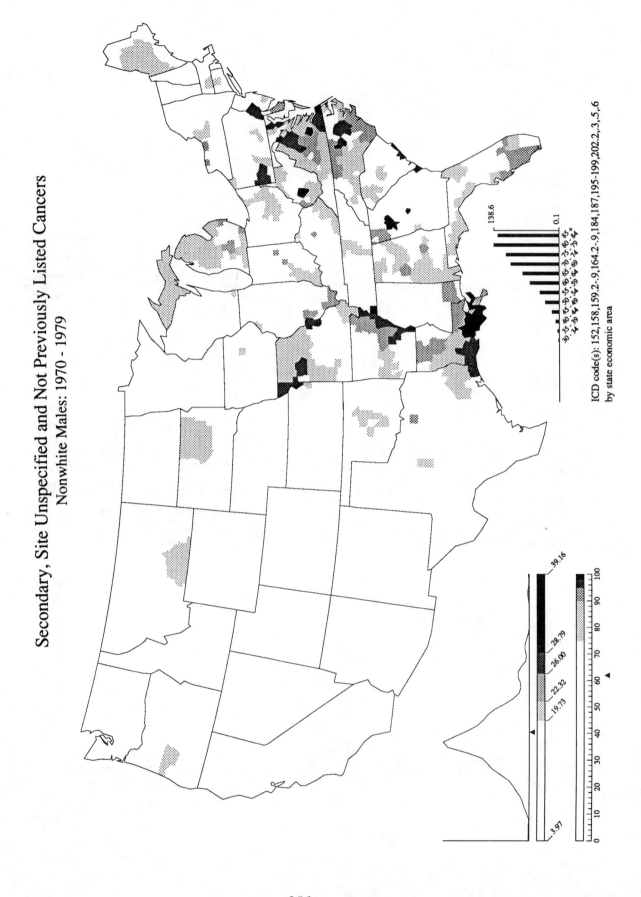

ICD code(s): 152,158,159.2-.9,164.2-.9,184,187,195-199,202.2,.3,.5,.6
by state economic area

Secondary, Site Unspecified and Not Previously Listed Cancers
Nonwhite Males: Relative Change

National Rates
1950 - 59:   17.9
1960 - 69:   18.4
1970 - 79:   18.1

ICD code(s): 152,158,159.2-.9,164.2-.9,184,187,195-199,202.2,.3,.5,.6
by state economic area

1950 - 59

98 - 99
95 - 97
90 - 94
75 - 89
0 - 74

1970 - 79

0. 75. 90. 95. 98. 99
    74   89   94   97   99

Secondary, Site Unspecified and Not Previously Listed Cancers
Nonwhite Females: 1950 - 1959

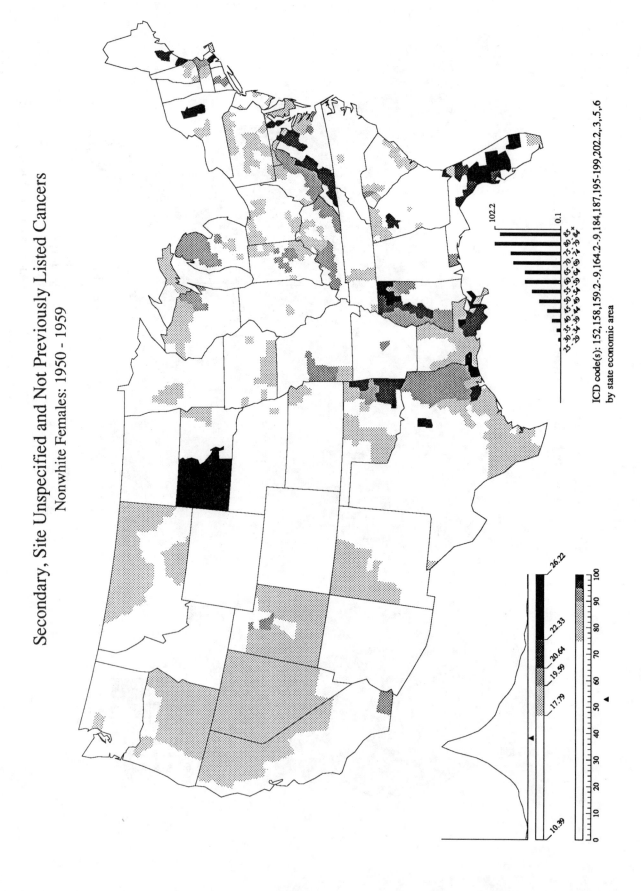

ICD code(s): 152,158,159.2-.9,164.2-.9,184,187,195-199,202.2,.3,.5,.6
by state economic area

358

Secondary, Site Unspecified and Not Previously Listed Cancers
Nonwhite Females: 1960 - 1969

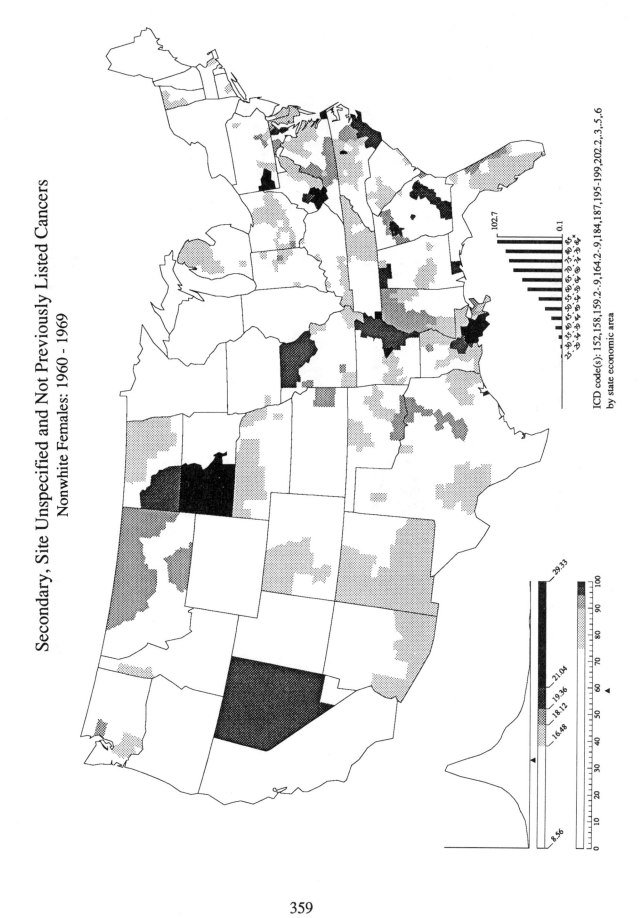

ICD code(s): 152,158,159.2-.9,164.2-.9,184,187,195-199,202.2,.3,.5,.6
by state economic area

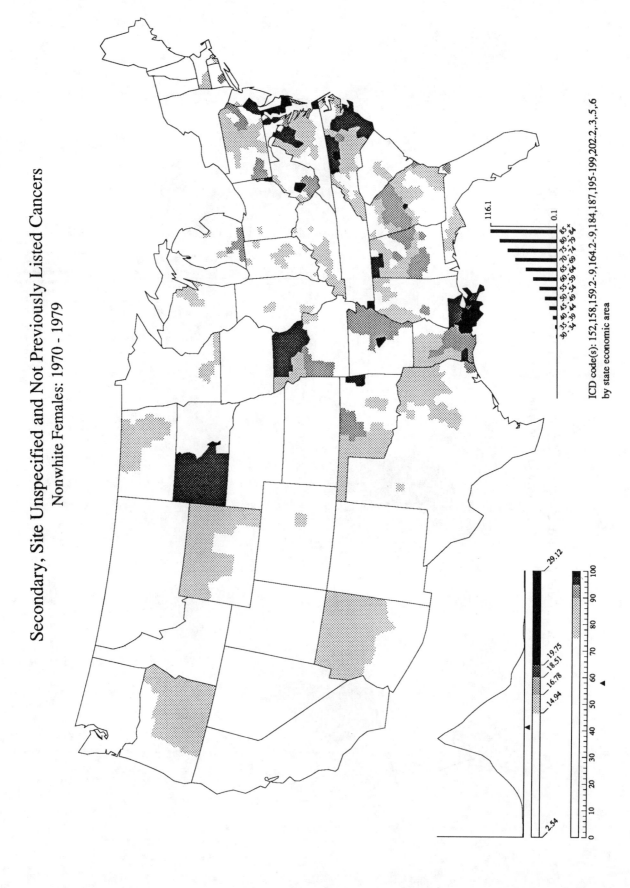

Secondary, Site Unspecified and Not Previously Listed Cancers
Nonwhite Females: 1970 - 1979

ICD code(s): 152,158,159.2-.9,164.2-.9,184,187,195-199,202.2,.3,.5,.6
by state economic area

Secondary, Site Unspecified and Not Previously Listed Cancers
Nonwhite Females: Relative Change

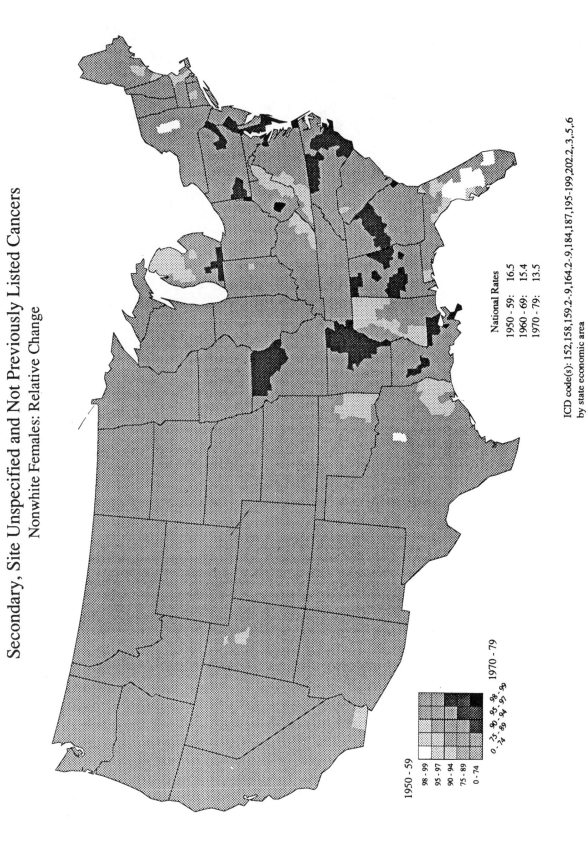

National Rates

1950 - 59:   16.5
1960 - 69:   15.4
1970 - 79:   13.5

ICD code(s): 152,158,159.2-.9,164.2-.9,184,187,195-199,202.2,.3,.5,.6
by state economic area

361

Counties of the United States
Number of Counties: 3072

State Economic Areas
Number of SEA's: 506

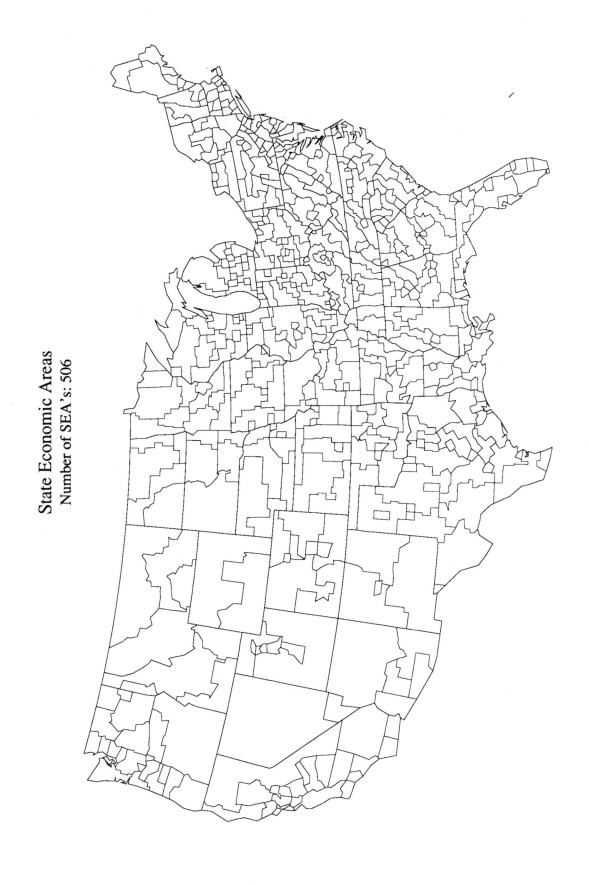